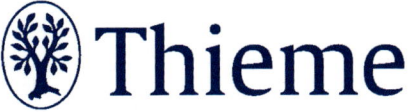

An Approach to Successful Tympanoplasty

B. M. Gupta, MS (ENT), DLO
Senior Otologist
Gupta ENT Hospital,
Nagpur, Maharashtra, India

Thieme
Delhi • Stuttgart • New York • Rio de Janeiro

Publishing Director: Ritu Sharma
Senior Development Editor: Dr. Nidhi Srivastava
Director-Editorial Services: Rachna Sinha
Project Manager: Shipra Sehgal
National Sales Manager: Bishwajit Kumar Mishra
Managing Director & CEO: Ajit Kohli

Thieme Medical and Scientific Publishers Private Limited.
A - 12, Second Floor, Sector - 2, Noida - 201 301, Uttar Pradesh, India, +911204556600
Email: customerservice@thieme.in
www.thieme.in

Cover design: © Thieme
Cover image source: © Thieme

Page make-up by RECTO Graphics, India

Printed in India

5 4 3 2 1

DOI: 10.1055/b000000989

ISBN: 978-93-95390-93-4
Also available as an e-book:
eISBN (PDF): 978-93-95390-96-5
eISBN (ePub): 978-81-966914-6-2

Contents

Videos

Video 1 Gelfoam patch test
https://www.thieme.de/de/q.htm?p=opn/
cs/23/11/22137972-93ff4a8b

Video 2 Endaural incision
https://www.thieme.de/de/q.htm?p=opn/
cs/23/11/22137959-f083c9c7

Video 3 Tympanoplasty type 1
https://www.thieme.de/de/q.htm?p=opn/
cs/23/11/22137960-e5e5257c

Video 4 Tympanoplasty with mastoid exploration
https://www.thieme.de/de/q.htm?p=opn/
cs/23/11/22137961-8e804aa4

Video 5 Canalplasty 1
https://www.thieme.de/de/q.htm?p=opn/
cs/23/11/22137962-7a9d5a66

Video 6 Canalplasty 2
https://www.thieme.de/de/q.htm?p=opn/
cs/23/11/22137963-d1e03f01

Video 7 Cartilage tympanoplasty
https://www.thieme.de/de/q.htm?p=opn/
cs/23/11/22137964-db027a3d

Video 8 Ossiculoplasty: Two cartilage technique from intact stapes
https://www.thieme.de/de/q.htm?p=opn/
cs/23/11/22137965-2a84b840

Video 9 Ossiculoplasty: Two cartilage technique from stapes footplate
https://www.thieme.de/de/q.htm?p=opn/
cs/23/11/22137966-ffe6506d

Preface

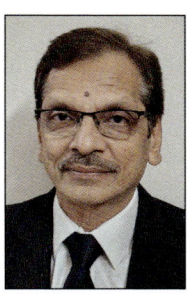

The inspiration for writing this book came to me during the period of lockdown when I had sufficient time. I wanted to share in this book the academic material along with my surgical experience which I accumulated over time.

This book contains various theoretical aspects of tympanoplasty, but a major part of this book covers many practical aspects which are very useful for junior consultants as well as for postgraduate students.

Most middle ear surgeries such as tympanoplasty and ossiculoplasty are very demanding and require a very systematic approach. Proper selection of cases, counseling of patients, preoperative preparation, surgical technique, and postoperative care are very important to make the surgery successful.

In this book, several surgical techniques have been shown with a series of photographs for the readers' better understanding. The photographs are very clear and self-explanatory.

The middle ear surgery is difficult as the surgeon is working in the depth with very important structures around. Hence, a thorough knowledge of the anatomy of the middle ear (temporal bone) is important, which junior surgeons can acquire by doing temporal bone dissections. The technique for ear surgery should be simple, safe, and reliable to give successful outcome. As the surgeon is working with high-speed burr and sharp instruments, working in the depth is dangerous. Hence, the surgical field should be widely accessible to avoid any accident.

In addition, the surgical field should be bloodless, which is achieved by appropriate use of adrenaline as well as by hypotensive anesthesia, especially in general anesthesia.

Each and every patient undergoing tympanoplasty should be prepared perfectly by thorough clinical examination including microscopic ear examination. Paper patch test with Gelfoam patch test should always be done to determine ossicular chain integrity including the status of the stapes. Each and every case should be treated like a project and all efforts should be made to make this project successful, which gives happiness and satisfaction to the patient as well as to the surgeon.

B. M. Gupta, MS (ENT), DLO

1 Classification of Tympanoplasty

Wullstein Classification (1956)

Tympanoplasty is classified into different types depending upon the defect in the middle ear system that needs to be repaired. There may be only perforation or there may be an associated ossicular chain defect (**Fig. 1.1**):

- Type I tympanoplasty: The tympanic membrane (TM) is grafted to an intact ossicular chain (intact lever mechanism).

- Type II tympanoplasty: The malleus and incus are partially eroded, reconstructed, and grafted (reconstructed lever mechanism).

- Type III tympanoplasty: The malleus and incus are completely absent. The TM is grafted to the stapes superstructure (no lever mechanism; only sound pressure transformation of the TM is present).

- Type IV tympanoplasty: The stapes superstructure is destroyed but the foot plate is mobile. The TM is grafted to a mobile foot plate (sound protection of one of the windows, usually the round window through the lower aeration pathways).

- Type V tympanoplasty: The TM is grafted to a fenestration in the horizontal semicircular canal.

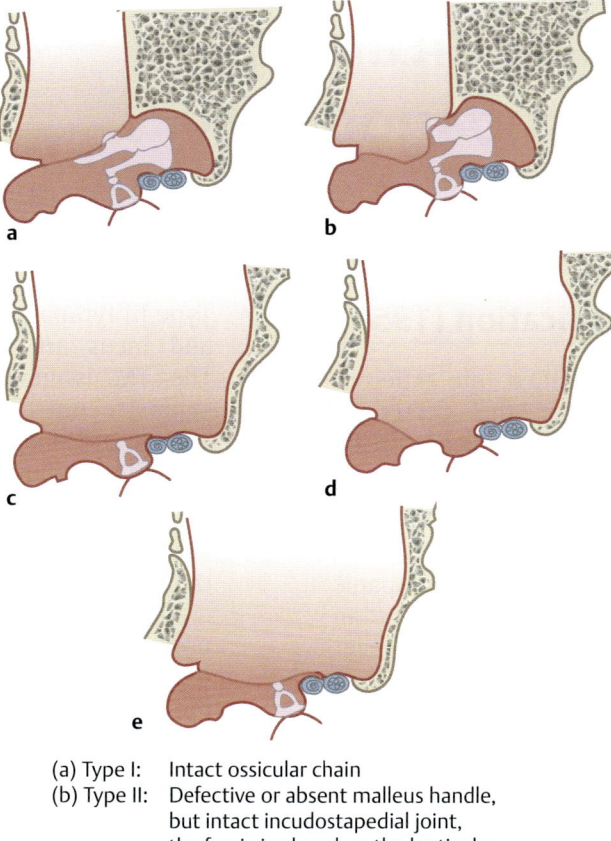

(a) Type I: Intact ossicular chain
(b) Type II: Defective or absent malleus handle,
               but intact incudostapedial joint,
               the fascia is placed on the lenticular
               process of the incus
(c) Type III: Myringoincudopexy
(d) Type IV: Sound protection
(e) Type V: Fenestration of the lateral ventricular canal

Fig. 1.1   Wullstein classification of tympanoplasty.

2 | Physiology of Hearing

Physiology of Hearing in Healthy Ear

The length of the handle of the malleus is more than that of the long process of the incus, creating a "lever ratio" of 1.3:1.

Similarly, the effective surface area of the tympanic membrane is larger than the surface area of the oval window, the ratio of which is 17:1. This is known as the "hydraulic ratio."

Hence, the total effect of lever ratio and hydraulic ratio is 17 × 1.3, which comes to 22. This is known as sound-pressure transformer ratio of the normal human ear, by which normal sound of large amplitude but small force is transformed into fluid-borne sound vibration of smaller amplitude but larger force, with around 27- to 30-dB gain.

Physiology of Hearing with Tympanic Membrane Perforation

Defect in the ossicular chain, especially the malleus and incus, affects the lever ratio and perforated eardrum affects the hydraulic ratio. Hence, deafness in a perforated eardrum is due to decreased transformer ratio. In addition, the following points should be noted:

- Direct stimulation of the round and oval windows leads to cancellation of the perilymphatic fluid waves.

- Sound pressure entering through the perforation acts on the medial surface of the tympanic membrane, against that on the lateral surface.

- All these lead to a 40- to 45-dB hearing loss.

- A good tympanoplasty restores the sound pressure transformer mechanism by constructing a normal tympanic membrane and proper ossicular chain connecting the normal tympanic membrane to the oval window.

- It also restores the sound protection for the round window by constructing a normal middle ear.

3 History of Tympanoplasty

As mentioned earlier, Wullstein, in the year 1953, described various surgical techniques to repair defects in the tympanic membrane and the ossicular chain caused by middle ear infection. In the same year, Zollner also described various surgeries to repair middle ear defects caused by chronic otitis media. The introduction of microscope in the same year improved the results of their surgery tremendously.

Earlier the grafting material used was partial-thickness skin graft. The problem with this grafting material was infection and necrosis. Later on, Zollner replaced partial-thickness skin graft by free full-thickness meatal skin graft with better results. Later on, in 1960, John Shea and Tabb started using vein graft as grafting material. In 1961, Heerman used the temporalis fascia as grafting material.

Ossiculoplasty material used in the beginning was plastic, which was associated with high failure rate. Hence, it was replaced by prosthesis made up of stainless steel and platinum. In 1960, homograft ossicles were also used but later discontinued due to risk of transmission of various infections. Various biocompatible alloplastic material like plastipore, polyethylene, polytetrafluoroethylene, hydroxylapatite, and titanium are used nowadays for ossiculoplasty.

4 Aim and Basic Principles of Tympanoplasty

The Basic Principles of Tympanoplasty Surgery

- Removal of disease from the middle ear cleft, especially irreversible mucosal disease.
- Repair of defect in the tympanic membrane and ossicles that have been damaged by disease to give normal and healthy middle ear.

For Successful Tympanoplasty We Need

- A vibrating membrane (tympanic membrane).
- A columella between vibrating membrane and functioning oval window (ossiculoplasty).
- Properly functioning windows, oval window, and round window on either side of the scala media of the cochlea.
- Good aeration (normal eustachian tube).

A Vibrating Membrane (Tympanic Membrane)

Perforated eardrum should be repaired to give good hearing and prevent recurrent infection via the following:

- External auditory meatus.
- Ascending infection from the nose via the eustachian tube. (It is easier for the infection to ascend up from the nose to the middle ear whenever there is a perforation in the tympanic membrane.)
- Very small size perforation in the tympanic membrane can be closed by repeated chemical cauterization.
- Moderate to bigger size perforation requires tympanoplasty.

Material of Choice

- Material of choice for grafting is temporalis fascia as it has low metabolic rate and good Survival chance. This is the most commonly used grafting material.
- It is available in plenty, both through endaural and postaural incision.

- It should be taken as high as possible over the surface of the temporalis muscle where it is thin.

- The common practice is to dry the fascia after harvesting it.

- In this dry state, it is easier to handle it, cut it, and place it properly and comfortably to repair the tympanic membrane defect.

- It soon absorbs the tissue fluid and recovers to normal appearance.

- It should not be heated as it gets devitalized leading to higher incidence of graft necrosis and graft failure.

The other material that can be used are the perichondrium, vein graft, and temporalis muscle squeezed and dried. These materials are very much useful in revision tympanoplasty when the temporalis fascia has already been used by a previous surgeon.

Even the cartilage with perichondrium can also be used as a graft material with equally good results. When nothing is available, the periosteum from the mastoid can be used as a graft.

The series of pictures in **Fig. 4.1** shows how to take out the perichondrium graft from the tragal cartilage.

Patent Eustachian Tube

- A normally functioning eustachian tube is essential for successful tympanoplasty. The functioning eustachian tube maintains an equal pressure on either side of the tympanic membrane.

- It is difficult to assess preoperatively the postoperative function of the eustachian tube.

- Valsalva manometry tympanometry gives an idea about eustachian tube function.

- A well-pneumatized temporal bone is an indicator of good ventilation of the middle ear in early childhood.

- If the eustachian tube is not functioning, surgery may not be successful, but negative tubal function is not an absolute contraindication for surgery as:

  ○ Tubal function can be restored by excising the scar tissue occluding the tympanic ostium of the eustachian tube during surgery.

  ○ After closure of the perforation, when the middle ear mucosa comes back to normal, the eustachian tube function improves.

Various causes of eustachian tube block especially in the nose like deviated nasal septum, hypertrophied turbinates, polypi, and adenoids should be taken care before performing tympanoplasty.

Nose, sinuses, and throat should be free from any septic focus. If the eustachian tube is permanently blocked due to adhesions, at present, there is no surgery to restore the patency of the eustachian tube.

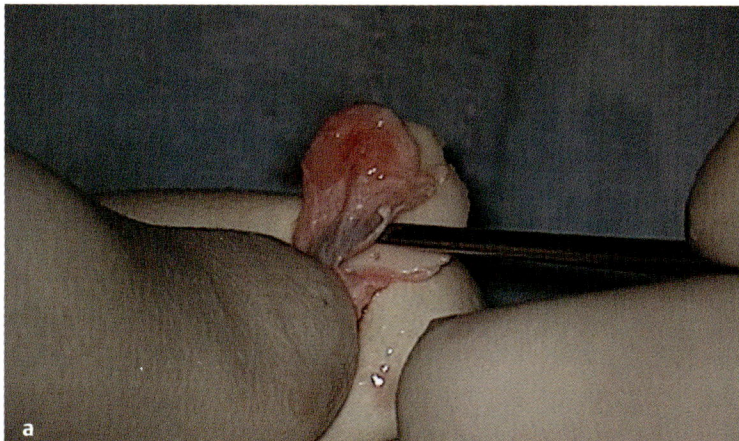

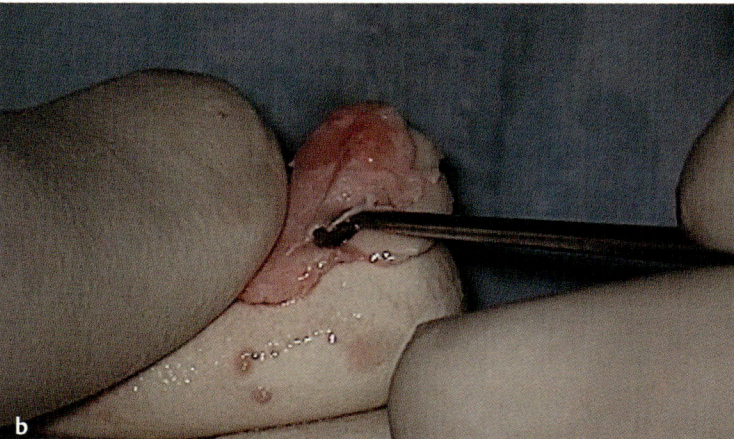

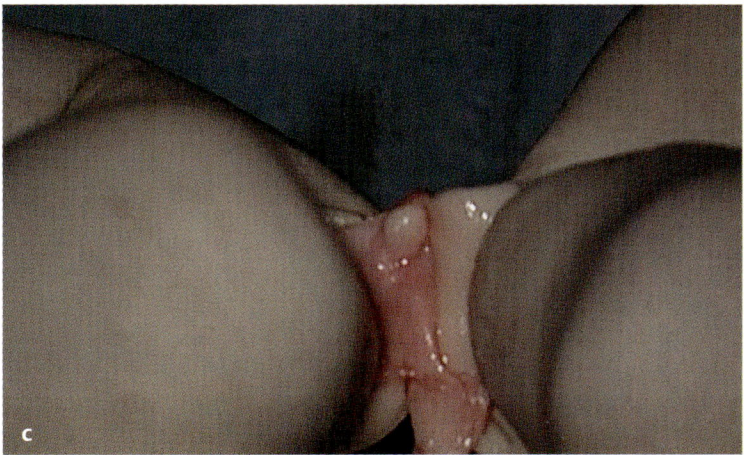

Fig. 4.1 **(a)** Big piece of tragal cartilage is taken out. By using the side knife, the perichondrium from one side of the cartilage is dissected. **(b)** Perichondrium dissection on one side of the cartilage is continued. **(c)** The perichondrium on one side of the tragal cartilage is separated by pulling it by fingers. *(Continued)*

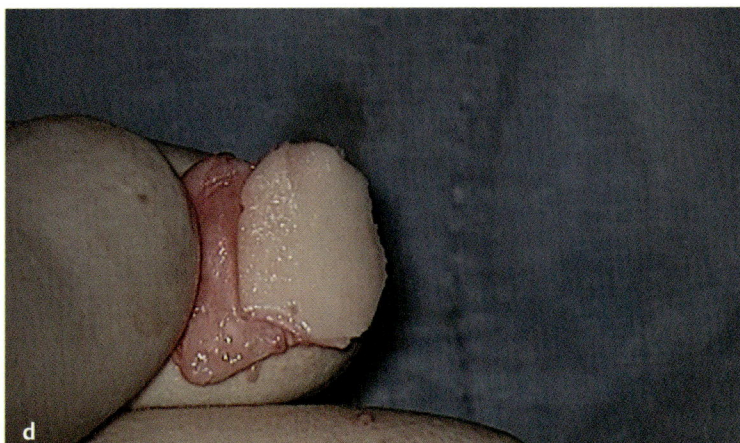

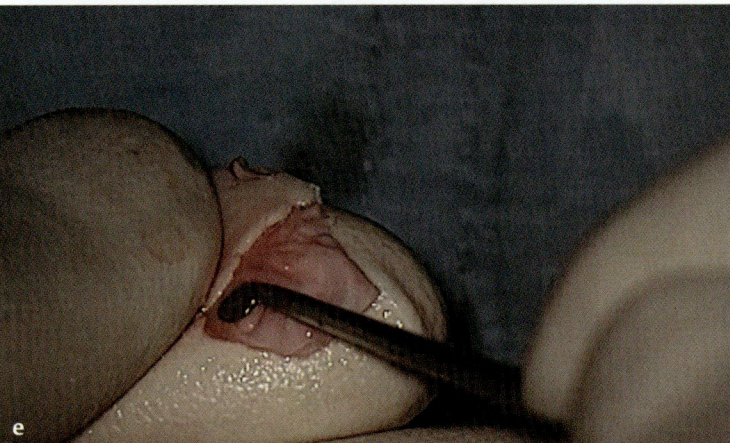

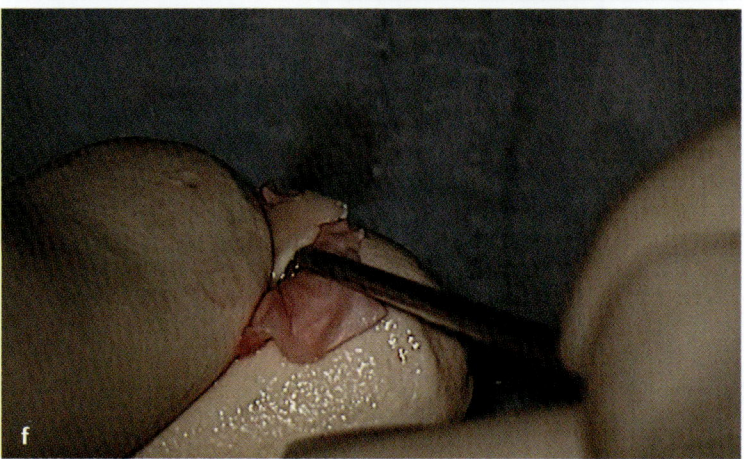

Fig. 4.1 *(Continued)* **(d)** The perichondrium from one side of the cartilage has been dissected and separated. **(e)** Perichondrium dissection at the lateral edge of the cartilage is continued on the other side of the cartilage and this perichondrium on other side is also dissected by a side knife. **(f)** The perichondrium on the other side of the cartilage is dissected by a side knife. *(Continued)*

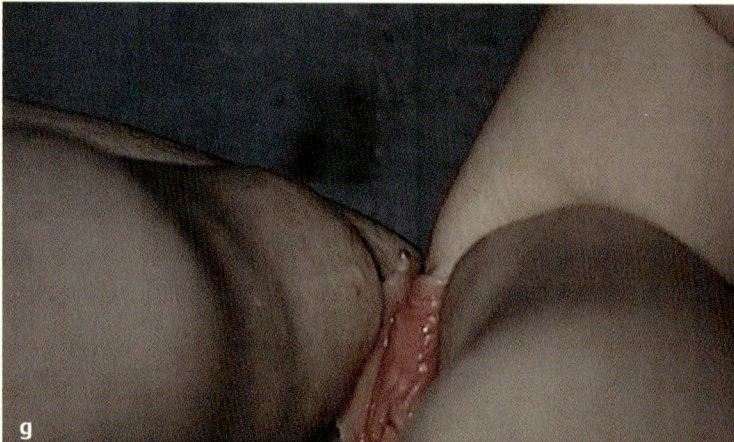

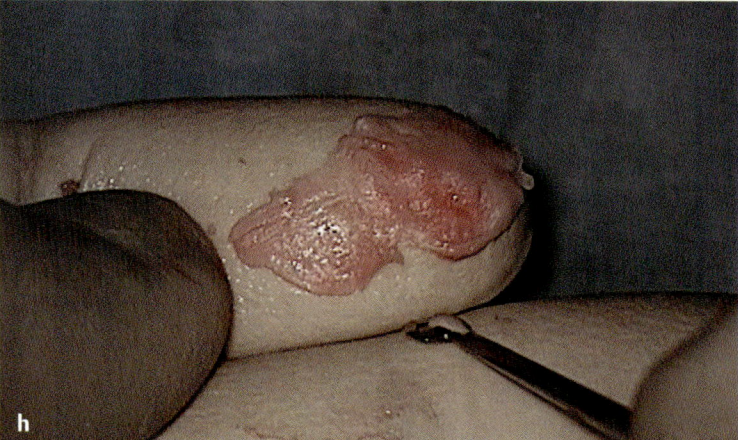

Fig. 4.1 *(Continued)* **(g)** The perichondrium on the other side of the cartilage is separated from the cartilage by pulling it by fingers. **(h)** Complete perichondrium has been dissected out from the cartilage. Now a big piece of perichondrium is available for grafting.

5 | Preoperative Ear, Nose, and Throat Examination

- Proper and complete ear, nose, and throat (ENT) examination is necessary before planning for surgery. Along with ear examination, the nose and throat should be examined for any pathology responsible for eustachian tube dysfunction. Any septic focus in the nose and throat should be taken care before tympanoplasty.

- Examination includes tuning fork test, audiogram, speech audiogram, and microscopic ear examination.

The degree of hearing loss depends upon the size of the perforation. Small perforation may not be associated with significant hearing loss. Larger perforations are associated with moderate to severe degree of conductive hearing loss depending upon the area of tympanic membrane involved.

Perforated tympanic membrane with ossicular discontinuity is associated with severe degree of conductive hearing loss up to 50 dB.

Perforated tympanic membrane is associated with an ascending type of air conduction curve in the audiogram with more loss for low frequency than for higher frequency. Hence, the degree of hearing loss and air bone gap gives an idea about the status of the middle ear, especially the status of the ossicular chain.

Patch Test

Before surgery is planned, the degree of hearing improvement after surgery is assessed by a patch test.

Routine patch test is done by closing the perforation by a piece of filter paper under a microscope. If there is an ossicular discontinuity like incus necrosis, there will not be any improvement in the hearing after placing the patch. This is confirmed by doing an audiogram before and after putting the patch.

This test will not tell anything about the stapes fixation.

Gelfoam Patch Test

In addition to the routine patch test, Gelfoam patch test is extremely useful in assessing the status of the stapes (**Fig. 5.1a–e**). Here, the audiogram is repeated, after keeping a moist Gelfoam in the middle ear through the perforation (**Fig. 5.1f**). This Gelfoam will touch the stapes.

If the stapes is normal and mobile, there will be good improvement in the hearing after placing the Gelfoam in the middle ear (like normal ossicular chain). If the stapes is fixed, this Gelfoam patch test will not

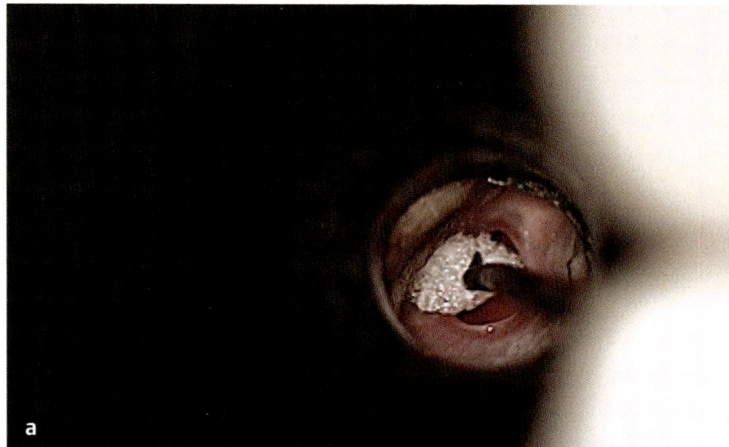

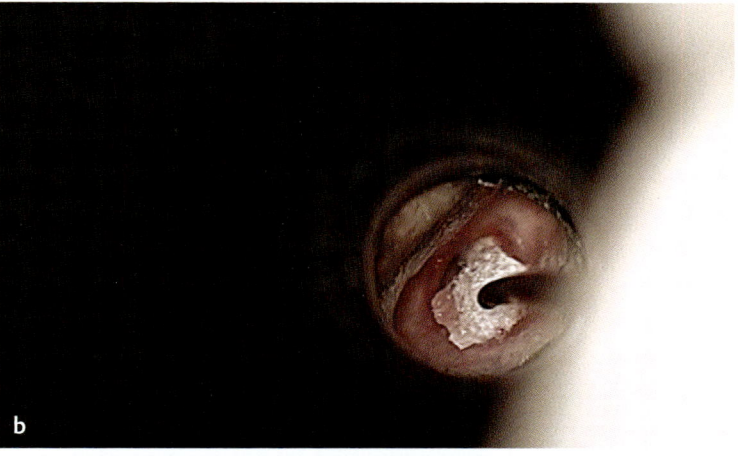

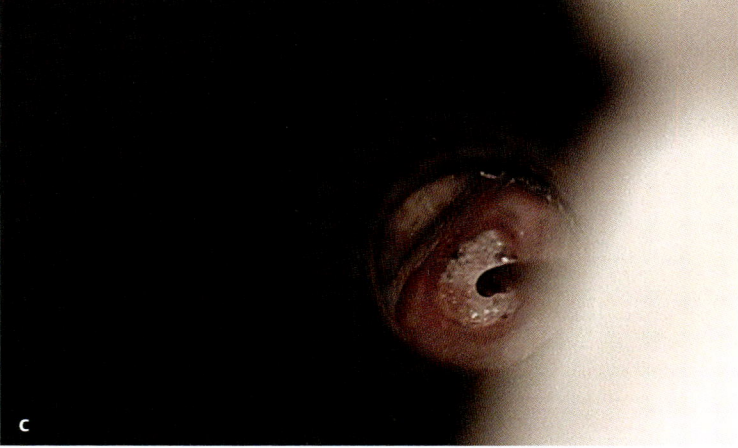

Fig. 5.1 **(a)** Large central perforation. Under microscope, Gelfoam is gently placed in the middle ear through the perforation. **(b)** Two or three small pieces of Gelfoam are placed in the middle ear. **(c)** Gelfoam is placed in the middle ear, touching the ossicular chain. *(Continued)*

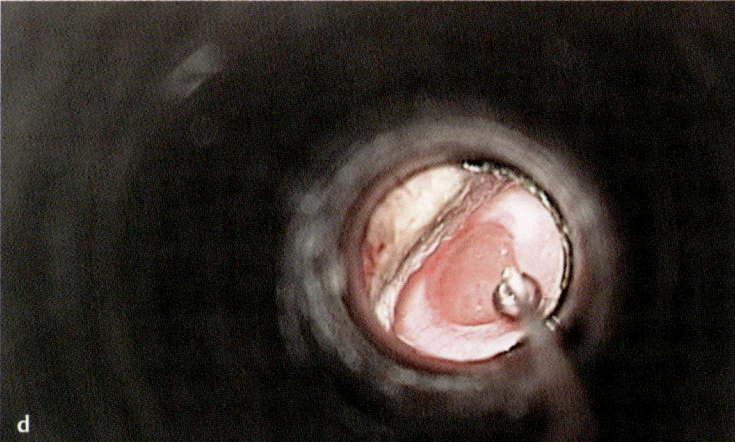

d

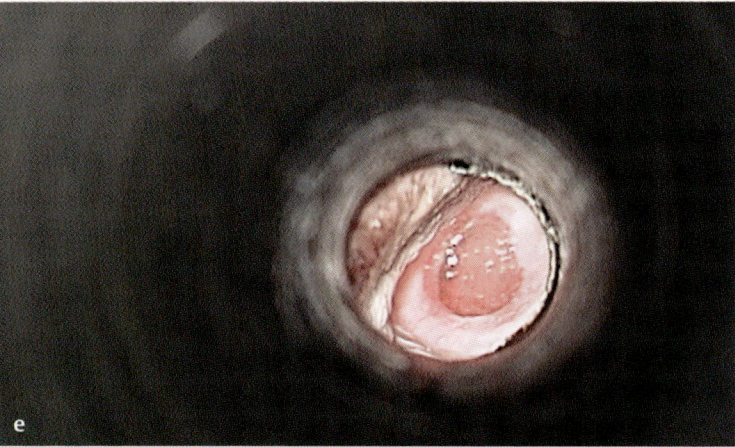

e

Fig. 5.1 *(Continued)* **(d)** Few drops of saline solution or antibiotic drops are instilled in the middle ear through the perforation. Gelfoam in the middle ear swells due to moisture. **(e)** Moist and swollen Gelfoam in the middle ear is touching the ossicular chain medially while also closing the perforation. An audiogram is repeated. **(f)** Gelfoam in the middle ear closing the perforation and touching the stapes leading to improvement in air conduction in the left ear.

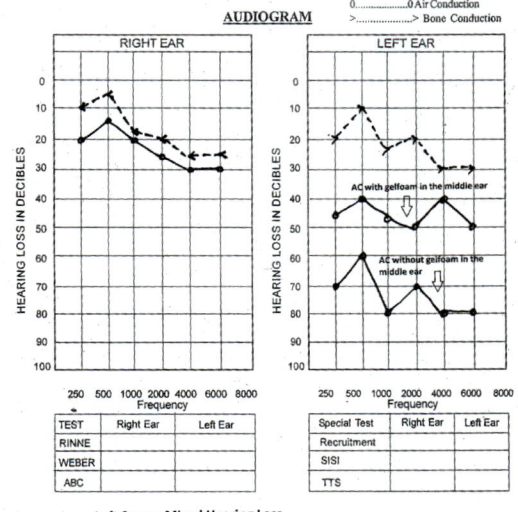

f

show any improvement in the hearing. This is negative Gelfoam patch test. When the Gelfoam patch test is negative, the patient should be told about the possibility of stapes fixation and they should be informed about the following before a surgery:

- There will not be any improvement in the hearing after surgery. On the contrary, there will be slightly decreased hearing after surgery even though myringoplasty is successful because the round window pathway is blocked by the reconstructed tympanic membrane.

- They should also be told about the possibility of a second-stage stapes surgery for its fixation.

Ear Selection

In general, there is a dictum that, in a bilateral disease, the worst ear should be selected first, but it is better if the ear in which there is a good improvement in the hearing with the patch test is operated on first than the ear with no improvement or little improvement in the hearing with the patch. A successful surgery helps the patient in gaining confidence, over the treating doctor and over himself.

Disease Activity during Tympanoplasty

- For a successful tympanoplasty, ideally the ear should be dry at the time of surgery.

- Earlier duration of keeping the ear dry for tympanoplasty was 6 months, but now dry ear is the only criteria; length of time is not important. Even the ear that remains wet with a tubotympanic discharge in spite of medical treatment can also be operated on as this discharge is allergic in these patients.

Informed Consent

All the patients should be informed before surgery regarding the disease process in the ear, various treatment options available, the exact nature of the surgery, associated risk of the surgery, and various complications.

In patients with suspected ossicular discontinuity and ossicular fixation, especially stapes fixation (confirmed by a Gelfoam patch test), they should always be informed about the possibility of a second-stage surgery.

6 Investigations

The following investigations should be done before surgery:

- X-ray of the mastoids: It is not essential to do X-rays of the mastoids before tympanoplasty, but as it is a very simple and cheap investigation, it should be done to know whether the mastoid is cellular or sclerosed. In an absolutely cellular mastoid (normal mastoid), there is no need to open the mastoid antrum.

X-ray of the mastoid gives an idea about the level of tegmen plate and sinus plate, which is helpful while opening the mastoid.

High-resolution computed tomography (HRCT) of the temporal bone is not needed in cases of tubotympanic disease. It is needed mainly in cases of unsafe otitis media (cholesteatoma).

- X-ray or CT scan of the paranasal sinus (PNS) should be done if sinusitis is suspected. The sinuses should be free from any infection.

- X-ray of the nasopharynx should be done in children to see for adenoids. If enlarged, it should be taken care of.

- General examination.

- Routine blood investigations.

- Electrocardiogram (ECG) is indicated to know about the fitness of the patient for surgery, especially in patients older than 45 years. If required, the patient should be shown to a physician.

- Chest X-ray should be done to confirm fitness of the patient.

- Xylocaine sensitivity tests.

- Anesthesia fitness.

- Preoperative antibiotics should be started 48 hours in advance.

- Culture and sensitivity of the discharge from the ear should be done if the ear is not getting dry.

7 Preparation and Position of the Patient

The side to be operated on is prepared by shaving around the pinna and cleaning by an antiseptic solution.

During surgery, the patient should lie down on the operating theater (OT) table in a comfortable supine position, with the head slightly turned on the opposite side. The part is cleaned and draped. In an obese patient, the head of the patient should be slightly lifted up by the pillow so that the shoulder does not come in between while working in the ear. In other patients, the neck of the patient is flexed and the head is extended at the atlanto-occipital joint. This brings the posterosuperior part of the tympanic cavity into proper view with better visualization of stapes, incudo-stapedial joint, and fallopian canal. The surgeon should sit comfortably on a cushioned stool or chair. His hands should rest on the patient's head or shoulder so that his hands are stable and do not get tired.

8 Anesthesia and Instruments Used for Tympanoplasty

Anesthesia

Anesthesia for tympanoplasty is either general or local. Most of the tympanoplasties are done under local anesthesia with sedation. General anesthesia is preferred in young, uncooperative, anxious patients. Local anesthetic agent (2% xylocaine with adrenaline 1 in 100,000) is infiltrated in the postaural region and in the external auditory meatus at the junction of the cartilaginous and bony meatus. Some infiltration is done at the incisura terminalis between the tragus and the ascending limb of the helix. The tragus is to be infiltrated if the surgeon is planning for removal of tragal cartilage (**Fig. 8.1a–f**).

If the surgery is done under local anesthesia, sedation given is a combination of injection pentazocine, injection Phenergan, and injection glycopyrrolate in proper doses. This is to be given intramuscularly, 45 minutes before surgery, supplemented by injection midazolam intravenously during surgery, if required, to reduce the anxiety of the patient and to sedate the patient.

General anesthesia is given in young, anxious, uncooperative patients. The choice of general anesthesia depends upon the anesthetist. Usually, hypotensive anesthesia is preferred to get dry bloodless field while operating. During general anesthesia, nitrous oxide gas is used. This nitrous oxide gas is released in the middle ear from the middle ear mucosa and pushes the graft and tympanomeatal flap laterally. Hence, there is a high possibility of graft getting displaced laterally, leading to graft failure. This supplementation of nitrous oxide gas should be withdrawn by the anesthetist just before the placement of the graft so that there is no chance of release of nitrous oxide in the middle ear after placement of the graft.

Local Anesthetic Agent (2% Xylocaine with Adrenaline 1 in 100,000) Is Infiltrated

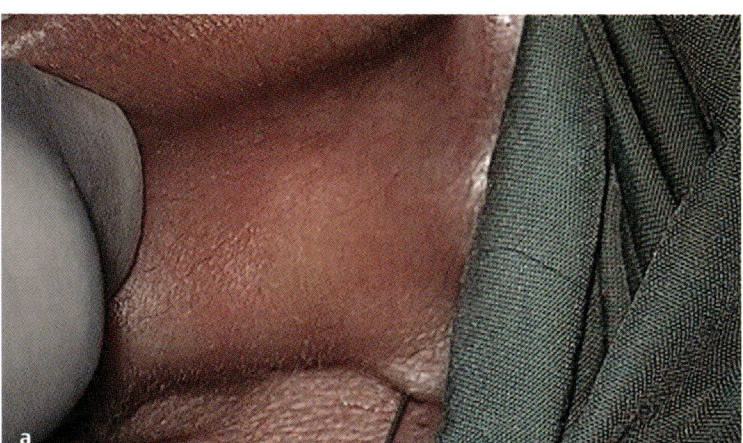

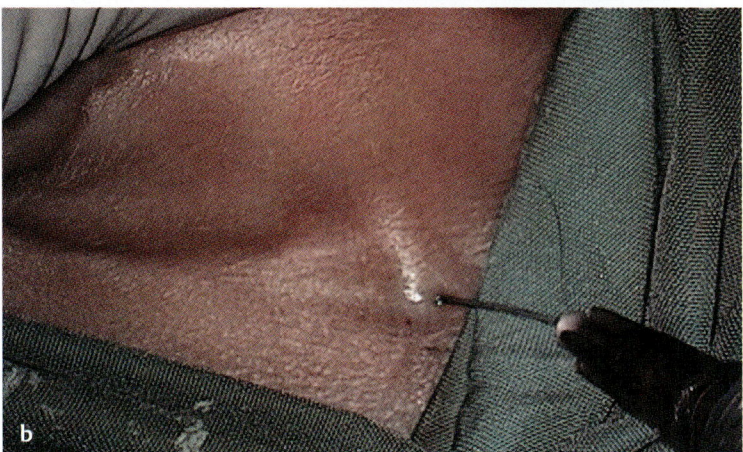

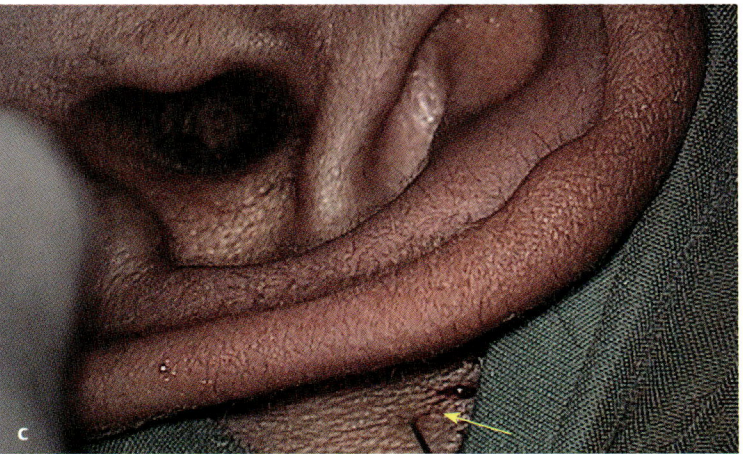

Fig. 8.1 **(a)** Infiltration of local anesthetic postaurally going toward the upper attachment of the pinna. **(b)** Infiltration of local anesthetic postaurally going toward the inferior attachment of the pinna. **(c)** Infiltration from the postaural region into the external auditory canal. The needle is inserted toward the external auditory canal medial to the pinna. *(Continued)*

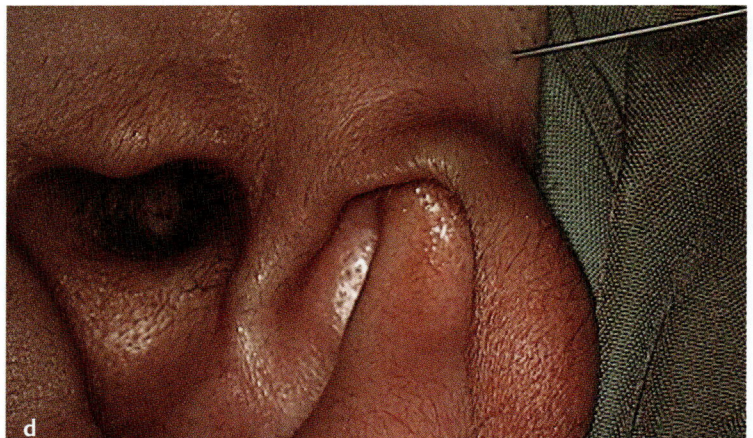

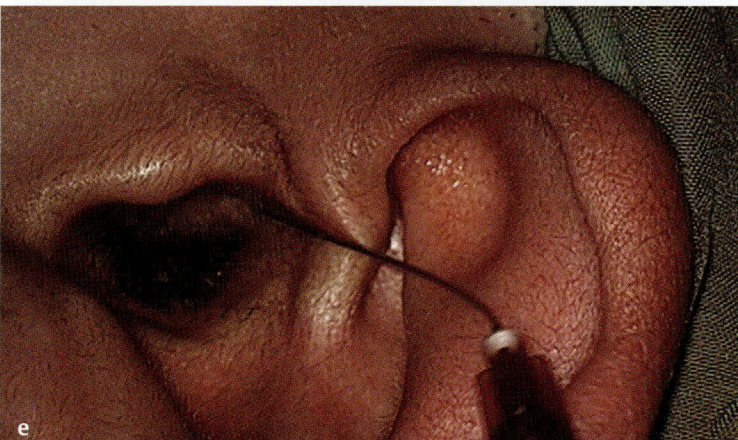

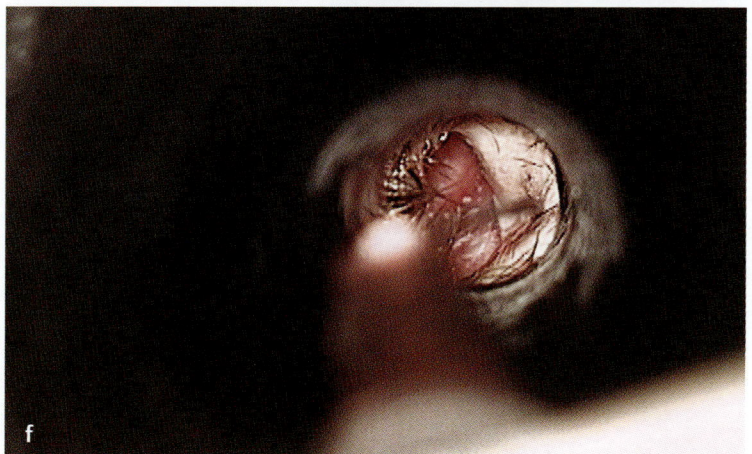

Fig. 8.1 *(Continued)*
(d) Infiltration is done between the tragus and the pinna.
(e) The anterior and inferior meatal wall is infiltrated by a local anesthetic agent.
(f) The posterior meatal wall is infiltrated.

Instruments used for tympanoplasty differ from surgeon to surgeon. Standard instruments which are common for every surgeon are shown in **Fig. 8.2**.

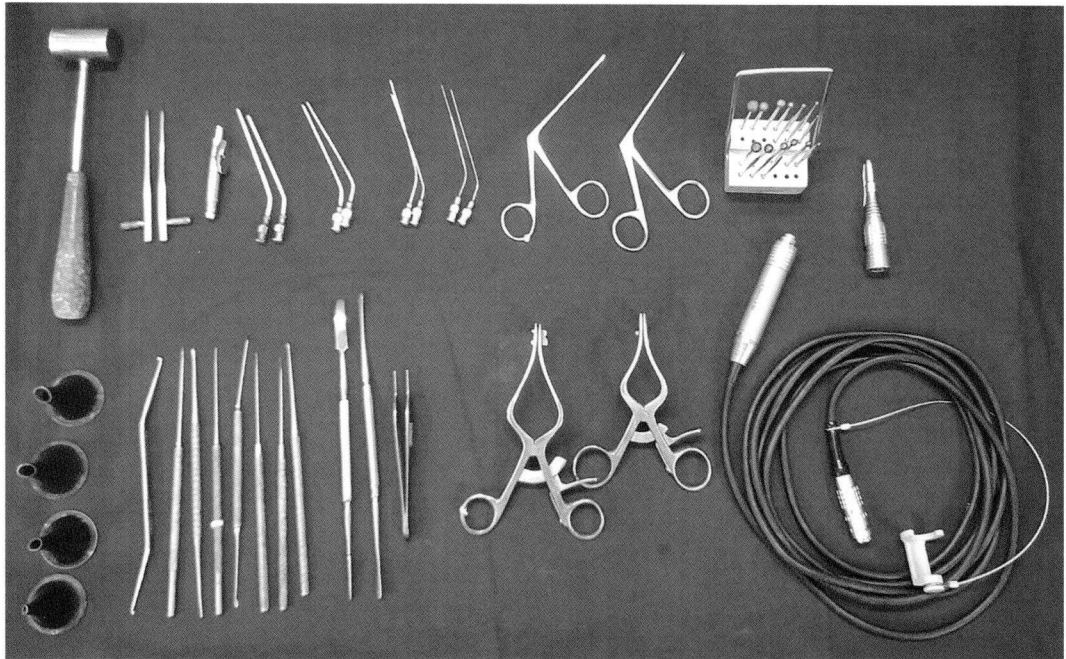

Fig. 8.2 Instruments used for tympanoplasty are standard with little variations from person to person. The most important instruments used for tympanoplasty are mastoid retractors, crocodile micro scissors and forceps, set of ear speculum, various picks, side and circular knife, drill machine (micro motor), handpiece with burrs and suction cannula. No doubt good operating microscope is a necessity.

9 | Incision

Incisions

Incision for tympanoplasty is either postaural or endaural.

Certain surgeons prefer endomeatal incision especially in patients with wide external auditory canal with no anterior meatal wall bulge. The mobility of cartilaginous external auditory canal with the pinna gives freedom to move the tip of the speculum to visualize the entire tympanic membrane. Here it is not possible to explore the mastoid, and separate incision is required to harvest the graft.

Endaural Incision

This is a small extra-cartilaginous incision having two parts (**Fig. 9.1**). The first part is a vertical incision that starts between tragus and helix and continues along the anterior margin of the ascending limb of the helix. The incision is deepened by cutting fibrous tissue between tragus and helix, exposing the temporalis fascia from which graft is harvested. The second part is a curved incision on the posterior meatal wall deep to the bone between the outer margin of the bony meatal wall and medial edge of the conchal cartilage superiory continued with the vertical incision (first incision). This incision is further deepened to the mastoid periosteum, which is incised and elevated pedicled posteriorly, thus exposing the mastoid. A self-retaining retractor is applied.

Postaural Incision

This incision starts from the upper attachment of the pinna going down along the postaural region toward the tip of the mastoid (**Fig. 9.2**). This is a bigger incision that gives wider access to the field of surgery. This incision in infants should stop at the middle of the postaural groove as in infants mastoid is not fully developed and the stylomastoid foramen with the facial nerve is superficial.

The temporalis fascia is exposed and the fascia graft is harvested. The mastoid periosteum is incised along the meatus and elevated up by using the periosteum elevator, pedicled onto the temporalis muscle. The mastoid is exposed, and a self-retaining mastoid retractors is applied.

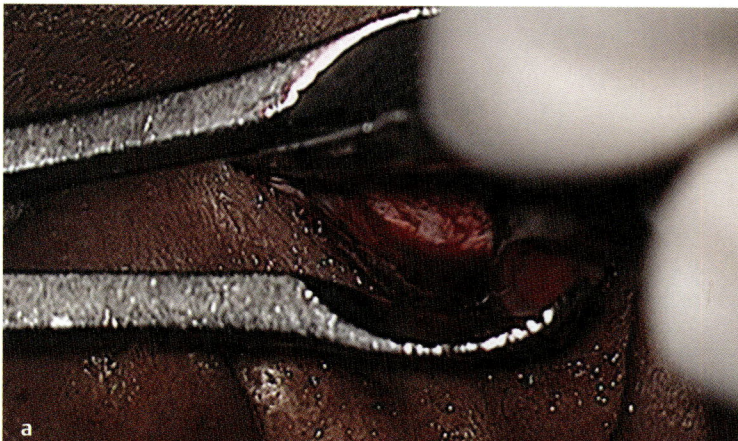

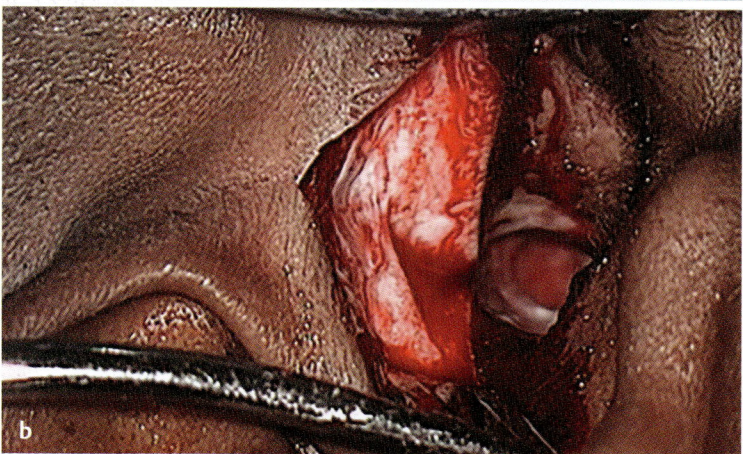

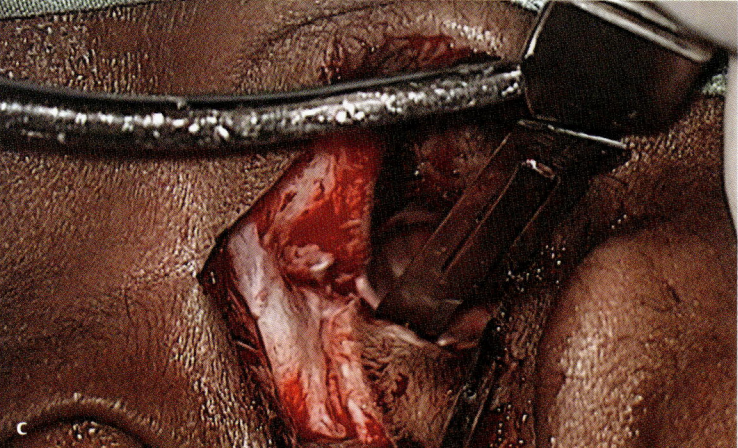

Fig. 9.1 **(a)** An endaural speculum is placed in the ear canal and vertical incision (first part of endaural incision) is given between tragus and ascending limb of helix. **(b)** Endaural retractor is applied to keep the incision opened. **(c)** A circular incision (second part of endaural incision) is given in the posterior canal wall to meet the first incision. *(Continued)*

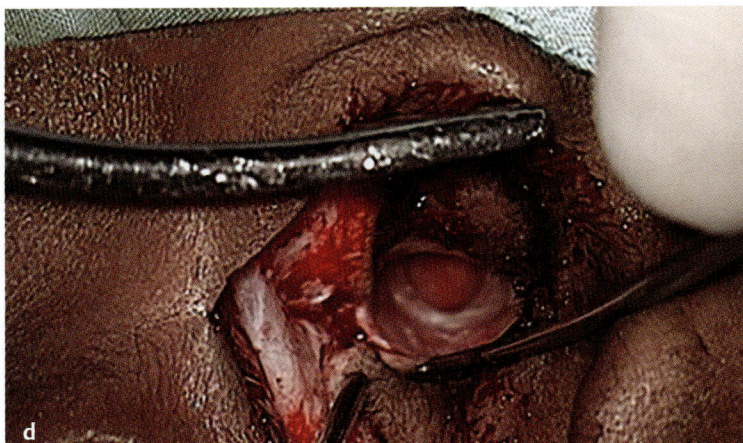

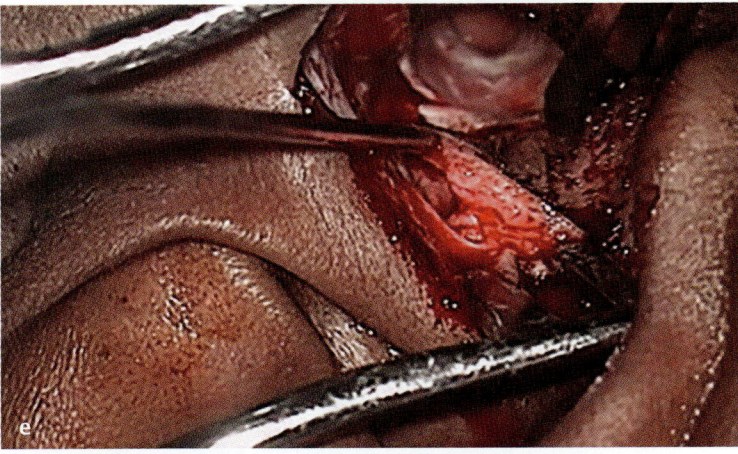

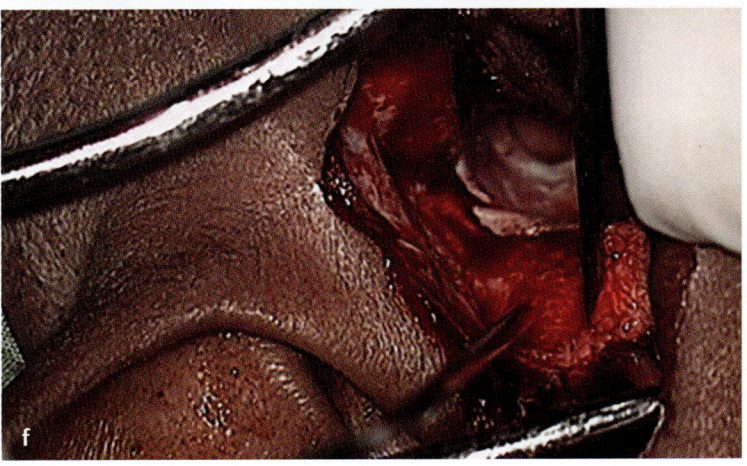

Fig. 9.1   *(Continued)*
(d) Posterior meatal wall skin is elevated. **(e)** Posterior meatal wall skin is elevated inferiorly. **(f)** Posterior meatal wall skin is elevated inferiorly by periosteum elevator, as low as possible to get good exposure. *(Continued)*

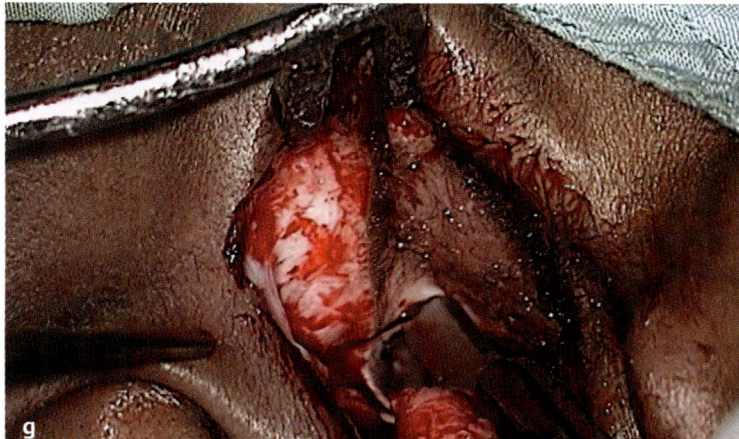

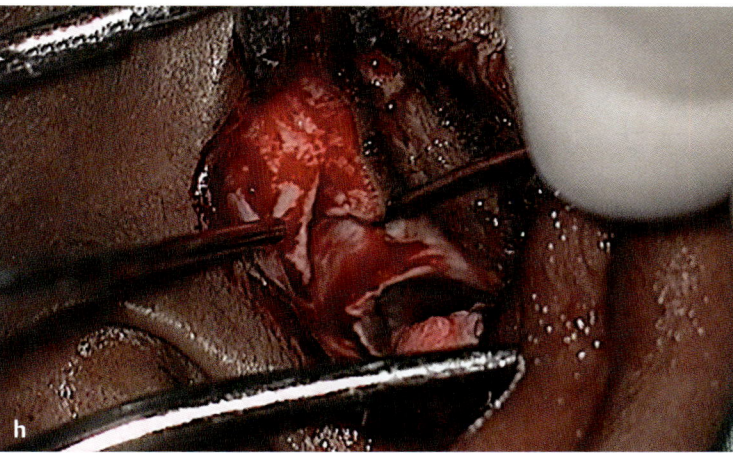

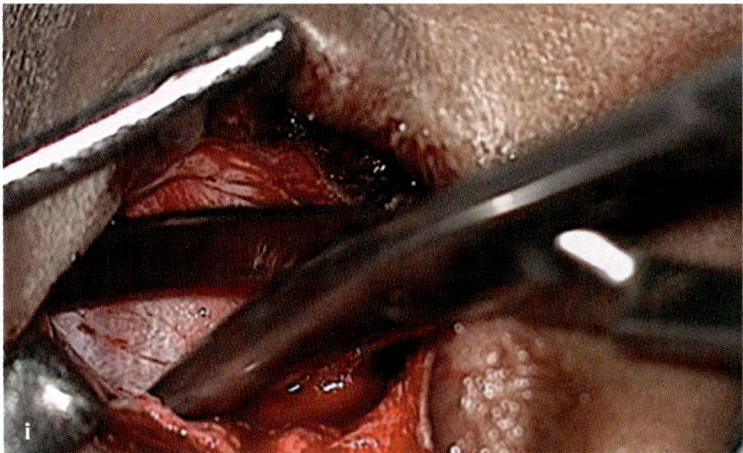

Fig. 9.1 *(Continued)* **(g)** Circular meatal wall skin incision is extended over the anterior bony meatal wall. **(h)** Anterior meatal wall skin is elevated laterally exposing the anterior bony meatal wall. **(i)** By dissection, temporalis fascia is exposed. *(Continued)*

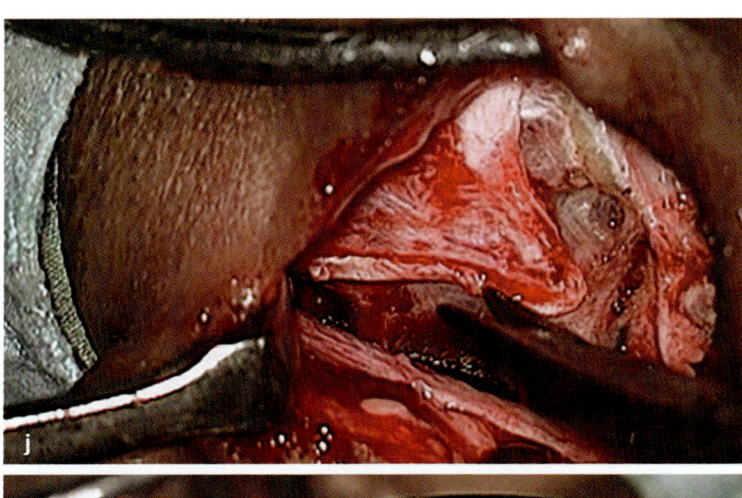

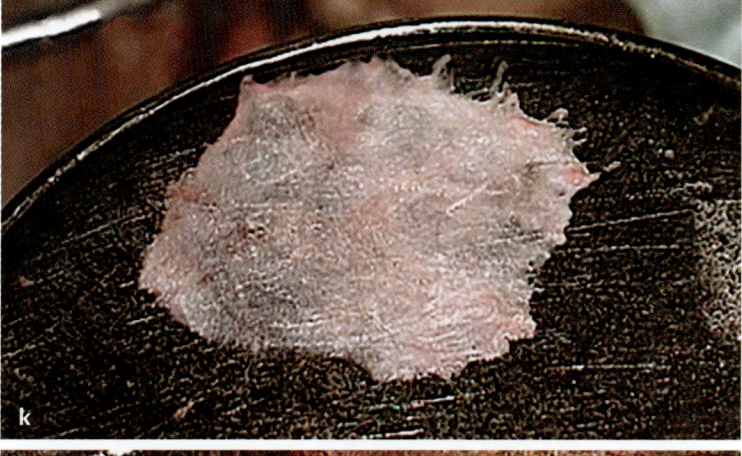

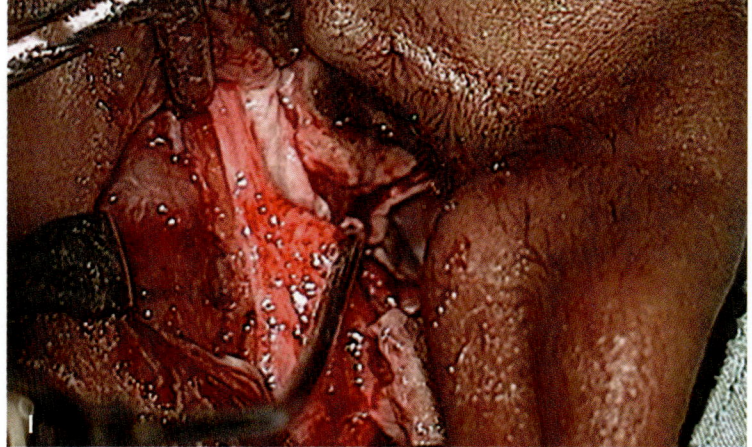

Fig. 9.1   *(Continued)*
(j) Temporalis fascia graft is harvested. **(k)** Temporalis fascia graft. **(l)** Periosteum over the mastoid is exposed by retractors. *(Continued)*

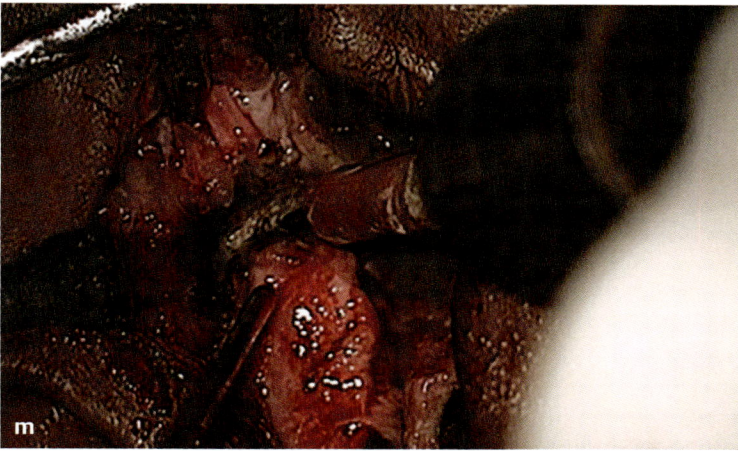

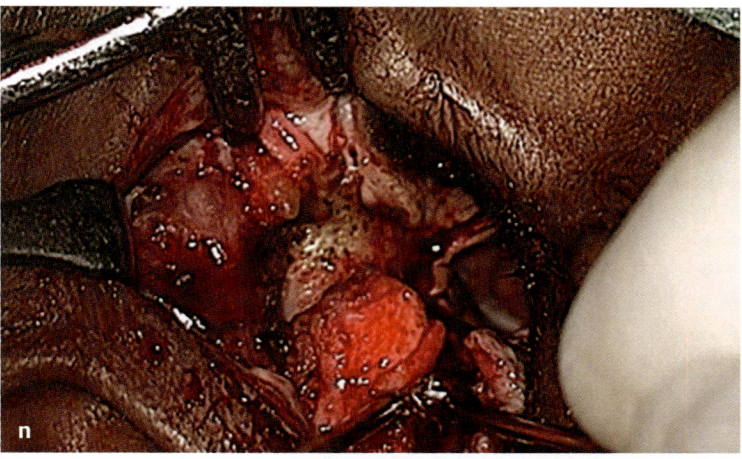

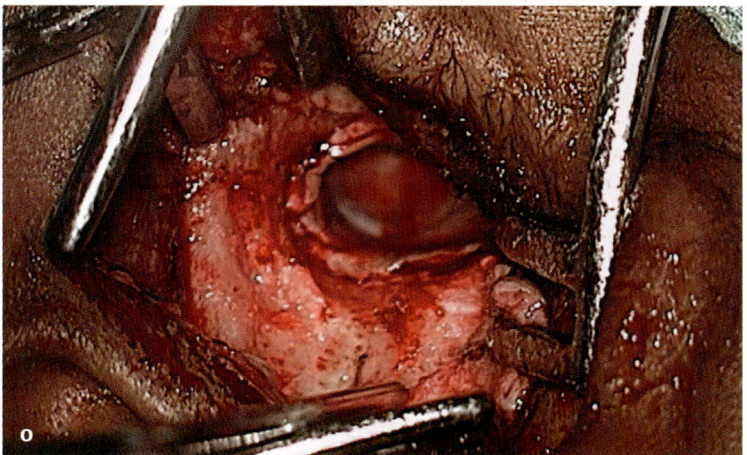

Fig. 9.1 *(Continued)* **(m)** Periosteum over the mastoid is incised. **(n)** Periosteum over the mastoid is separated and dissected, pedicled posteriorly, and is dissected as posterior as possible to expose the mastoid completely, may be up to the tip. **(o)** Retractors are applied exposing the mastoid and meatus with tympanic membrane nicely for tympanoplasty and mastoidectomy

Comparison between Postaural and Endaural Incision

Postaural (Fig. 9.2)	Endaural (Fig. 9.3)
Big incision	Very small incision
Lot of tissue dissection	Minimum tissue dissection
Consumes more time	Quick opening and closing
Cuts postaural sensory nerves	Not cutting any sensory nerves
Postoperative pain and edema are more	Minimal pain and edema

Postaural (Fig. 9.2)	Endaural (Fig. 9.3)
Risk of wound gaping	No risk of wound gapping
Big incision mark	Very small incision mark
More chances of keloid formation	Very less chances of keloid formation

There are many advantages of an endaural incision over a postaural incision. Hence, why to go for the bigger postaural incision when surgery can be successfully done through the smaller endaural incision (**Fig. 9.4**).

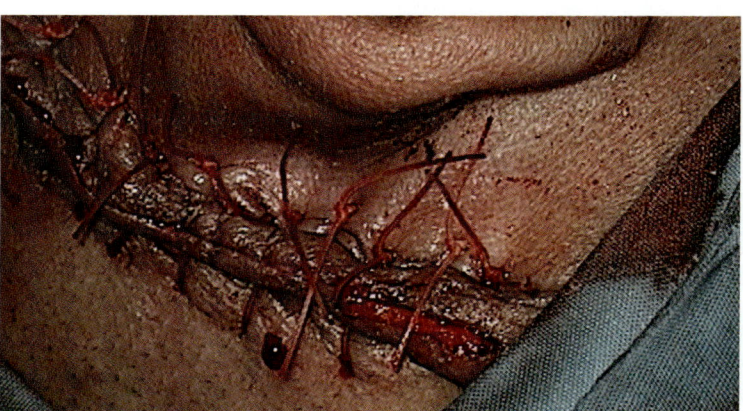

Fig. 9.2 Postaural incision: big incision, lots of tissue dissection, lots of suturing, and more postoperative pain.

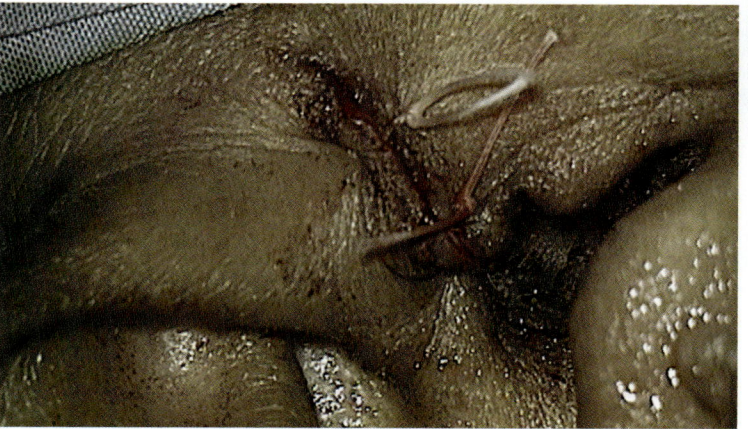

Fig. 9.3 Endaural incision: small incision, minimum tissue dissection, minimum suturing, and minimum postoperative pain.

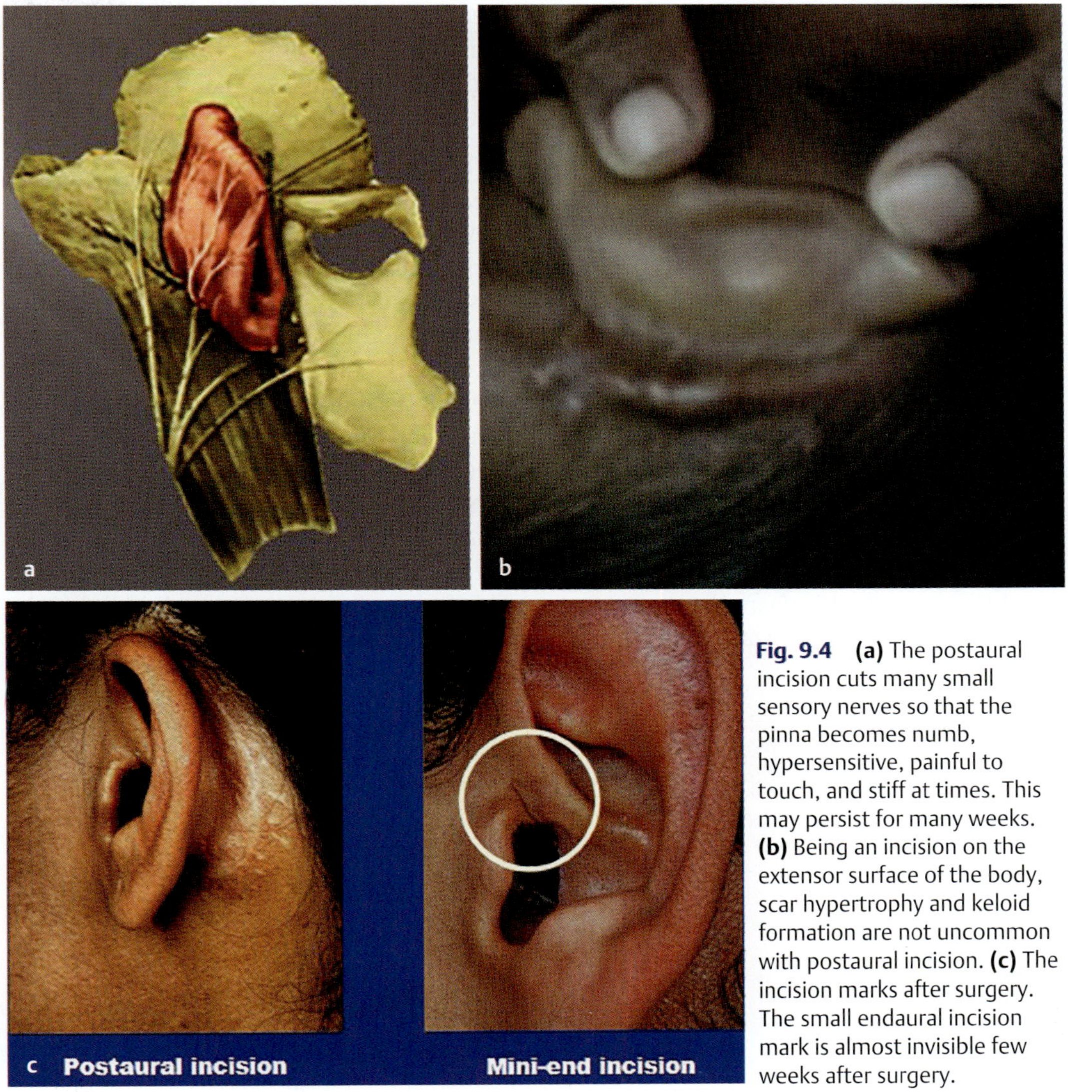

Fig. 9.4 **(a)** The postaural incision cuts many small sensory nerves so that the pinna becomes numb, hypersensitive, painful to touch, and stiff at times. This may persist for many weeks. **(b)** Being an incision on the extensor surface of the body, scar hypertrophy and keloid formation are not uncommon with postaural incision. **(c)** The incision marks after surgery. The small endaural incision mark is almost invisible few weeks after surgery.

Meatal Skin Flaps

There are a lot of diversities in elevating the meatal skin lining of the inner two-third of the bony meatus. The meatal skin is elevated either as a pedicled flap or as a free graft before doing a bony framework or before placing the graft. The pedicled skin flaps are preferred over the free graft. This meatal skin flap may be pedicled either superiorly or inferiorly or on the tympanic membrane as in Lempert's tympanomeatal flap. Whatever flaps are used, they are dissected gently and safely placed in the meatus to prevent them from any injury either by any instrument or by burr.

The skin of the superior bony meatal wall is said to be rich in blood supply, and it should be conserved for faster postoperative healing and faster epithelization of the bony meatus. Hence, it is termed a "vascular strip." These are all theoretical possibilities and surgery should be planned accordingly after considering all these factors.

The ultimate conclusion is that the meatal skin, whatever way it has been elevated, should be conserved during surgery and reposited back into its original position so that at the end the complete external auditory canal is lined by the skin for faster healing and epithelization. It also prevents granulation tissue formation in the canal and prevents postoperative meatal stenosis. If the skin is falling short following canalplasty, the postaural skin is taken out as a free full-thickness skin graft to cover the raw areas in the external auditory canal. This free graft is taken up well in lining the external auditory canal for faster healing.

10 Technique of Tympanoplasty

Surgery is done either by an onlay technique or by an underlay technique.

In the earlier days, the onlay technique was more popular, but later the underlay technique became more popular as various advantages of the technique over the onlay technique were realized.

Onlay Technique

In this technique, the graft is placed lateral to the tympanic membrane remnants after removal of the epithelial layer and is placed medial or lateral to the handle of the malleus.

Underlay Technique

In this technique, the graft is placed medial to the tympanic membrane remnants with the annulus and medial to the handle of malleus. The success rate will be high with this technique with a 360-degree elevation of tympanomeatal. Here, the graft is supported by the bony meatal wall, which results in a high success rate.

Interlay Technique

In the interlay technique, the epithelial layer is separated from the endothelial layer. This separation is possible anteriorly and inferiorly and not possible posteriorly.

Hence, the graft is placed interlay anteriorly and underlay posteriorly.

The full cuff (360-degree) interlay technique was developed by Dr. A.B.R. Desai with a high success rate, and there are many followers to his full cuff interlay technique.

The onlay technique for repairing tympanic membrane perforation has been replaced by the underlay technique because of various problems with the onlay techniques, which are the following:

- Lateralization of the graft: Here the graft falls away from the handle of the malleus, away from the tympanic membrane remnants.

- Blunting of the anterior sulcus: Here the anterior sulcus becomes thick and blunt due to formation of granulations with healing with fibrosis, as the anterior sulcus in not skin lined (**Fig. 10.1**).

- Epithelial pearl: The squamous epithelium remaining deep to the fascia leads to the formation of the epithelial pearl.

The underlay technique gives highly successful results:

- There are no chances of medialization of the graft, as the graft is well supported by the bony meatal wall on all the sides.

- There are no chances of blunting of the anterior sulcus, as the anterior sulcus is skin lined.

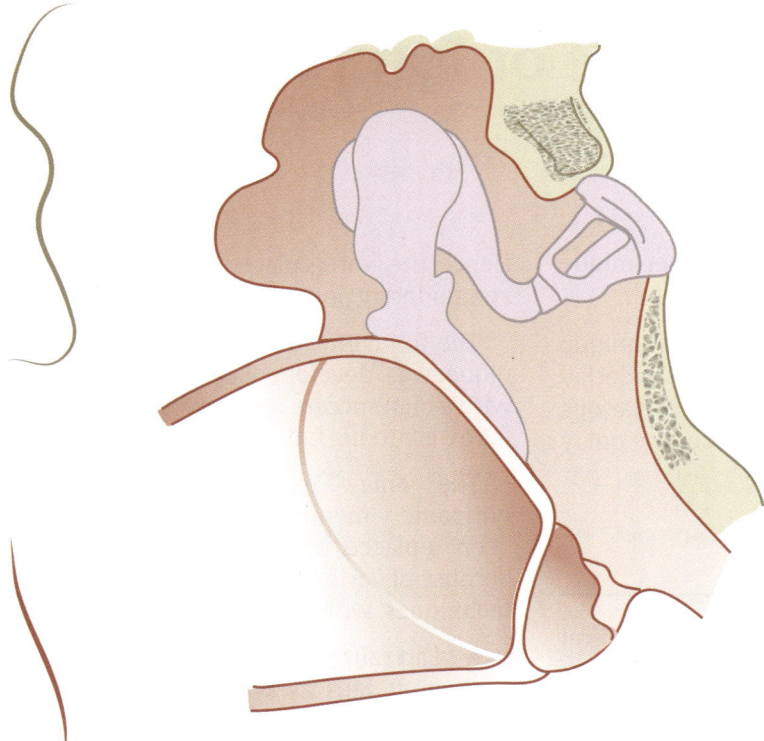

Fig. 10.1 Blunting of the annulus.

- There is no chance of lateralization of the graft, as the graft is medial to the handle of the malleus.

- There is no chance of epithelial pearl formation.

- While placing the underlay graft, the middle ear is entered by elevating the tympanomeatal flap. Once the middle ear is entered and the eustachian tube is visualized, its patency can be checked.

During healing, the endothelium from the edges of the perforation can grow over the graft.

Migration of this endothelium from the edges of the perforation over the fascia graft leads to granular myringitis, which can be prevented by destroying the endothelium, at the edges of the perforation by chemical cauterization.

For chemical cauterization, 50% trichloroacetic acid (TCA) or 30% silver nitrate should be used.

Cauterization also freshens the edges of the perforation; hence, there is no need to remove the margins of perforation.

Surgical Technique

Case 1: Type 1 Tympanoplasty

Surgery is done either under local or general anesthesia (**Figs. 10.2–10.36**). Either postaural or endaural incision is made. Whatever anesthesia or incision is selected, the basic technique remains the same. The ultimate aim is to achieve successful hearing results.

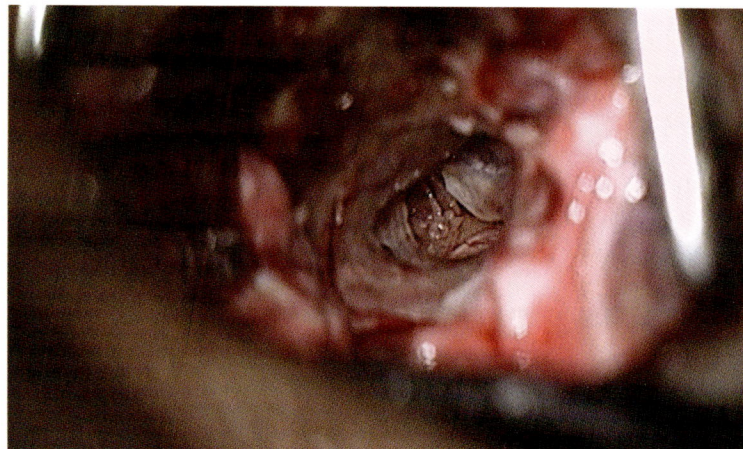

Fig. 10.2 Large central perforation. Tympanoplasty is done via an endaural incision. Bulging anterior bony canal wall hiding the anterior margin of perforation.

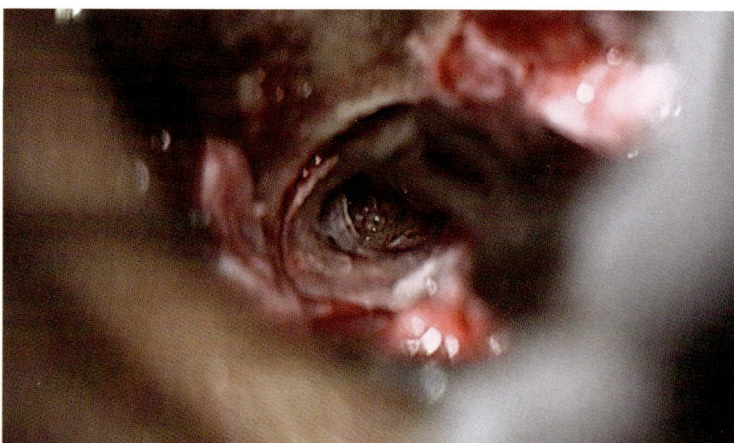

Fig. 10.3 A 360-degree circumferential meatal wall skin incision is made.

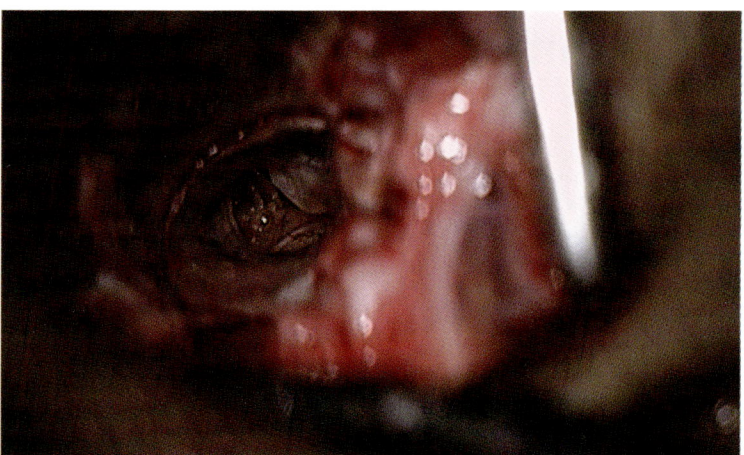

Fig. 10.4 A 360-degree circumferential meatal wall skin incision is completed.

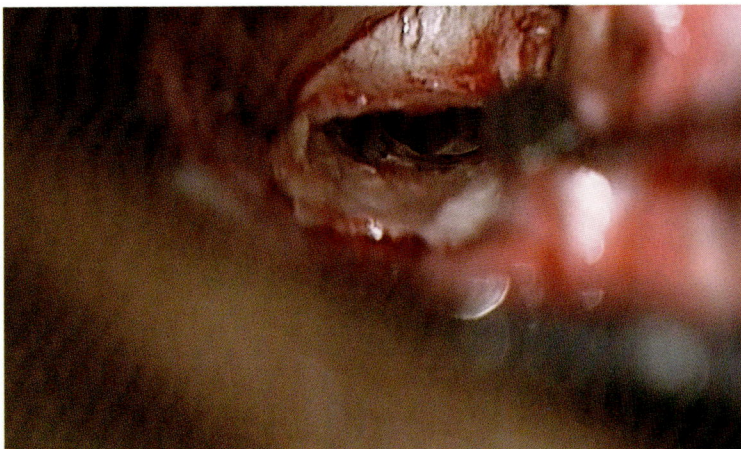

Fig. 10.5 Circumferential tympanomeatal flap is elevated.

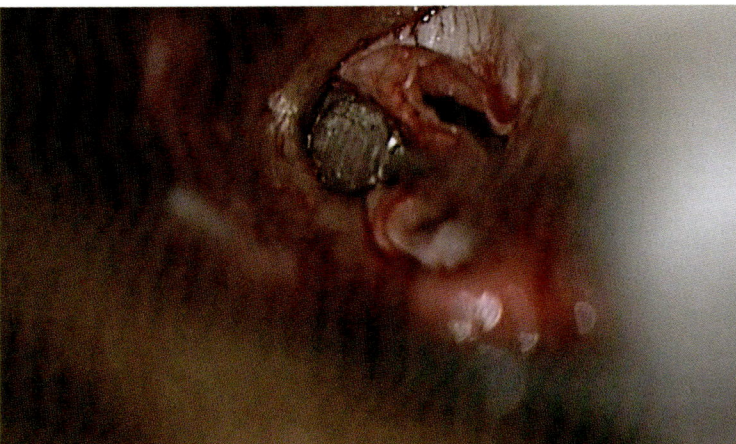

Fig. 10.6 Elevation of the anterior and inferior meatal wall skin is made by a circular knife.

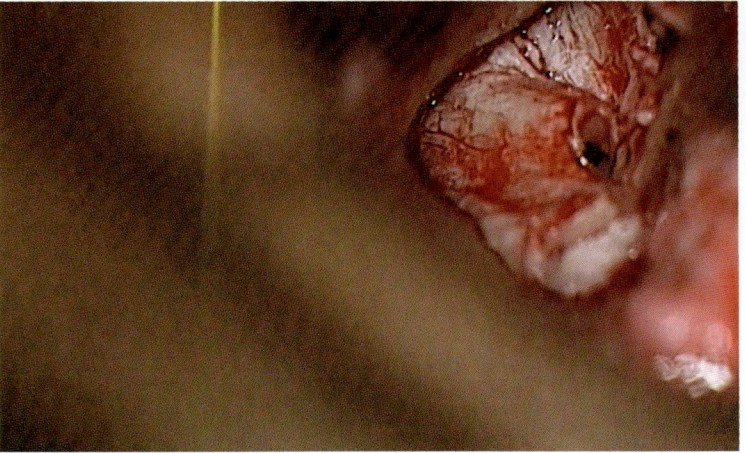

Fig. 10.7 Elevation of the anterior and inferior meatal wall skin is continued up to the annulus.

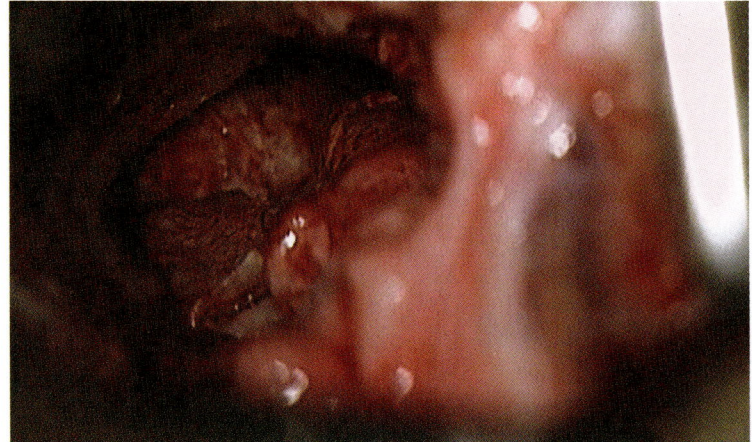

Fig. 10.8 Elevation of the anterior and inferior meatal wall skin is done up to the annulus. Bulging anterior and inferior bony meatal wall is hiding the annulus.

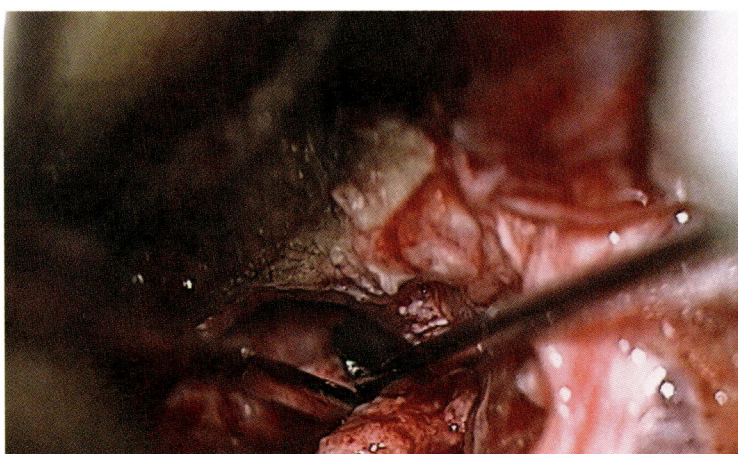

Fig. 10.9 Superior meatal wall skin is elevated up to the neck of the malleus.

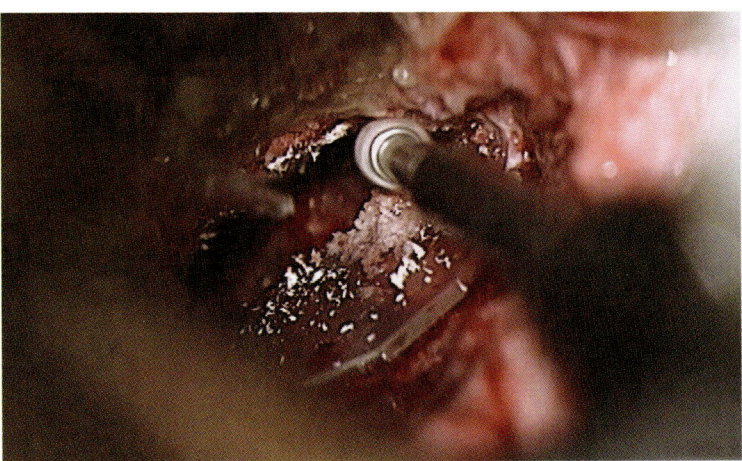

Fig. 10.10 Bulging superior and anterior bony meatal wall is reduced by canalplasty. Tympanomeatal flap is protected by a thick sheet of silastic.

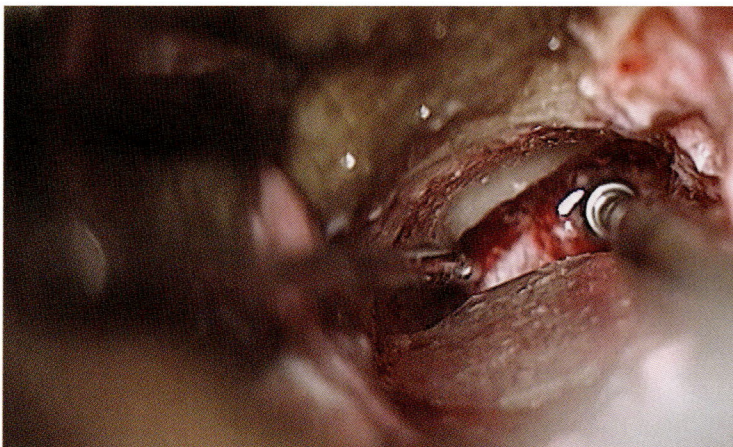

Fig. 10.11 Bulging bony anterior meatal wall is reduced by canalplasty to expose the annulus.

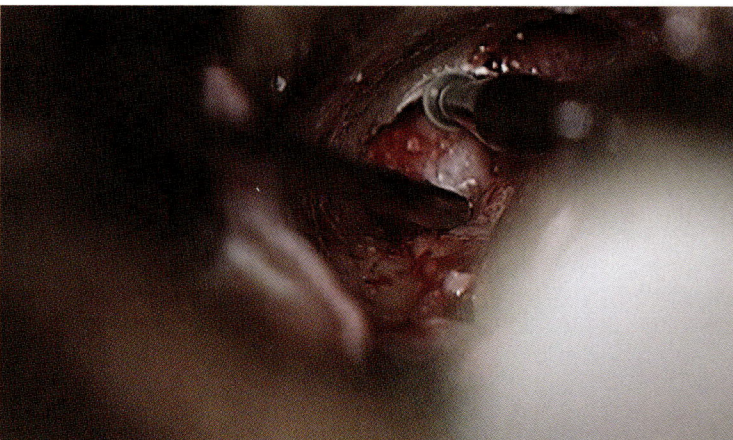

Fig. 10.12 Bulging anterior bony meatal wall is further reduced by canalplasty to expose the annulus.

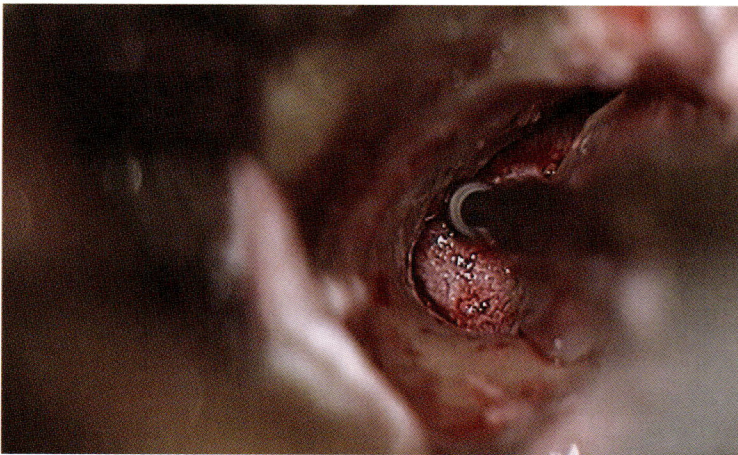

Fig. 10.13 Diamond burr is used to reduce the medial part of the canal wall to prevent injury to tympanomeatal flap.

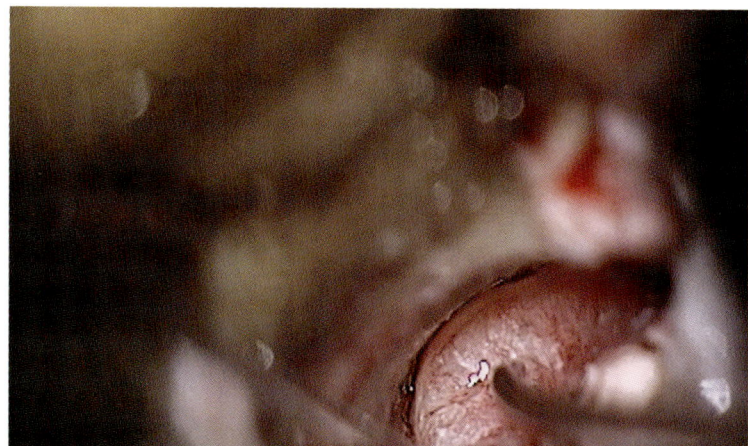

Fig. 10.14 The annulus is exposed after canalplasty.

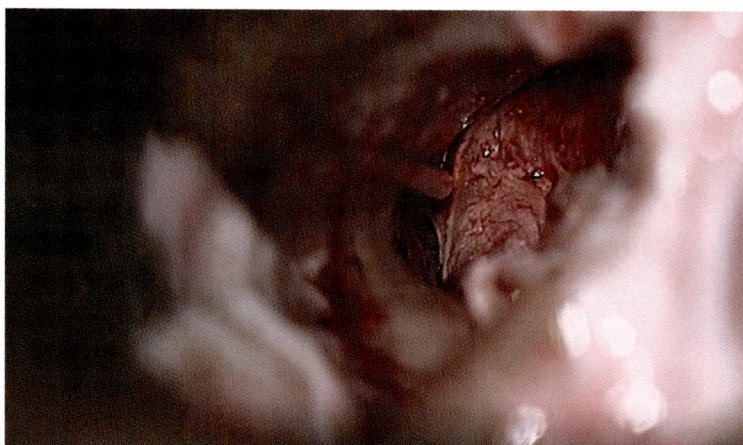

Fig. 10.15 The anterior annulus is elevated from the tympanic sulcus.

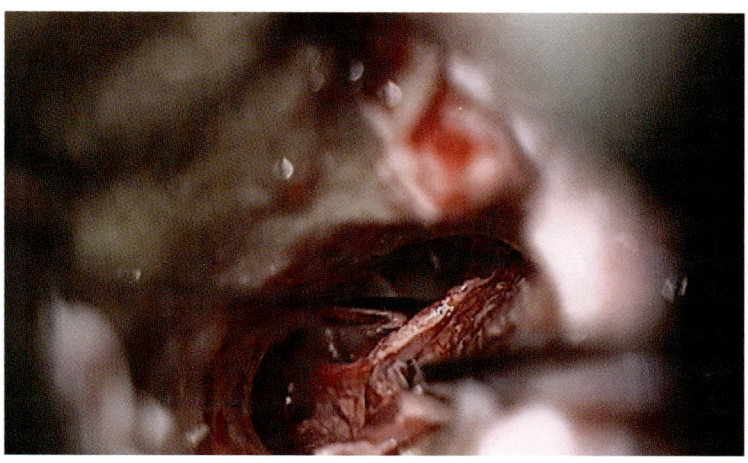

Fig. 10.16 Annulus elevation from the tympanic sulcus is continued up to the neck of the malleus.

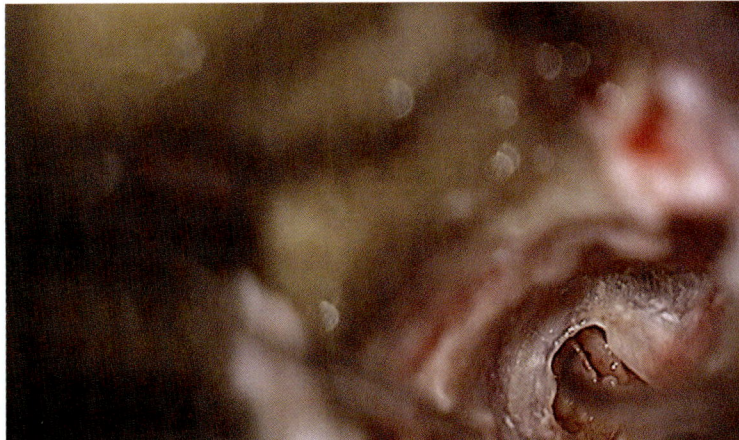

Fig. 10.17 Anterior part of the tympanic membrane, which was not seen earlier, is now completely exposed after canalplasty.

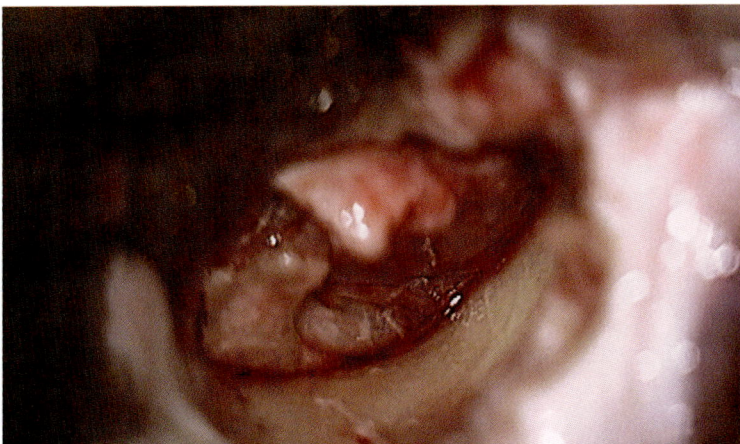

Fig. 10.18 Posterior tympanomeatal flap is elevated up to the annulus.

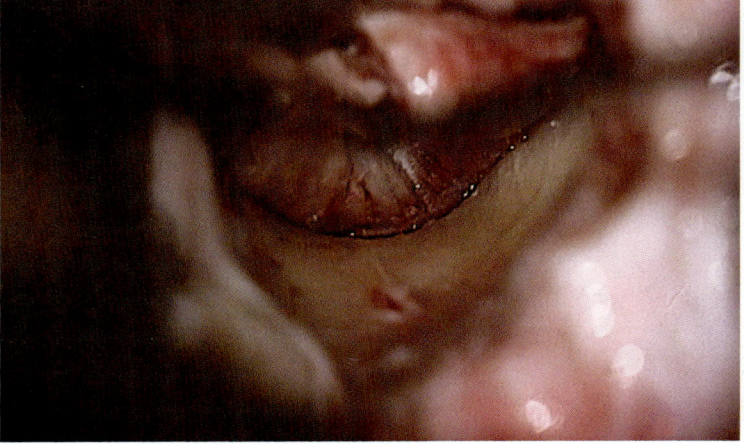

Fig. 10.19 The posterior annulus is exposed completely.

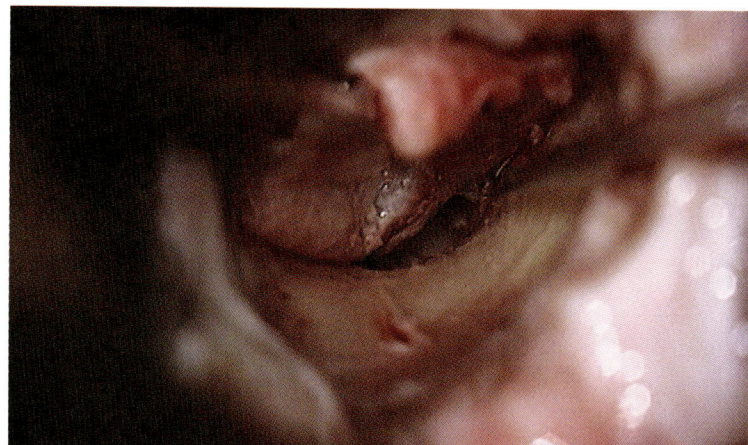

Fig. 10.20 Tympanic cavity is entered after elevating the tympanic annulus from the sulcus.

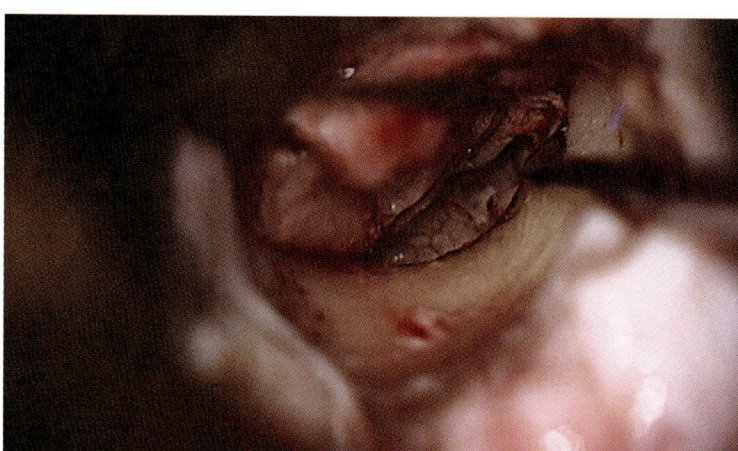

Fig. 10.21 The middle ear is entered, and the malleus handle and the incus are exposed.

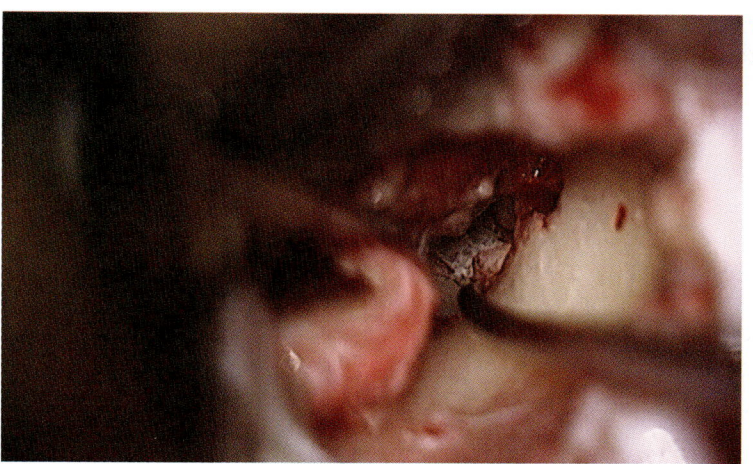

Fig. 10.22 Mobility of the stapes is confirmed.

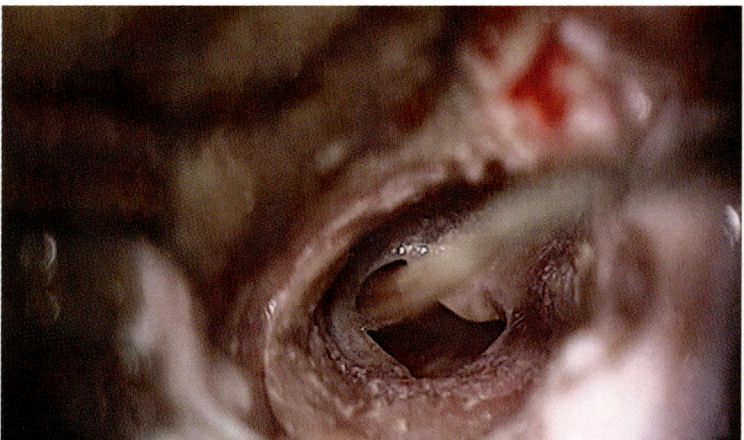

Fig. 10.23   Margins of the perforation is freshened by chemical cauterization by using 50% trichloroacetic acid (TCA).

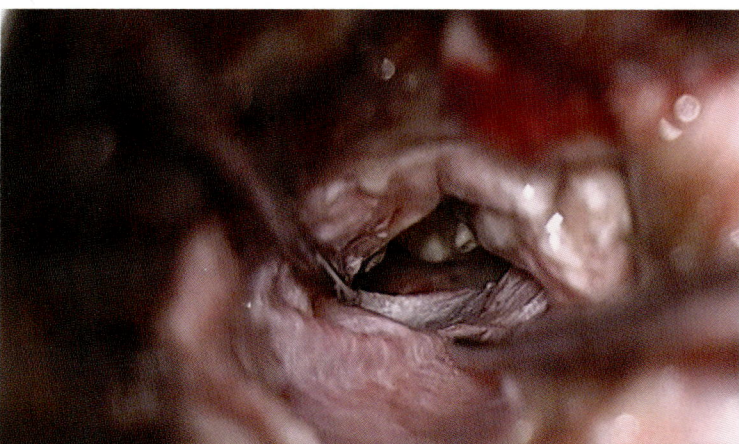

Fig. 10.24   An underlay graft (fascia) is placed.

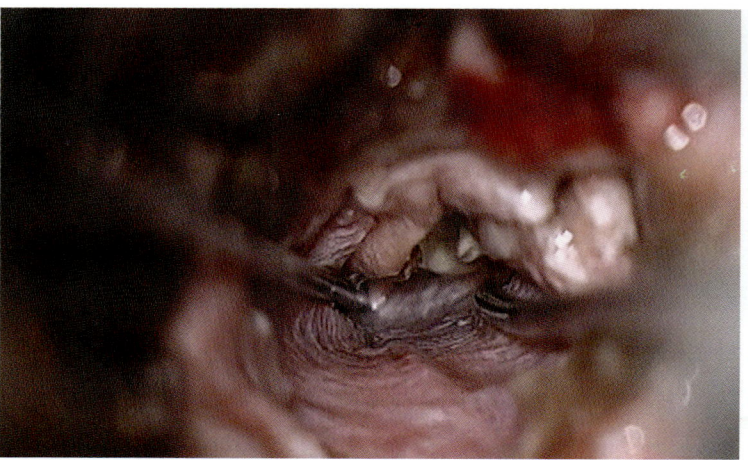

Fig. 10.25   An underlay graft is placed medial to the handle of the malleus.

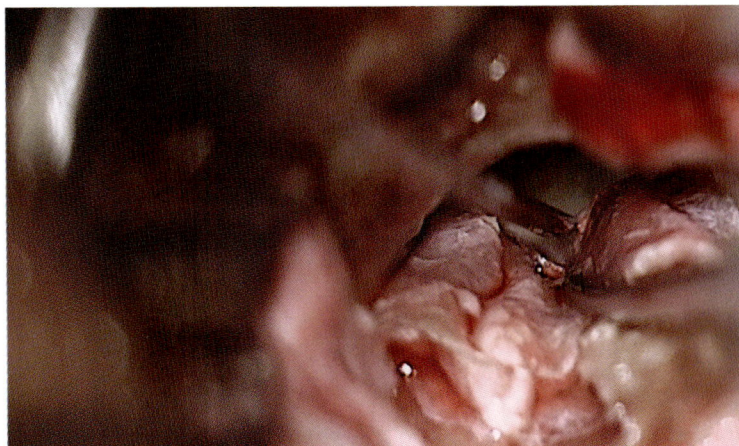

Fig. 10.26 Anterior tympanomeatal flap is lifted to pull the graft anteriorly lying medial to the handle of malleus, to rest it on the anterior and superior bony meatal wall to prevent medialization of the graft.

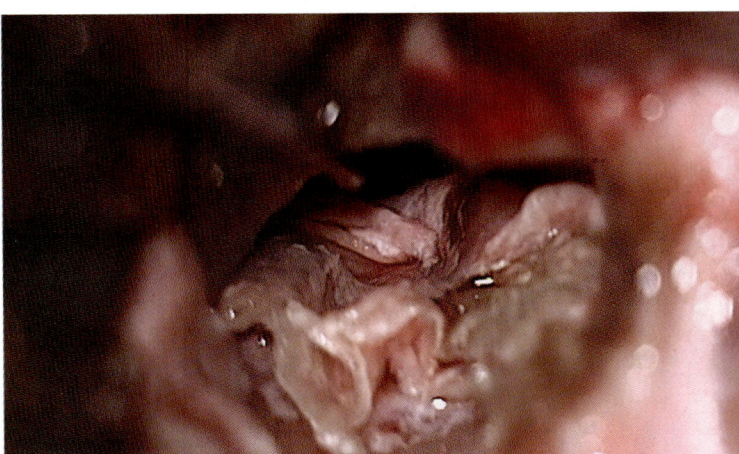

Fig. 10.27 The graft is pulled anteriorly under the anterior tympanomeatal flap lying medial to the handle of the malleus, to rest it on the anterior and superior bony meatal wall to prevent medialization of the graft.

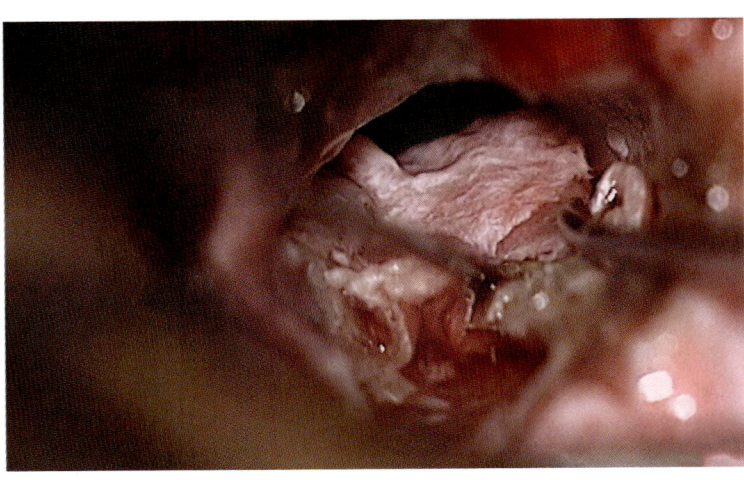

Fig. 10.28 The graft is pulled adequately anteriorly under anterior the tympanomeatal flap lying medial to the handle of the malleus, to rest it on the anterior and superior bony meatal wall to prevent medialization of the graft.

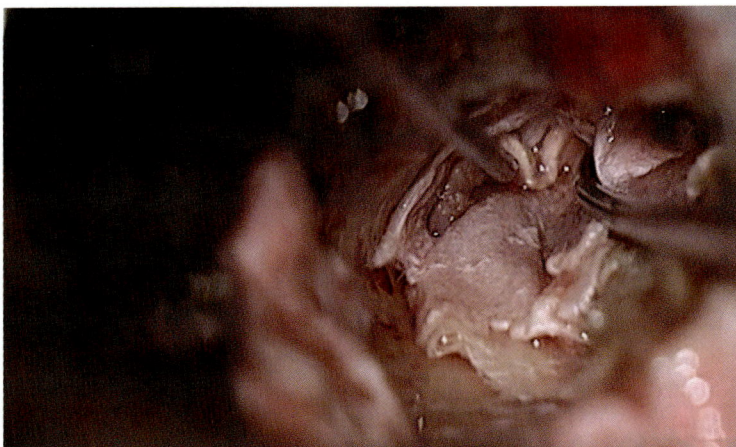

Fig. 10.29 After placing the graft on the meatal wall circumferentially, the annulus is reposited back into its original position, that is, into the tympanic sulcus area.

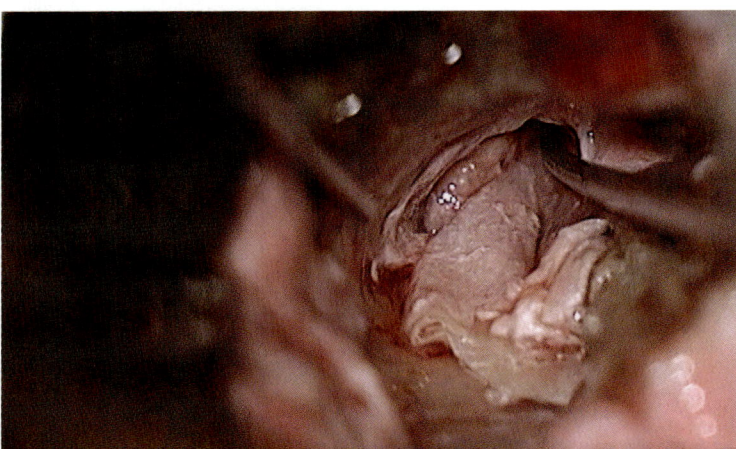

Fig. 10.30 Graft is resting on the bony meatal wall circumferentially and attempt is made to reposit the annulus into its original position.

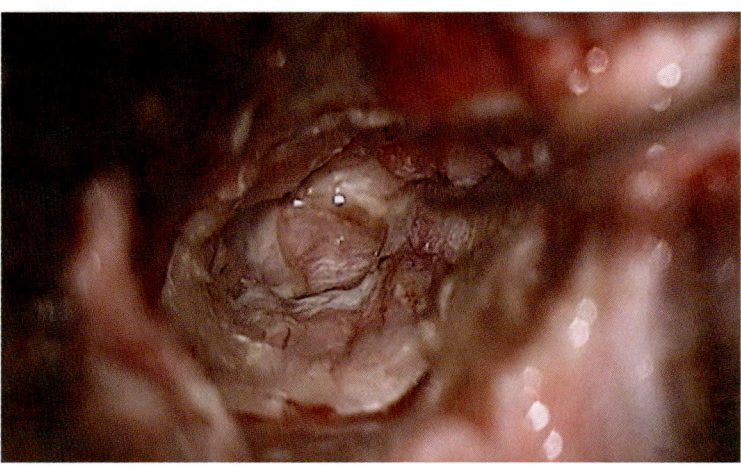

Fig. 10.31 Tympanomeatal flap is reposited back into its original position so that anteroinferior tympanomeatal angle is maintained and it is skin lined; hence, there is no chance of blunting of the anterior sulcus.

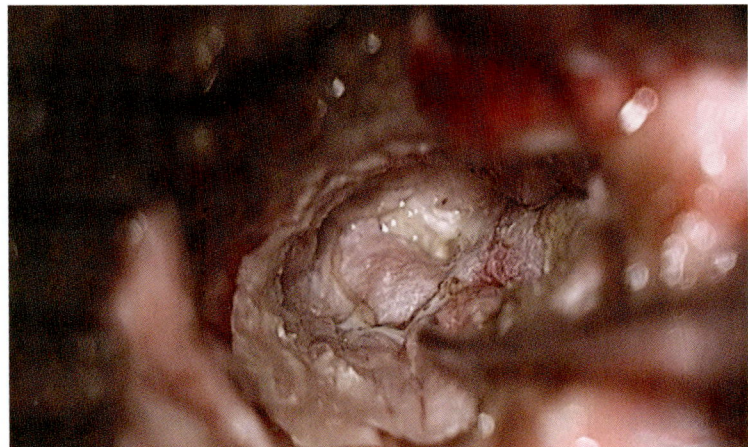

Fig. 10.32 Finally perforation is closed by an underlay graft, which is well supported by the bony meatal wall on all the sides.

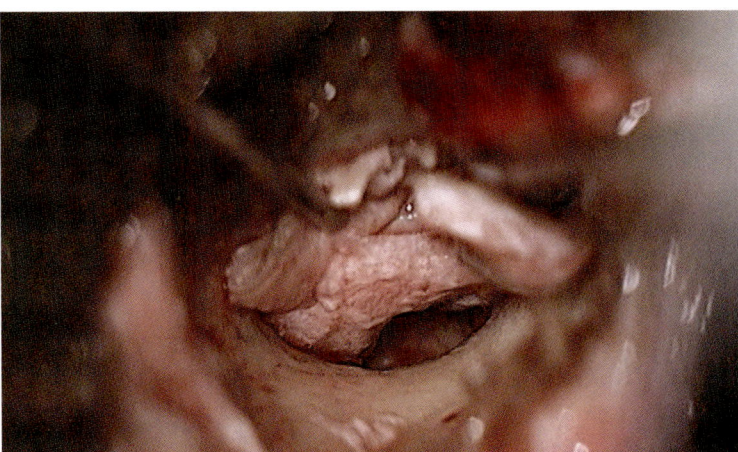

Fig. 10.33 Posterior tympanomeatal flap is elevated to reconfirm the placement of the graft on the posterior and inferior meatal wall.

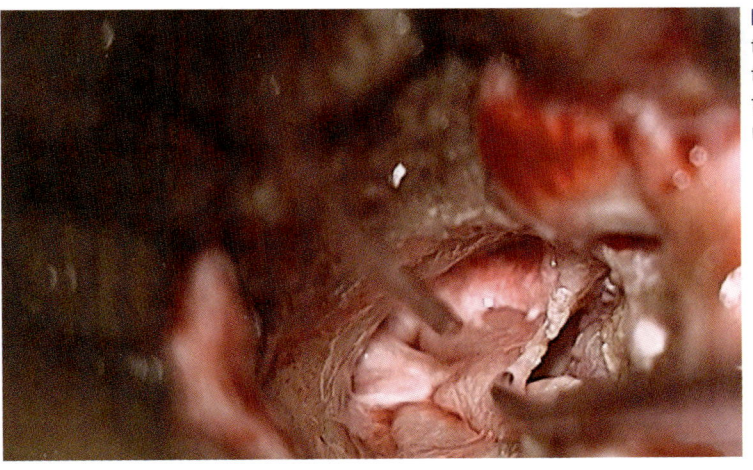

Fig. 10.34 Anterior tympanomeatal flap is elevated to confirm the placement of the graft on the anterior bony meatal wall.

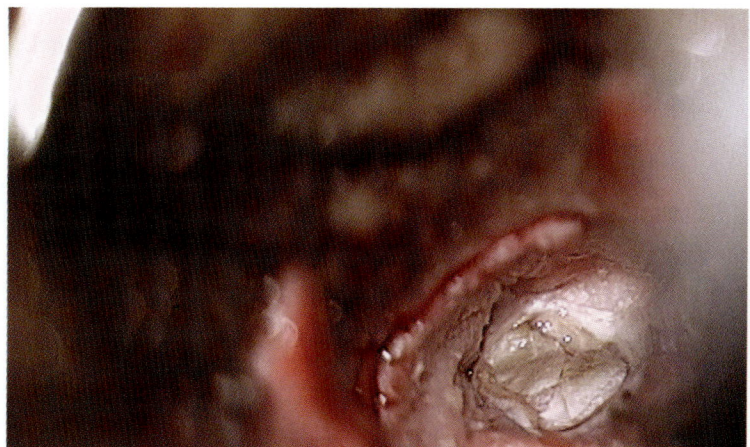

Fig. 10.35   The graft is covered by pieces of meatal skin for fast epithelialization.

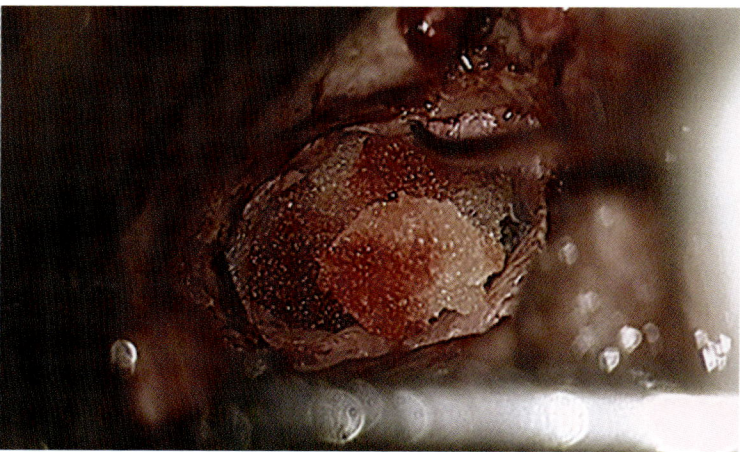

Fig. 10.36   Gelfoam is placed in the external auditory canal and the incision is closed.

Case 2: Tympanoplasty in a Case with Intact but Eroded Lenticular Process of the Incus

Continuity of the ossicular chain is maintained. The eroded lenticular process is covered by **Y**-shaped cartilage to prevent further pressure erosion of the lenticular process of the incus by retracted tympanic membrane (long-term ossicular continuity is maintained; **Figs. 10.37–10.51**).

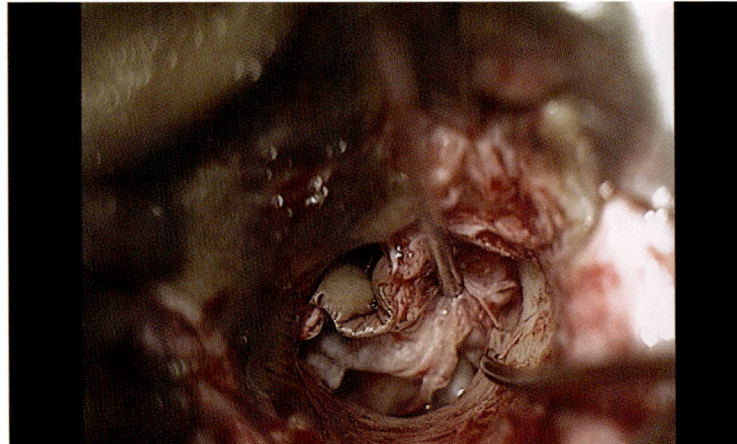

Fig. 10.37 The middle ear is entered after elevating the tympanomeatal flap.

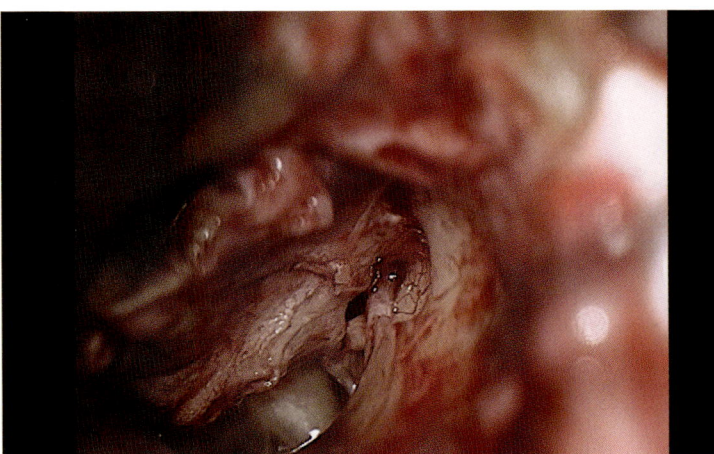

Fig. 10.38 The lateral surface of the incus lenticular process is eroded, but continuity is maintained. The stapes is intact and mobile.

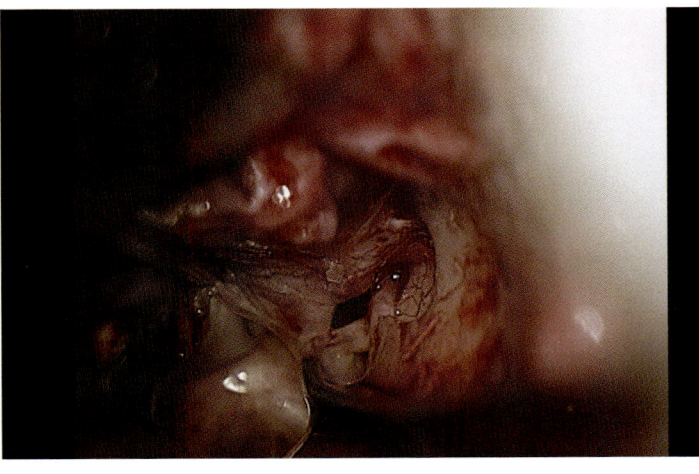

Fig. 10.39 The tympanic membrane is adherent to the incus lenticular process, which is eroded. Attempt is made to dissect the tympanic membrane from the incus lenticular process by sharp pick without any tear.

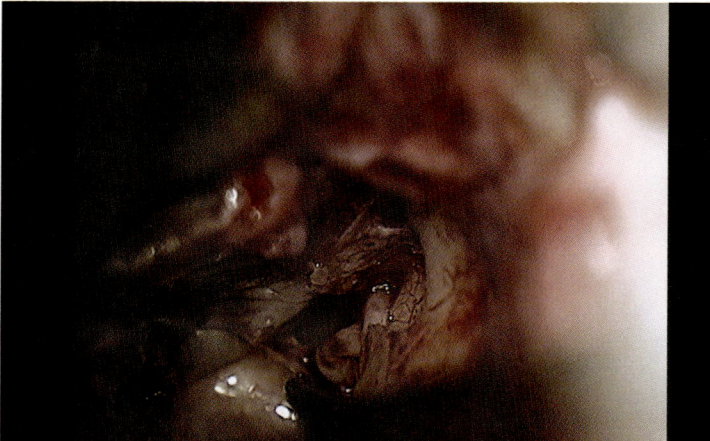

Fig. 10.40   The tympanic membrane is gently dissected from the incus lenticular process by sharp pick without any tear in the tympanic membrane. Few mucosal bands are separated.

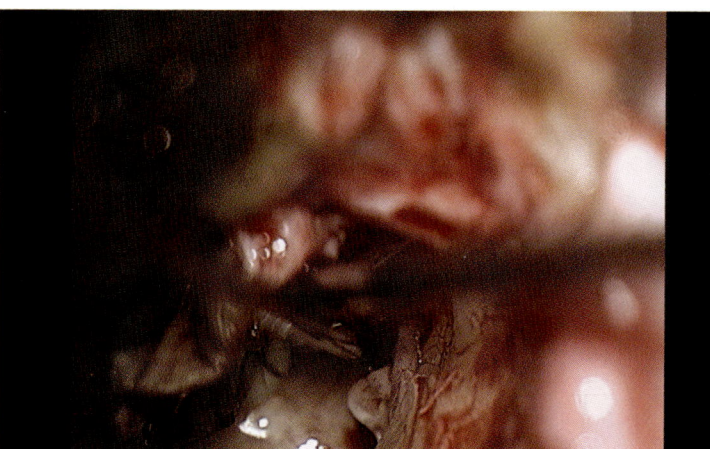

Fig. 10.41   The tympanic membrane has been gently dissected. Ossicular chain continuity is maintained, but the incus lenticular process is eroded on its lateral side. The middle ear is healthy.

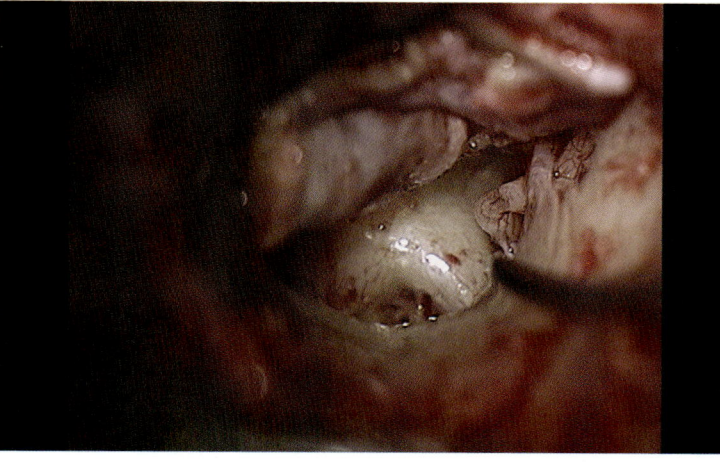

Fig. 10.42   The ossicular chain is intact and mobile. Round window reflex is present. Middle ear mucosa is normal and healthy.

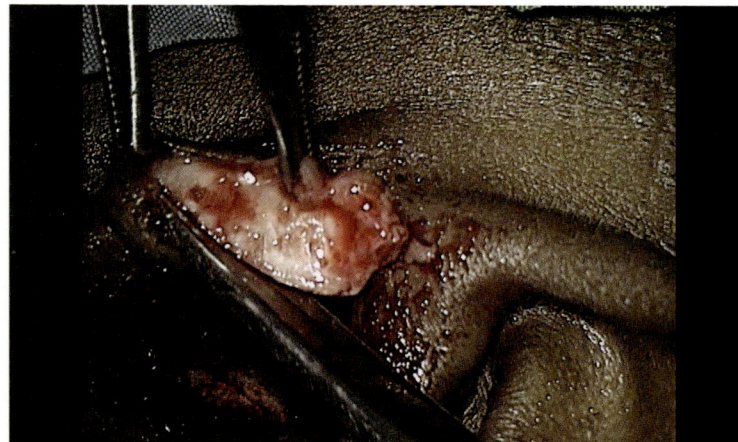

Fig. 10.43 A small piece of cartilage with the perichondrium is removed from the tragus.

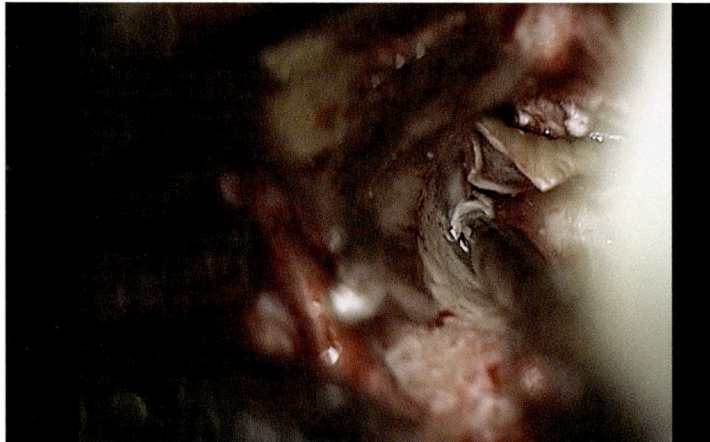

Fig. 10.44 A groove is made at the level of the inferior sulcus for placement of the cartilage.

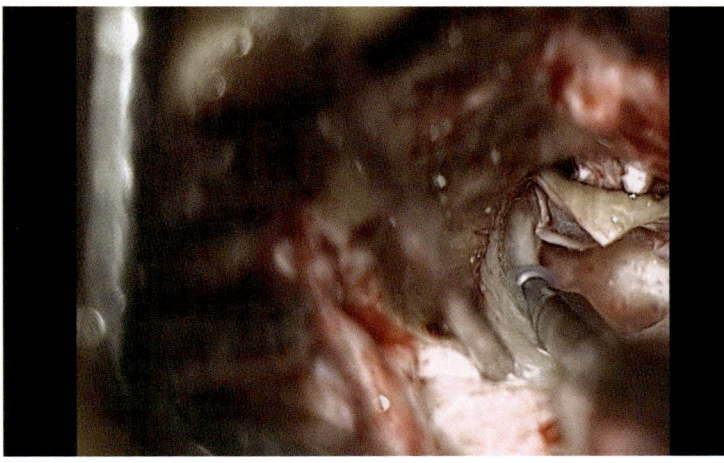

Fig. 10.45 The groove is further deepened for the cartilage to rest on it.

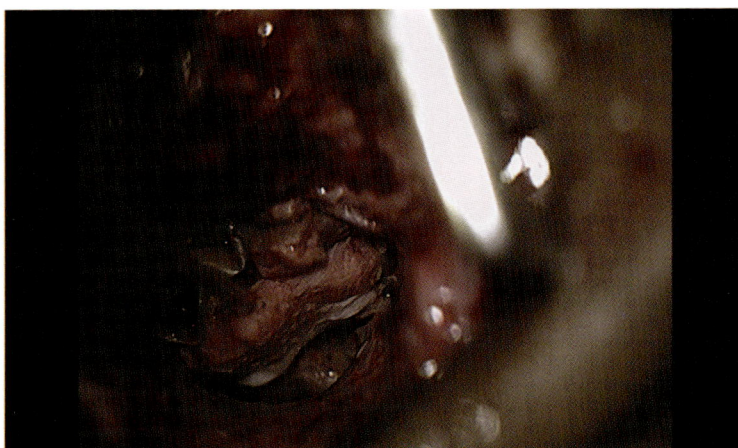

Fig. 10.46 The underlay graft is placed.

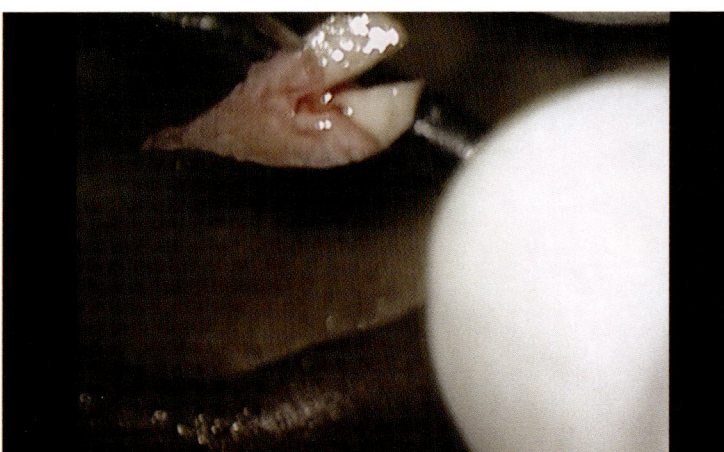

Fig. 10.47 A Y-shaped cartilage with the perichondrium is prepared from the tragal cartilage piece.

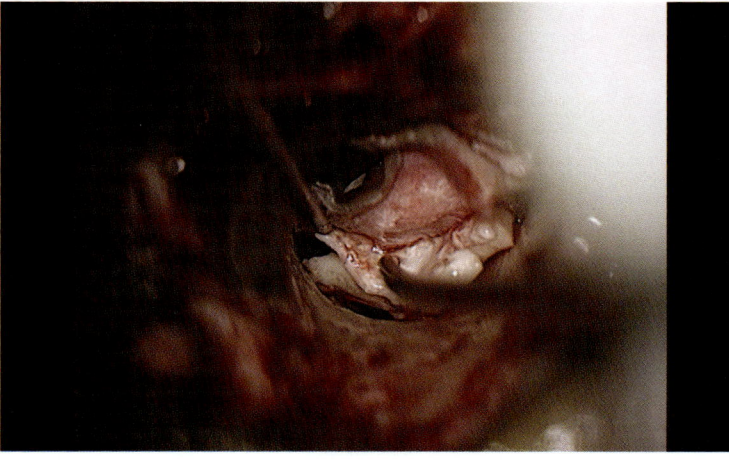

Fig. 10.48 A Y-shaped cartilage is placed horizontally in the middle ear.

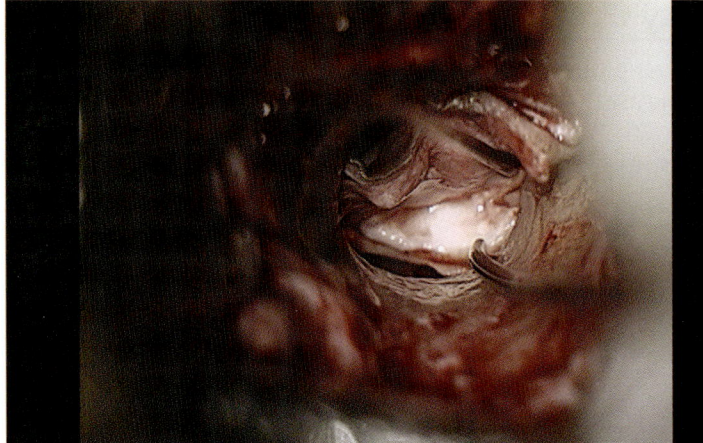

Fig. 10.49 A **Y**-shaped cartilage is placed horizontally in the middle ear with its lower end resting in the groove at the level of the inferior sulcus with its upper **Y**-shaped end encircling the incus lenticular process to prevent future retraction and adhesion of the tympanic membrane to the incus, to avoid further erosion of its long process.

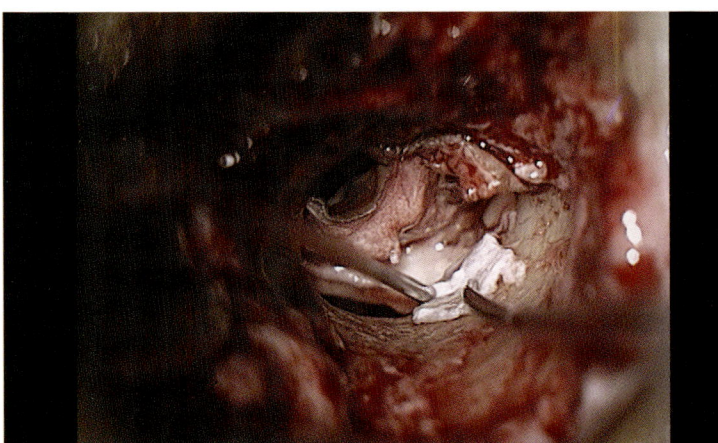

Fig. 10.50 The postero-superior part of the tympanic cavity is reinforced by the perichondrium to prevent any retraction pocket in future.

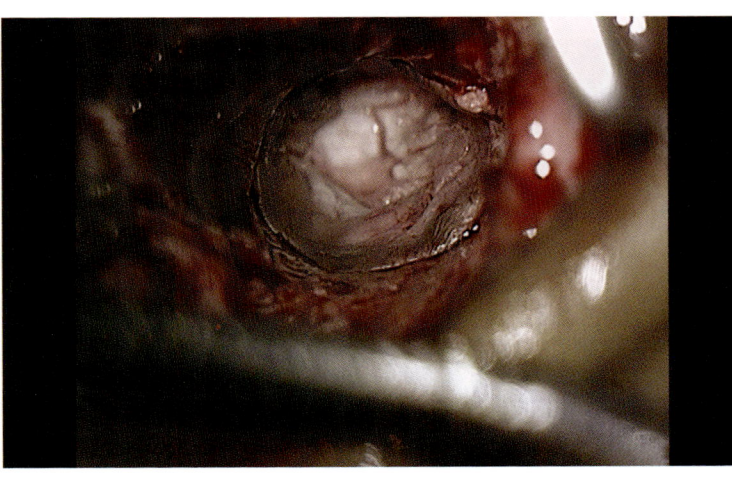

Fig. 10.51 The tympano-meatal flap is reposited back.

Case 3: Type 1 Tympanoplasty

Details of the tympanoplasty in a patient with subtotal perforation with 360-degree elevation of the meatal wall cuff in case 3 are presented in **Figs. 10.52–10.77**.

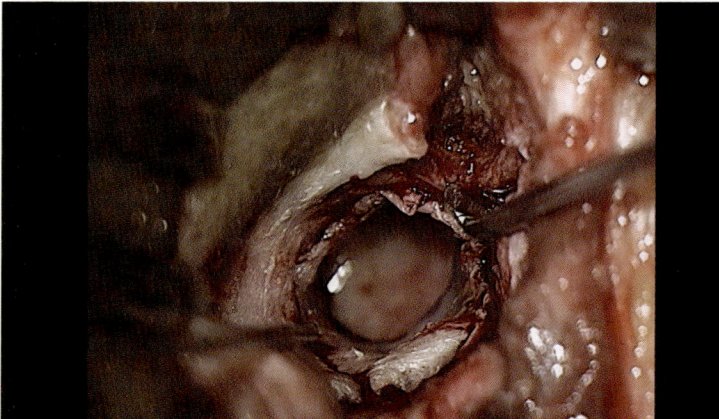

Fig. 10.52 Endaural incision, fascia graft, and circumferential meatal wall skin incision are given.

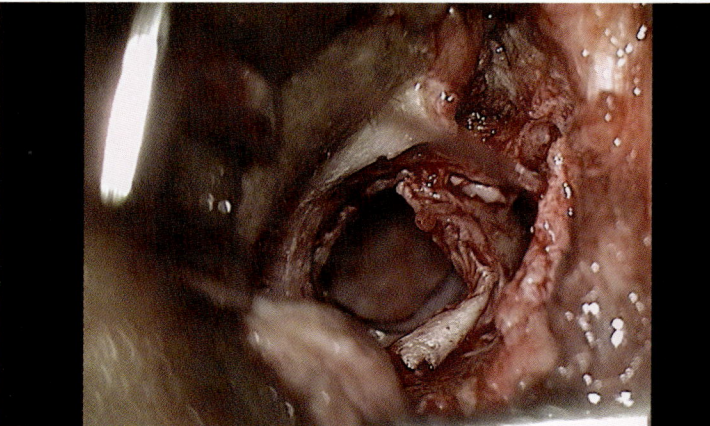

Fig. 10.53 The postero-superior tympanomeatal flap is elevated.

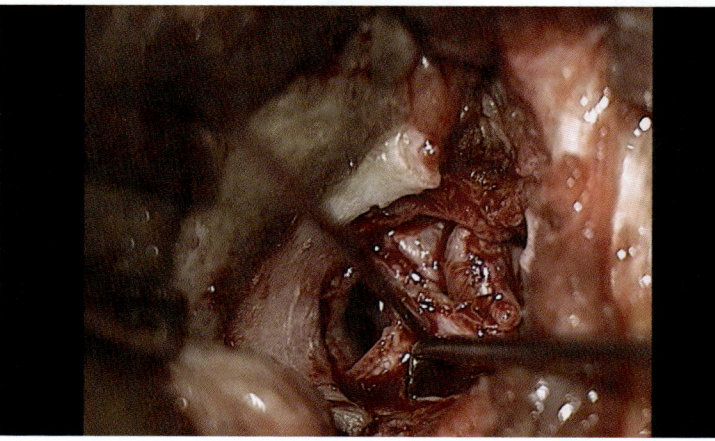

Fig. 10.54 The inferior tympanomeatal flap is elevated.

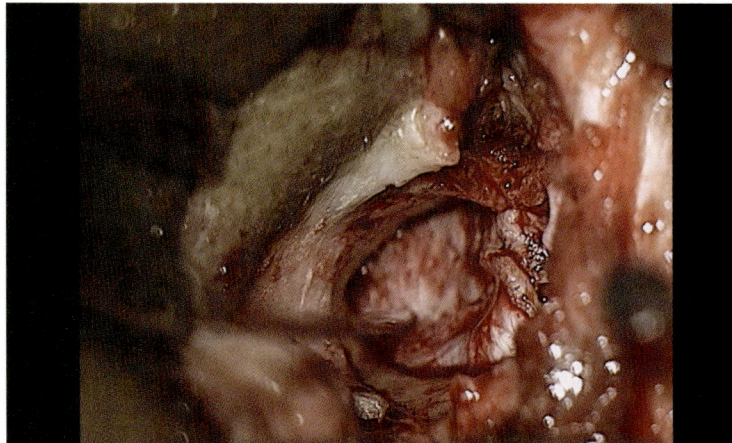

Fig. 10.55 The anterior tympanomeatal flap is elevated.

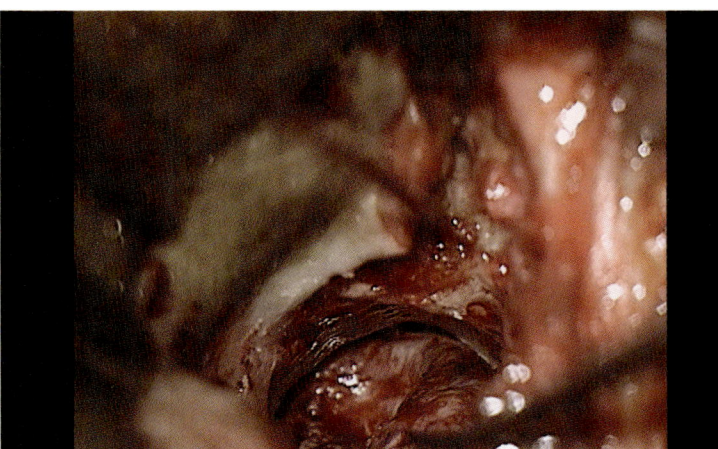

Fig. 10.56 The anterior tympanomeatal flap elevation is continued till the annulus.

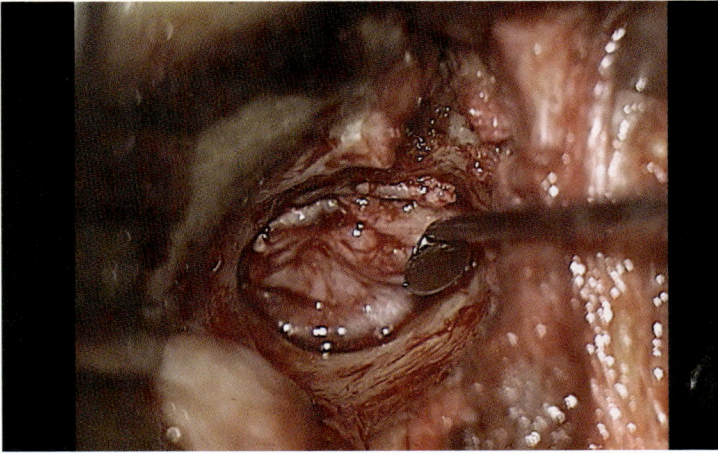

Fig. 10.57 The posterior tympanomeatal flap is elevated and elevation is continued till the annulus.

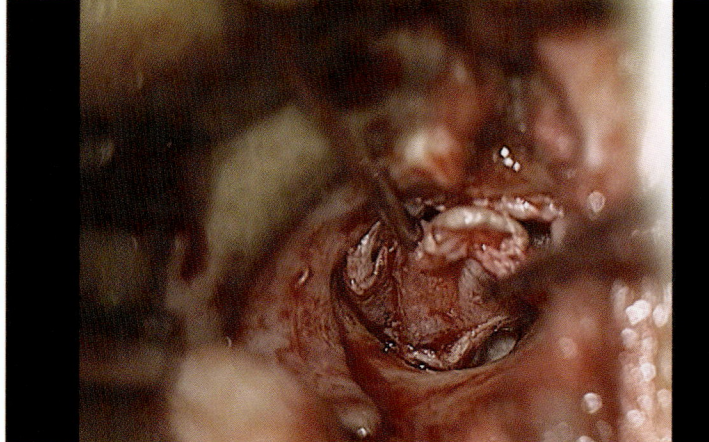

Fig. 10.58 The posterior tympanomeatal flap is elevated. The annulus is elevated from the sulcus and the middle ear is entered.

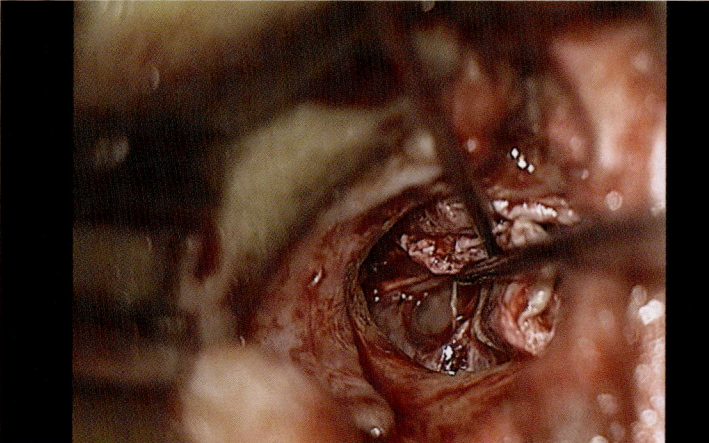

Fig. 10.59 The inferior annulus is elevated from the sulcus.

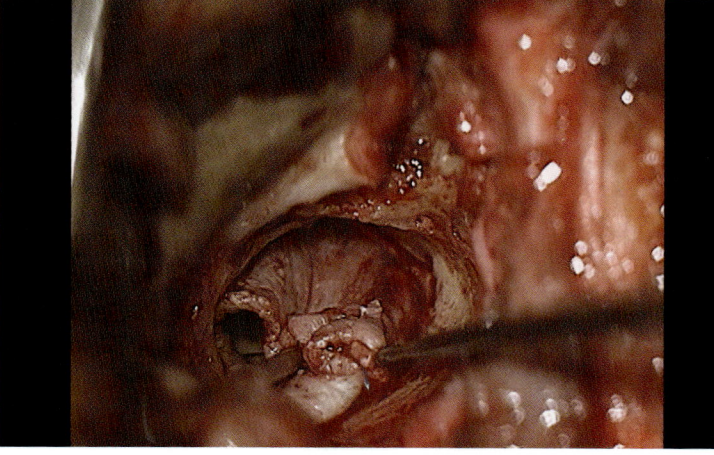

Fig. 10.60 The anterosuperior tympanomeatal flap elevation is continued up to the annulus.

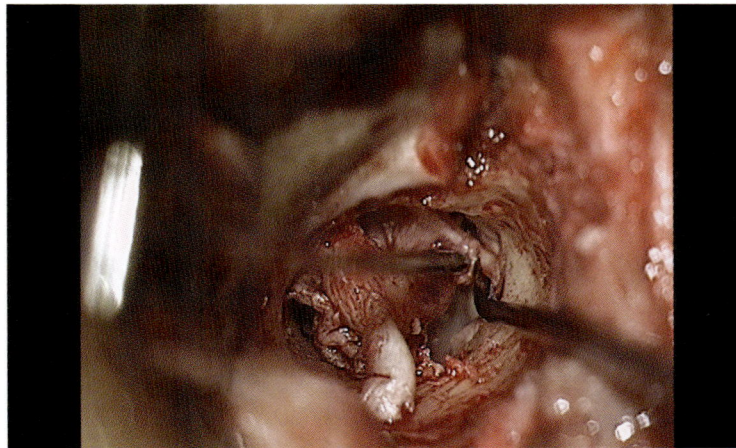

Fig. 10.61 The annulus is elevated from the sulcus anterior and posterior to the neck of the malleus.

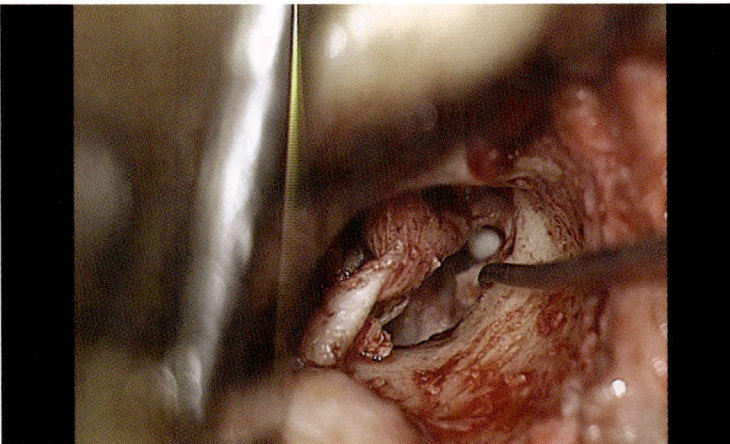

Fig. 10.62 The incus and stapes are examined for mobility and continuity.

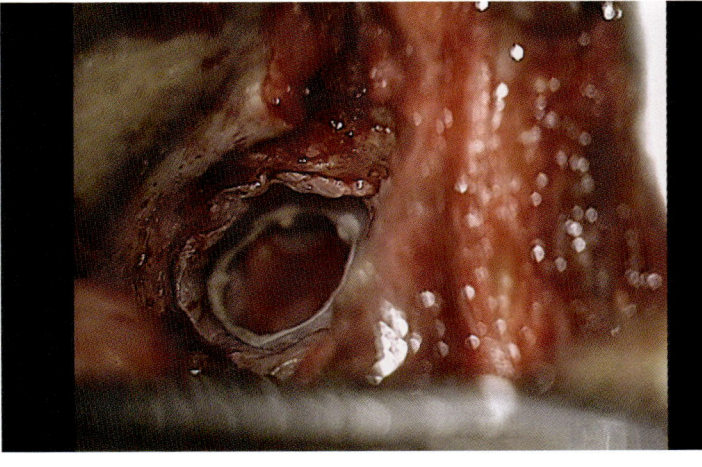

Fig. 10.63 Margins of the perforation are cauterized by 50% trichloroacetic acid (TCA).

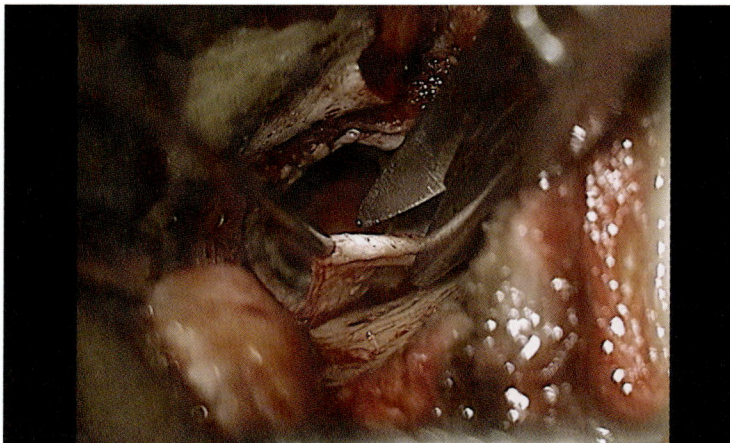

Fig. 10.64 A small piece of meatal skin is excised.

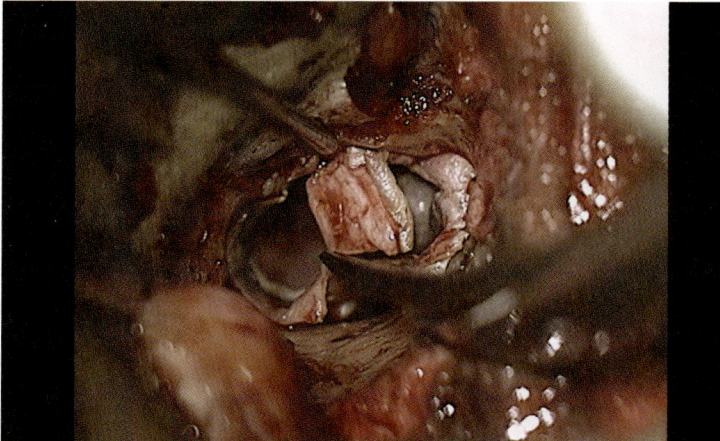

Fig. 10.65 A small piece of meatal skin is excised to be placed over the graft.

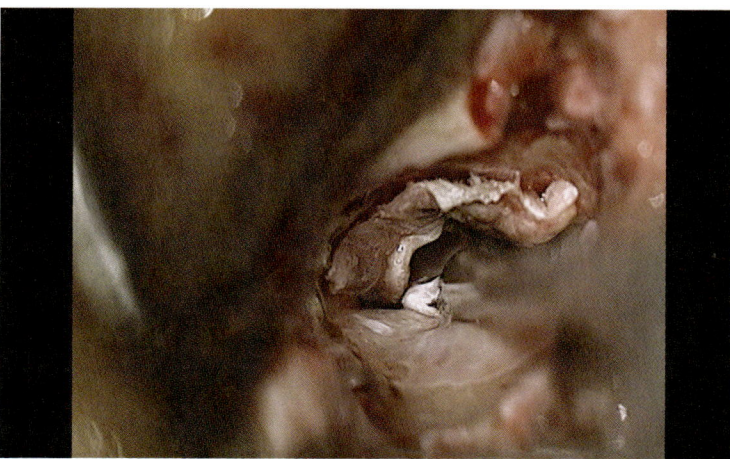

Fig. 10.66 The graft is placed in the middle ear.

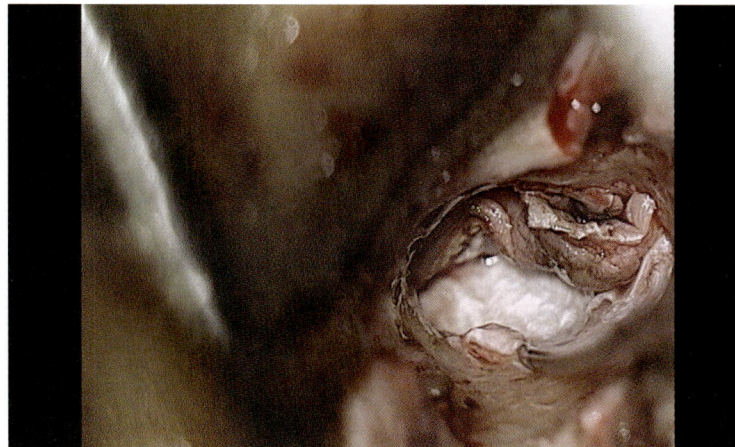

Fig. 10.67 The graft is placed in the middle ear medial to the handle of the malleus.

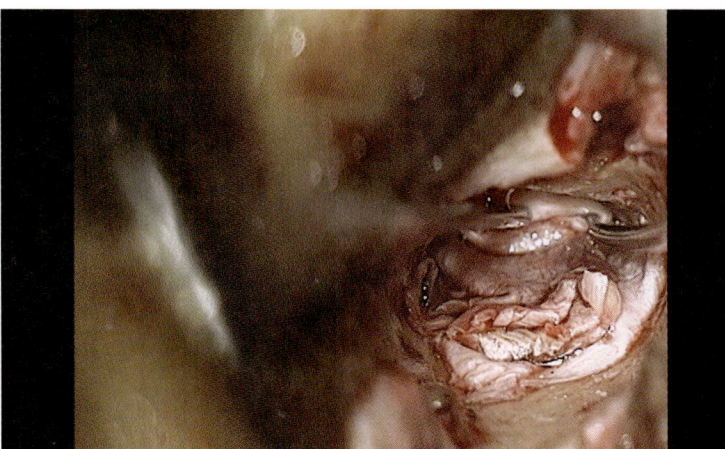

Fig. 10.68 The graft is pulled anteriorly between the annulus and the sulcus.

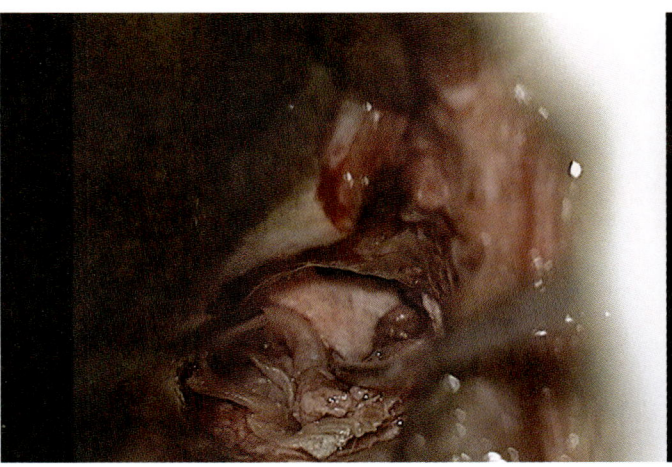

Fig. 10.69 The graft is pulled anteriorly between the annulus and the sulcus to be supported by the anterior bony meatal wall.

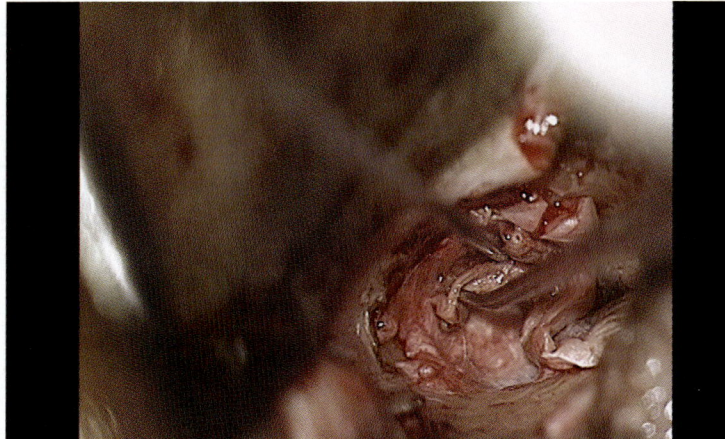

Fig. 10.70 The graft is supported inferiorly by the inferior bony meatal wall, and the inferior annulus is reposited back into its original position.

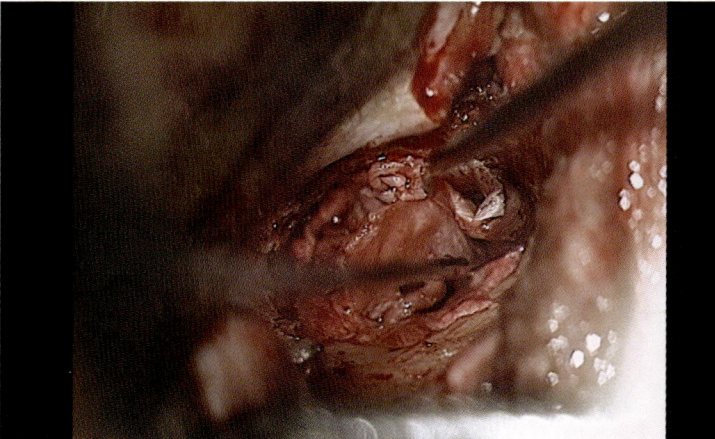

Fig. 10.71 The posterior part of the graft is supported by the posterior meatal wall.

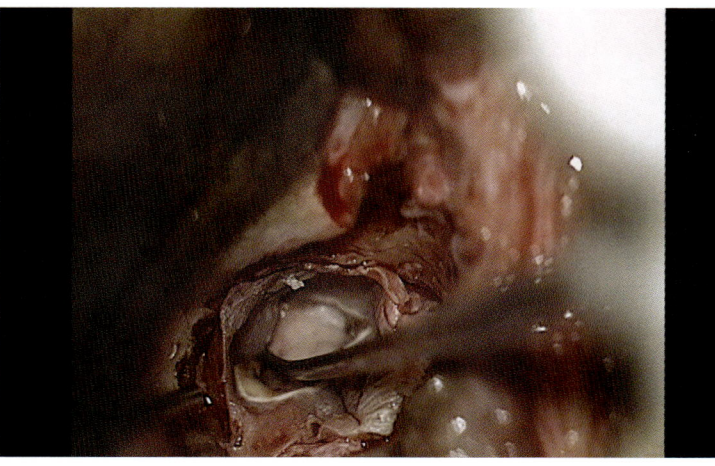

Fig. 10.72 The tympano-meatal flap is reposited back into its original position.

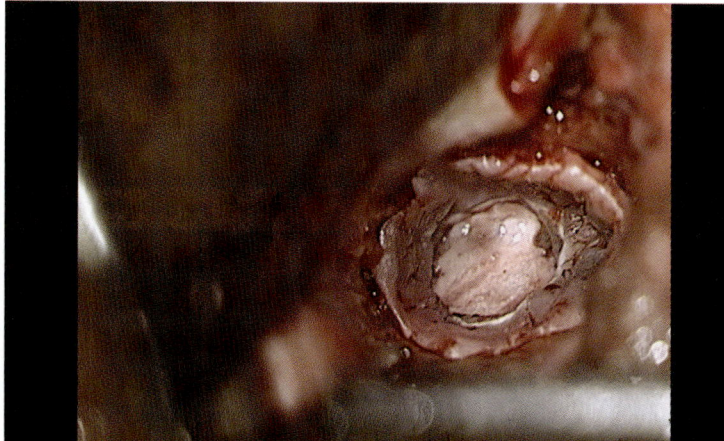

Fig. 10.73 The tympano-meatal flap is reposited back into its original position. The anterior tympanomeatal angle is skin lined to prevent blunting.

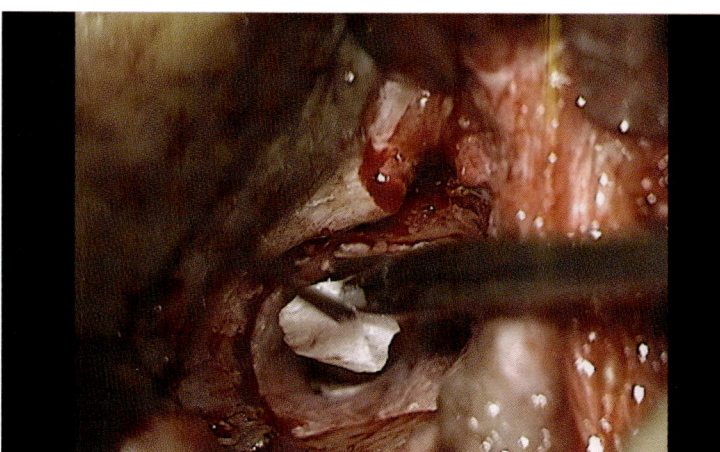

Fig. 10.74 The meatal skin piece is to be placed over the graft.

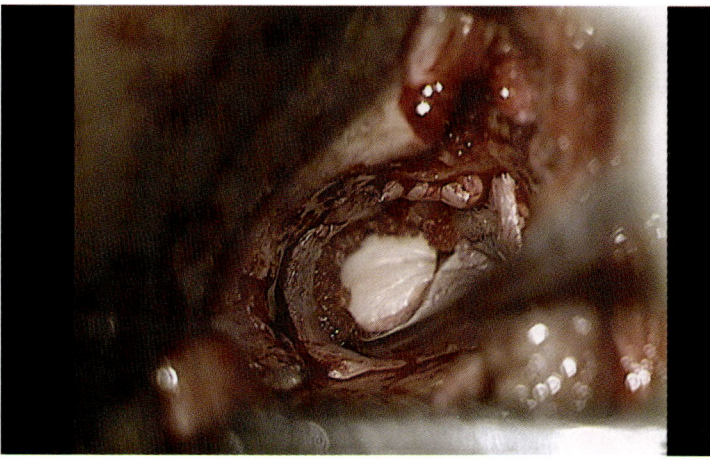

Fig. 10.75 The graft is covered by the meatal skin piece for fast epithelialization.

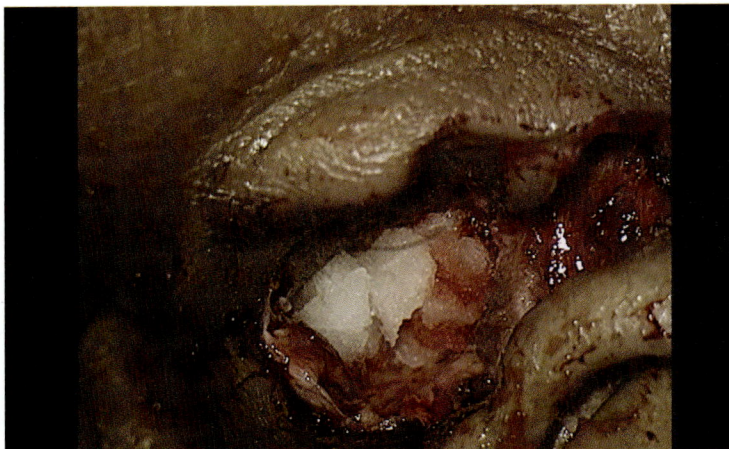

Fig. 10.76 Gelfoam is placed in the external auditory canal.

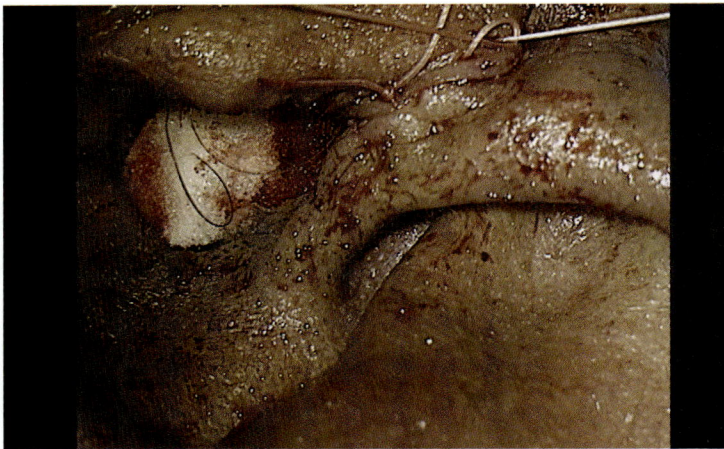

Fig. 10.77 Incision is closed by two stitches.

Case 4: Tympanoplasty in the Cases with Very Thin (Narrow) Anterosuperior Margin of Perforation

Graft reinforcement is done by the tympanomeatal flap rotation technique (**Figs. 10.78–10.90**).

In patients having subtotal perforation or very thin (narrow) anterosuperior perforation margins, good overlapping of the graft is necessary for a successful surgery.

The area of the anterosuperior narrow margin of the perforation can be increased by complete 360-degree elevation and mobilization of the tympanomeatal flap, dissecting the tympanic membrane from the handle of the malleus except at the tip, so that the whole tympanomeatal flap with the tympanic membrane can be rotated clockwise in the right ear and anticlockwise in the left ear, to increase the area of the anterosuperior drum margin. By doing that, there will be good overlapping of the fascia at the anterosuperior perforation margins

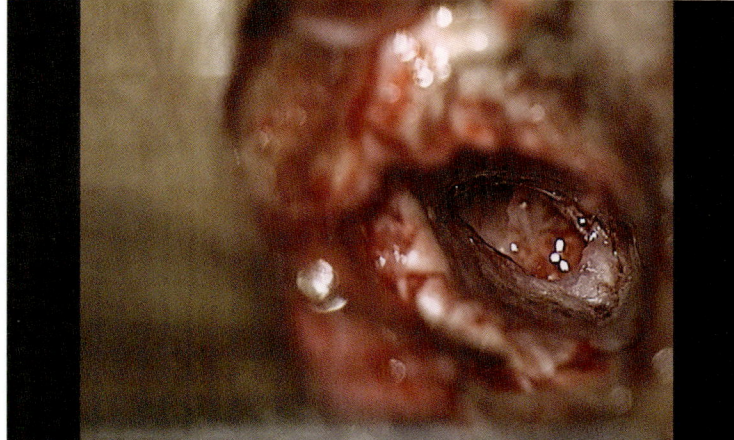

Fig. 10.78 Right ear endaural incision, fascia graft, perforation in the anterior part of the tympanic membrane with very thin (narrow) anterosuperior margins of the perforation.

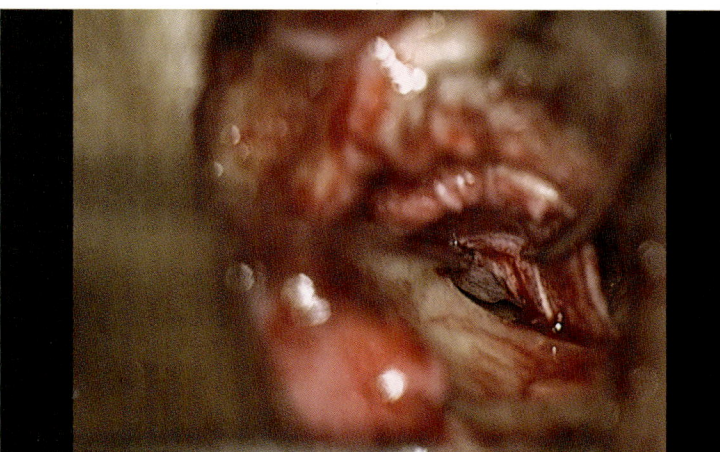

Fig. 10.79 The posterior tympanomeatal flap is elevated.

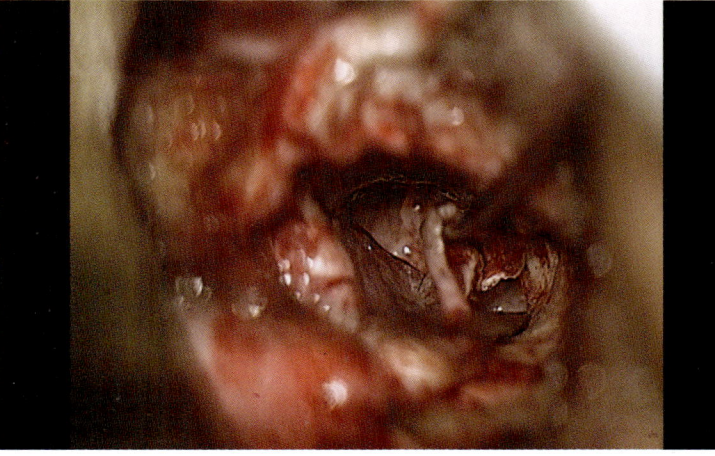

Fig. 10.80 The inferior tympanomeatal flap is elevated.

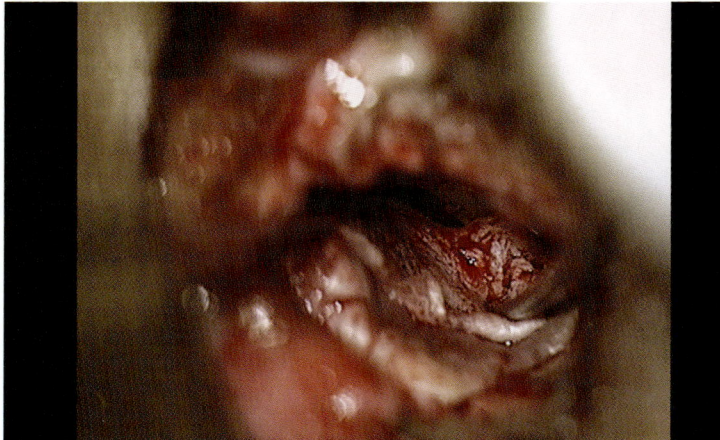

Fig. 10.81 The anterior tympanomeatal flap is elevated.

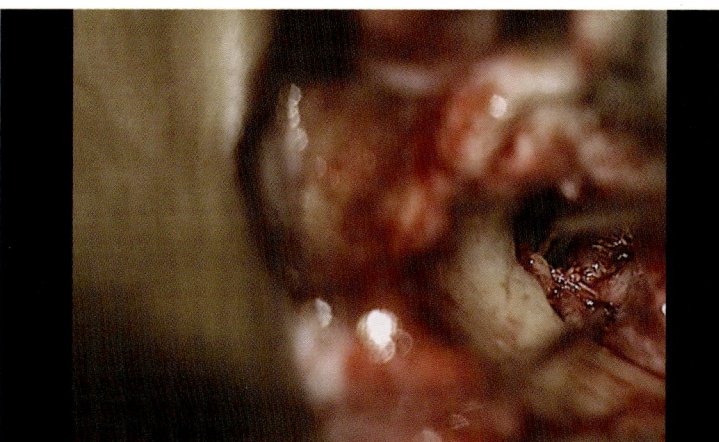

Fig. 10.82 The superior tympanomeatal flap is elevated and continued up to the lateral process of the malleus.

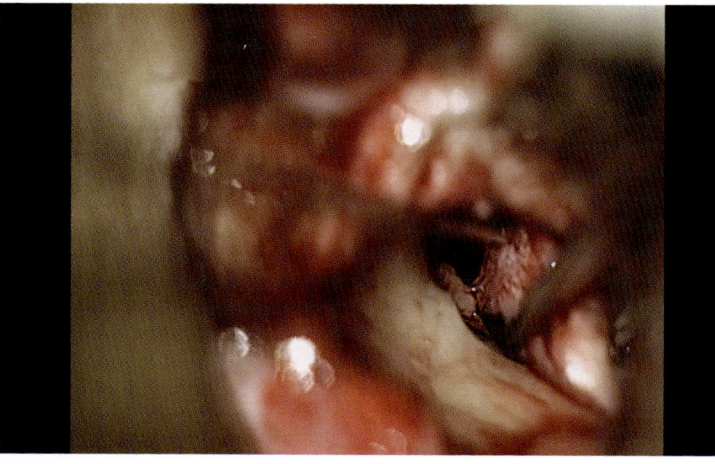

Fig. 10.83 The tympanic membrane is gradually dissected from the handle of the malleus.

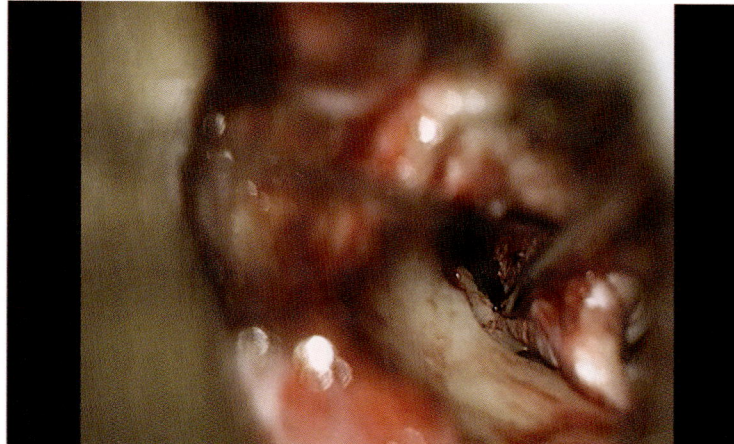

Fig. 10.84 The tympanic membrane is completely separated from the handle of the malleus except at the tip where it remains attached to the tip of the handle of the malleus.

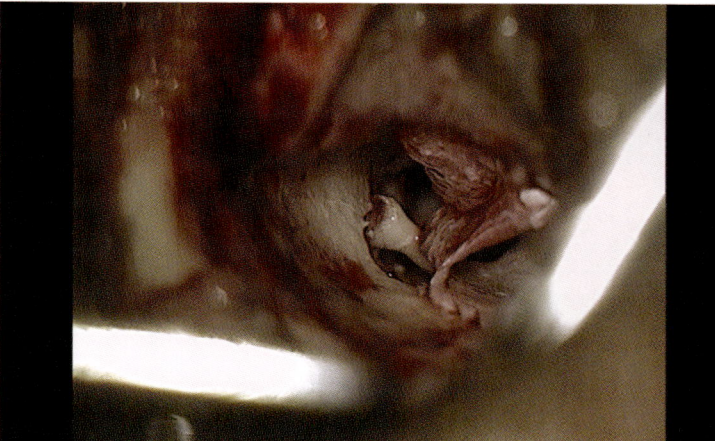

Fig. 10.85 Tympanic membrane is completely separated from the handle of malleus except at the tip (under higher magnification).

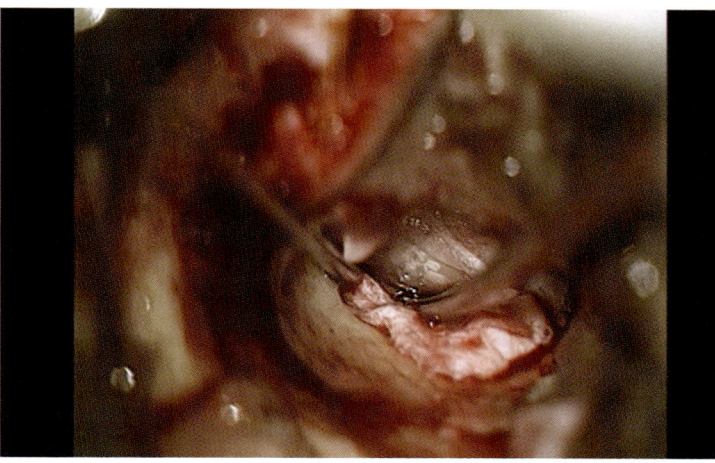

Fig. 10.86 The underlay graft is placed under the posterior tympanomeatal flap.

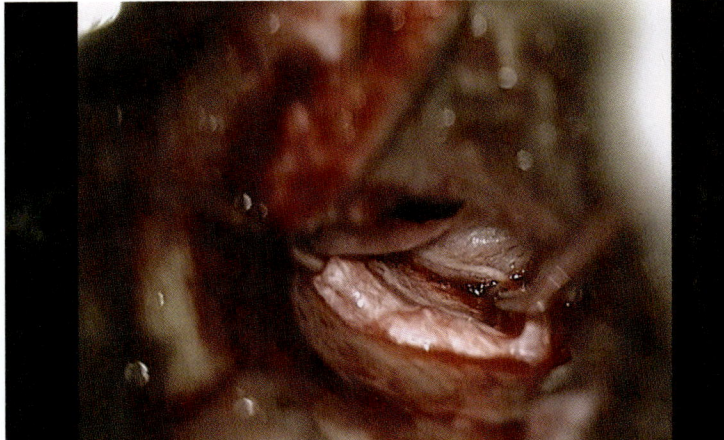

Fig. 10.87 The graft is slided under the handle of the malleus to be pulled anteriorly under the anterior tympanomeatal flap.

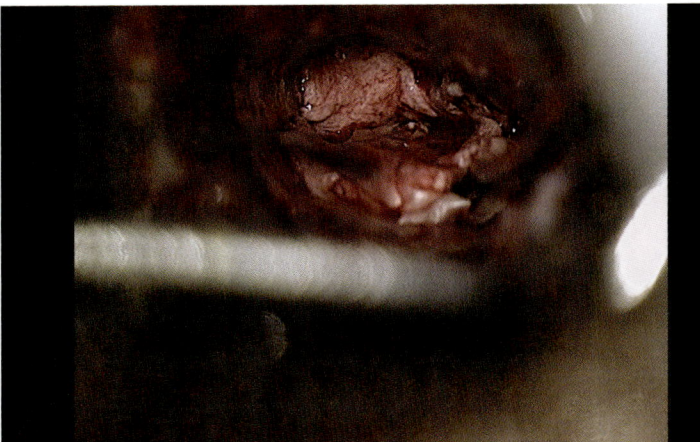

Fig. 10.88 Graft is pulled anteriorly under the anterior tympanomeatal flap anterior to the neck of the malleus resting on the anterosuperior bony meatal wall.

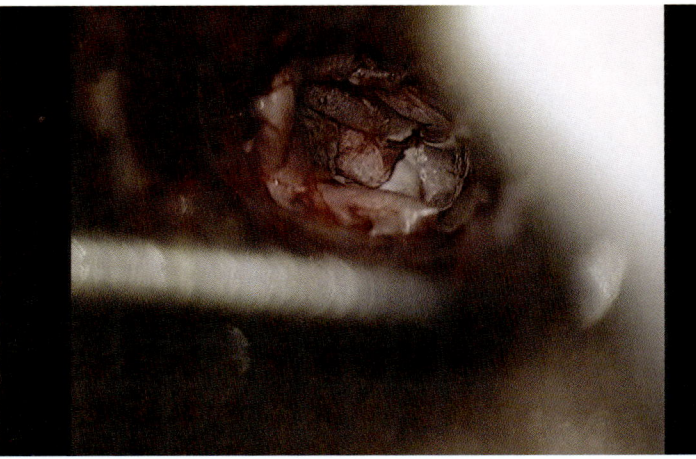

Fig. 10.89 Completely mobilized tympanomeatal flap is rotated in a clockwise direction to create a wider anterosuperior perforation margin to have good overlapping of the graft by a wider tympanomeatal flap leading to high success rate in tympanoplasty.

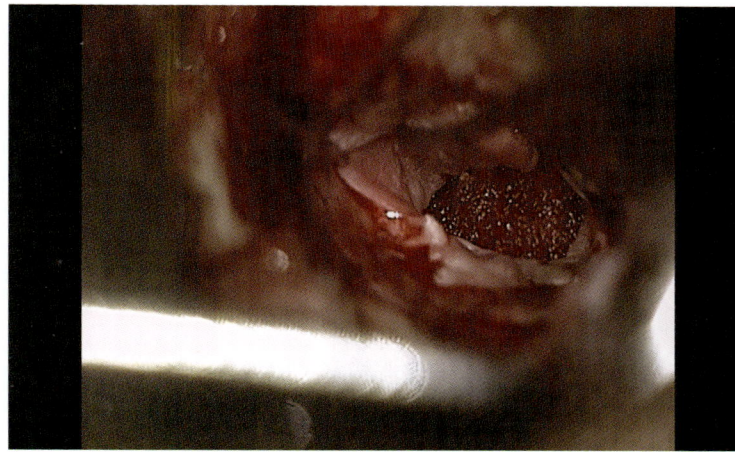

Fig. 10.90   Gelfoam is to be placed in the external auditory canal and the incision is to be closed.

by wider tympanomeatal flap, to get better surgery results. In addition to this, the anterosuperior part of the underlay graft anterior to the neck of the malleus, along with the malleus handle, is reinforced by covering it by a small second piece of graft before repositing the tympanomeatal flap. The purpose of this reinforcement is to create good bonding between the first graft and the malleus handle to ensure success.

Case 5: Tympanoplasty in a Similar Patient Having Subtotal Perforation with Very Thin (Narrow) Anterosuperior Margin of Perforation

Graft reinforcement is done by the tympanomeatal flap rotation technique (case 2; **Figs. 10.91–10.105**).

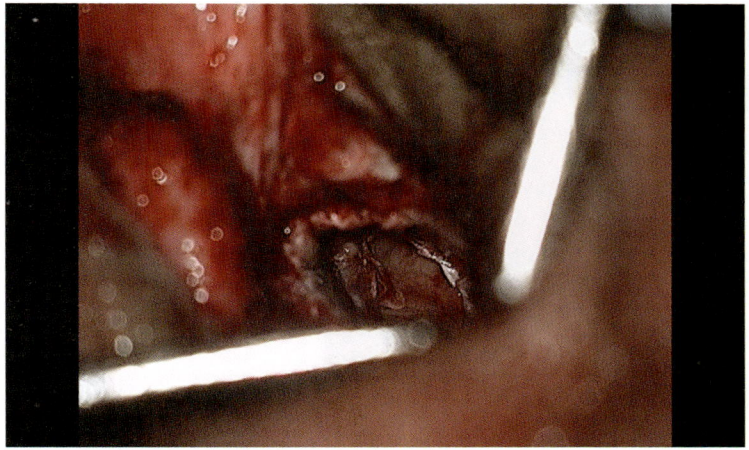

Fig. 10.91   Endaural incision. The fascia graft is harvested, retractors are applied, and subtotal perforation is seen.

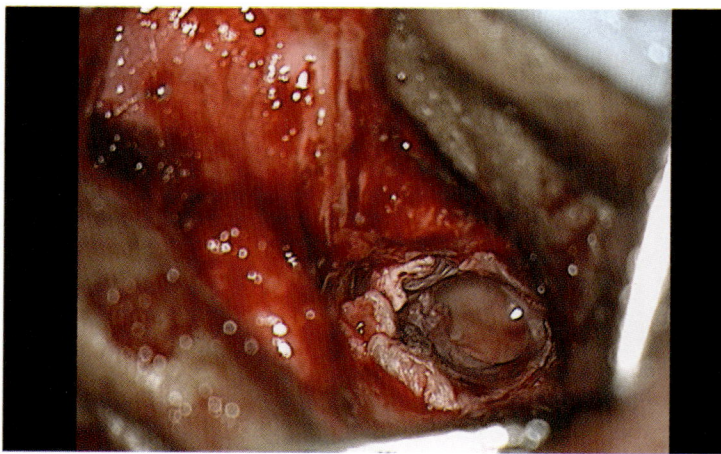

Fig. 10.92 Subtotal perforation is seen.

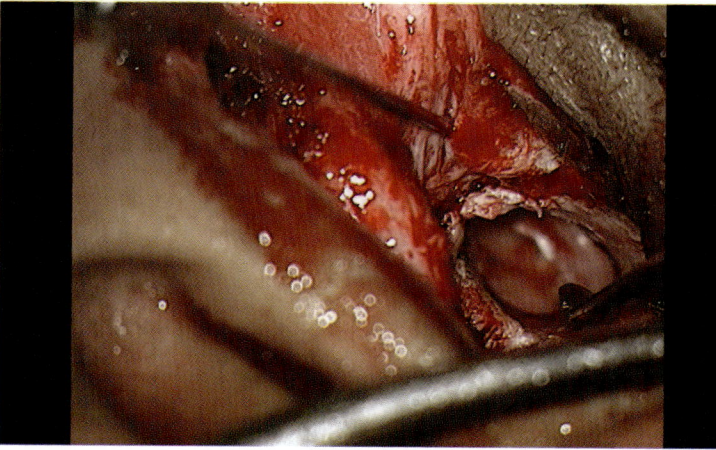

Fig. 10.93 Circumferential (360-degree) meatal wall incision is made.

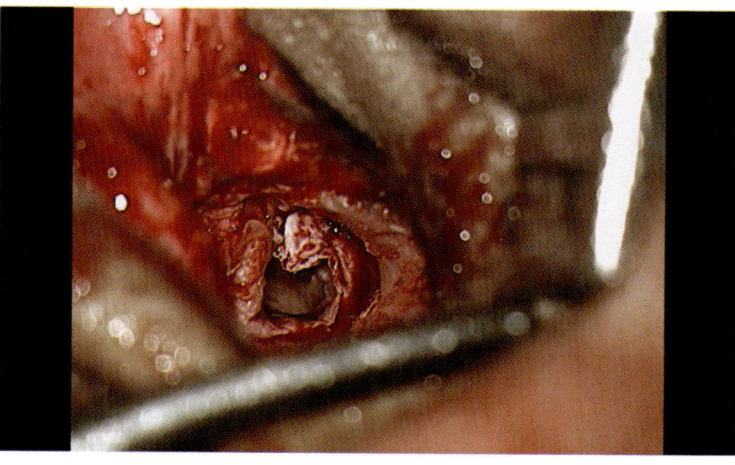

Fig. 10.94 360-degree meatal wall skin is elevated till the annulus.

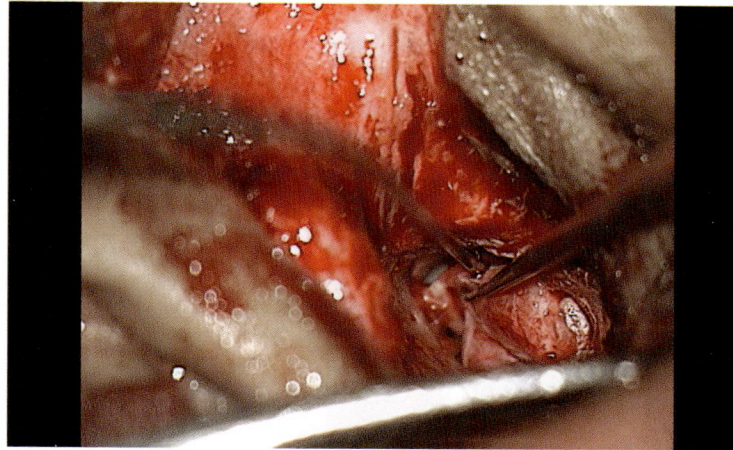

Fig. 10.95 The superior tympanomeatal flap is elevated, continued up to the lateral process of the malleus.

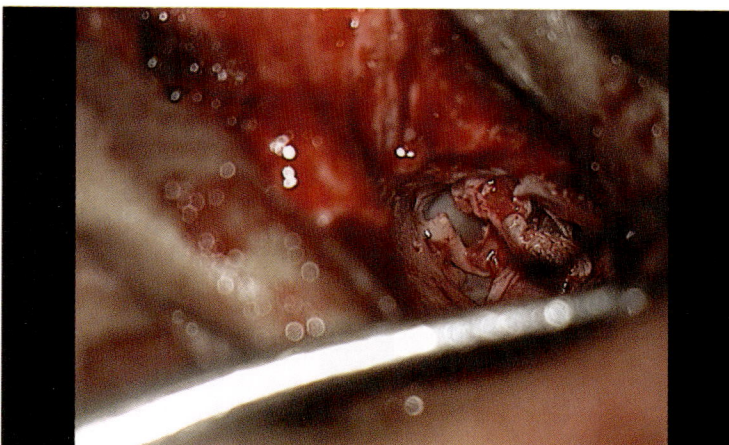

Fig. 10.96 The tympanic membrane is completely separated from the handle of the malleus except at the tip.

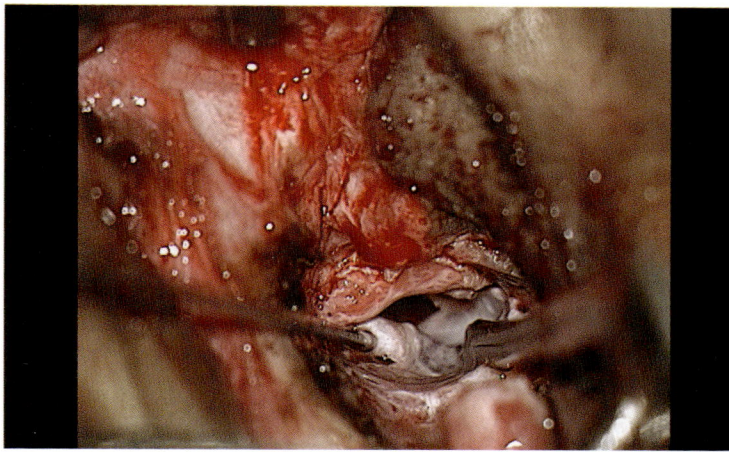

Fig. 10.97 The underlay graft is placed.

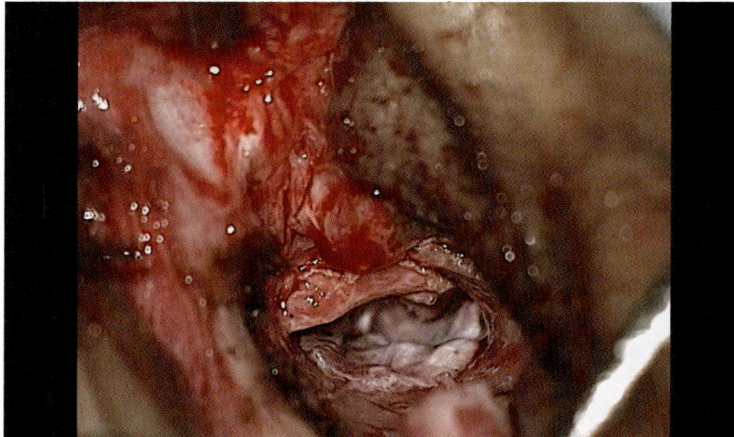

Fig. 10.98 The graft is slided anteriorly medial to the handle of the malleus.

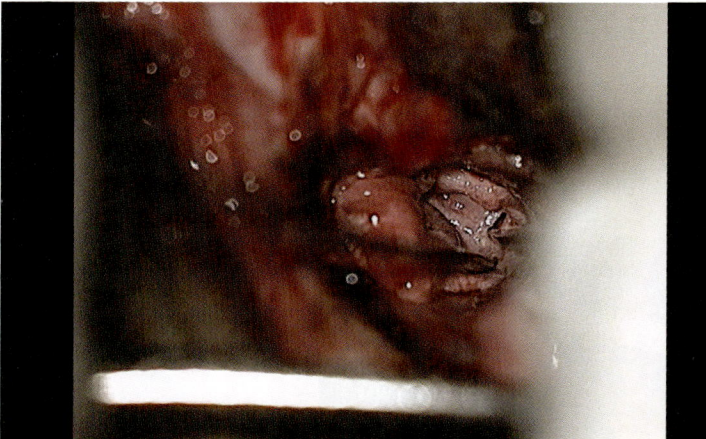

Fig. 10.99 The graft is supported anteriorly by the anterior bony meatal wall under the anterior tympanomeatal flap.

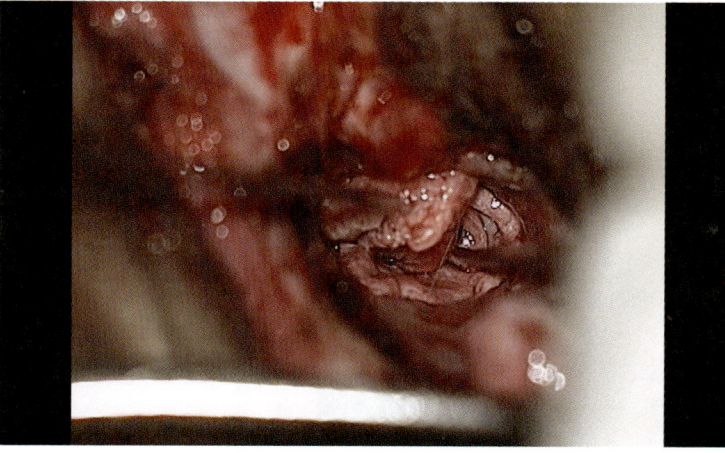

Fig. 10.100 The graft is pulled superiorly anterior to the neck of the malleus.

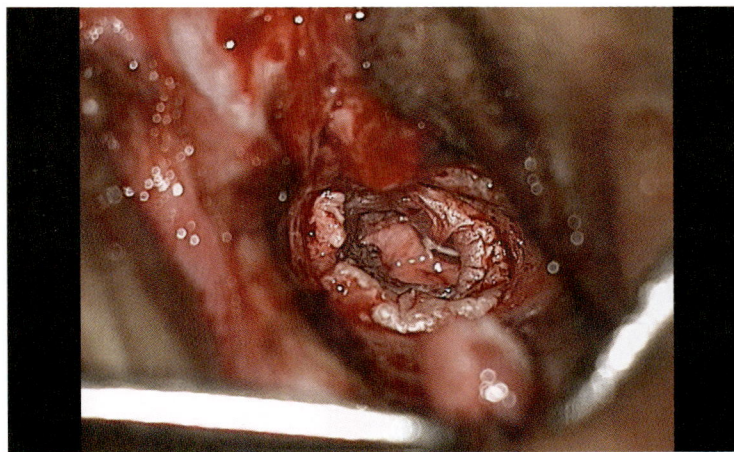

Fig. 10.101 The tympanomeatal flap is reposited back.

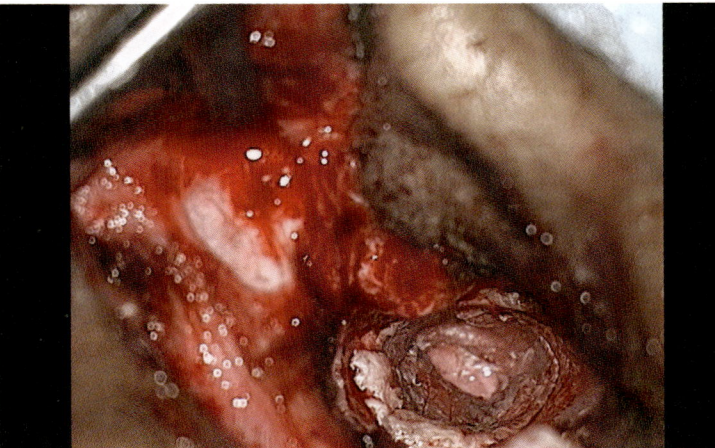

Fig. 10.102 Completely mobilized tympanomeatal flap is rotated in a clockwise direction to create wider anterosuperior perforation margin to have good overlapping of the graft by a wider tympanomeatal flap.

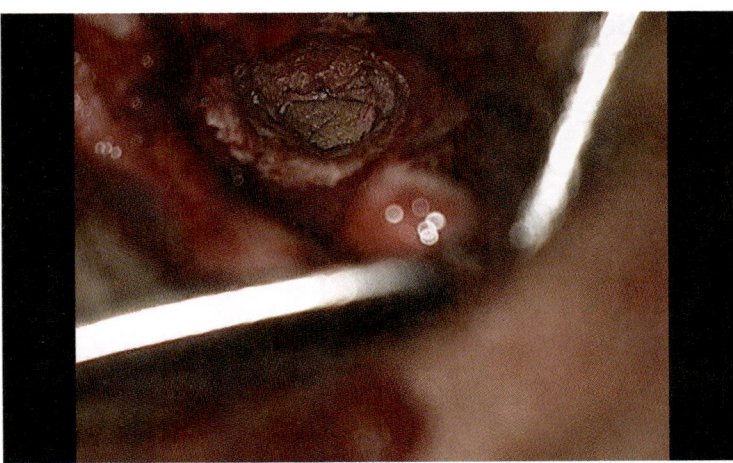

Fig. 10.103 The graft is covered by full-thickness skin harvested from the postaural region.

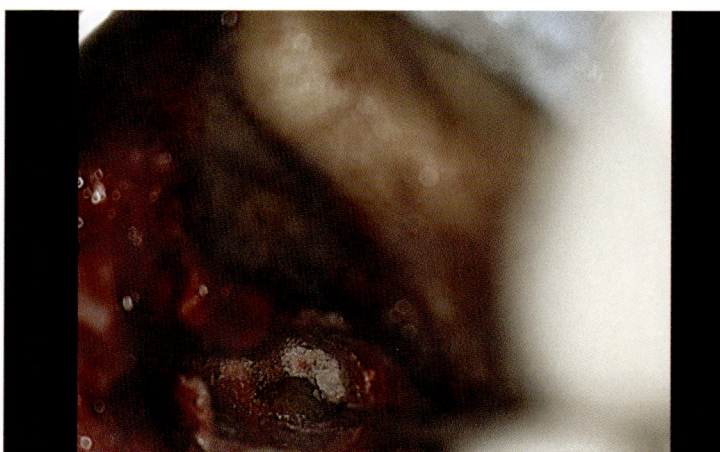

Fig. 10.104 Gelfoam is placed in the external auditory canal.

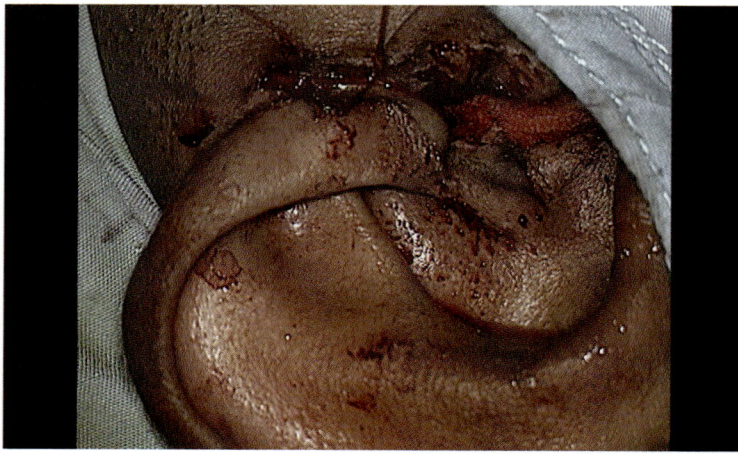

Fig. 10.105 Incision is closed.

Case 6: Tympanoplasty in a Patient with Subtotal Perforation of Tympanic Membrane with Very Narrow Drum Margins (Free Graft Technique)

The patient needs complete 360-degree elevation of the tympanomeatal flap as a free graft with placement of the fascia graft followed by repositioning of the tympano-meatal flap for better overlapping of the tympanomeatal flap over the fascia graft (**Figs. 10.106–10.120**).

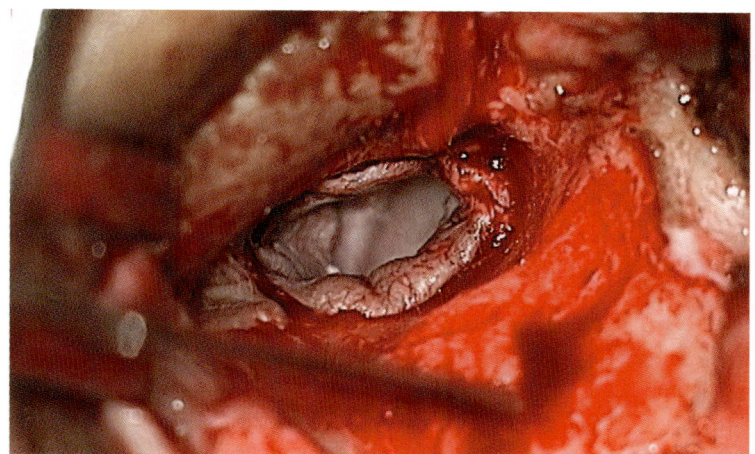

Fig. 10.106 Subtotal perforation of the tympanic membrane.

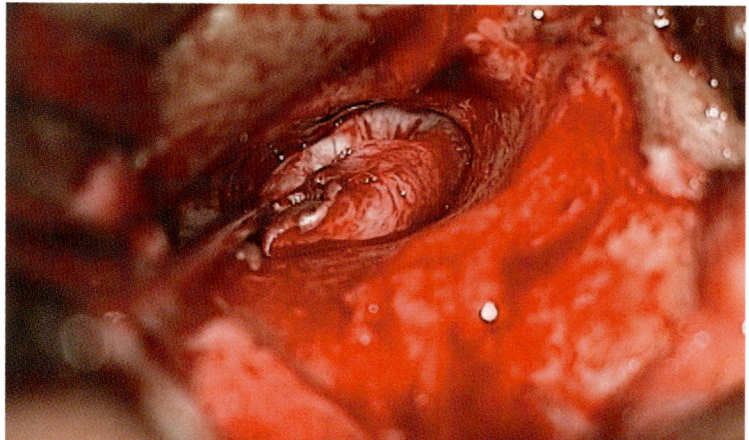

Fig. 10.107 Complete 360-degree elevation of the tympanomeatal flap is done.

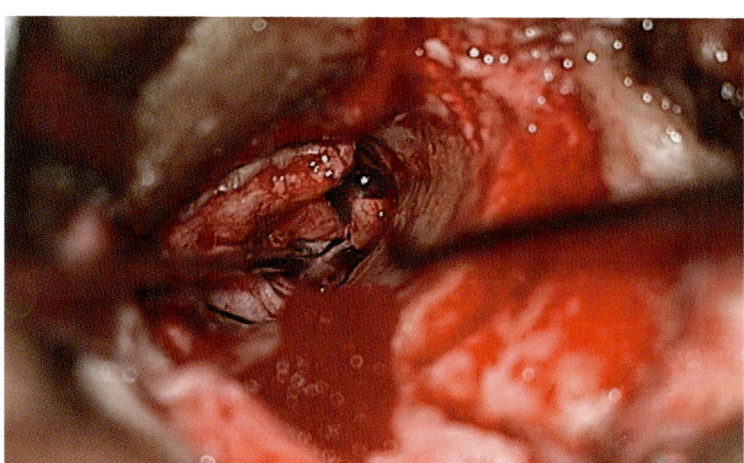

Fig. 10.108 Complete tympanomeatal flap is separated from the handle of the malleus. The tip of the handle of the malleus is destroyed.

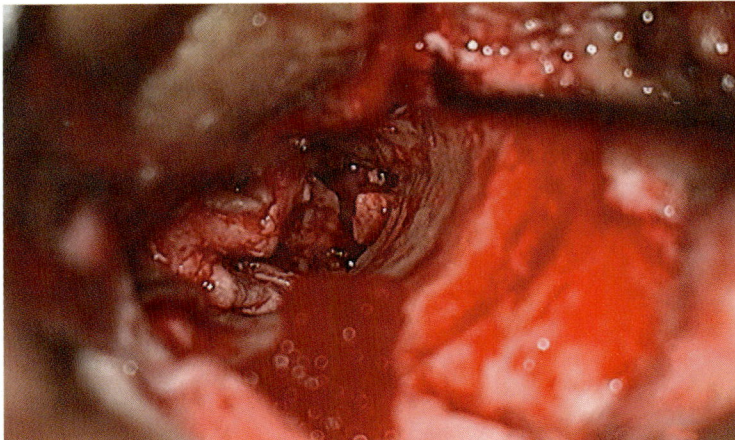

Fig. 10.109 Complete tympanomeatal flap is freed from all the sides to be removed as a free graft.

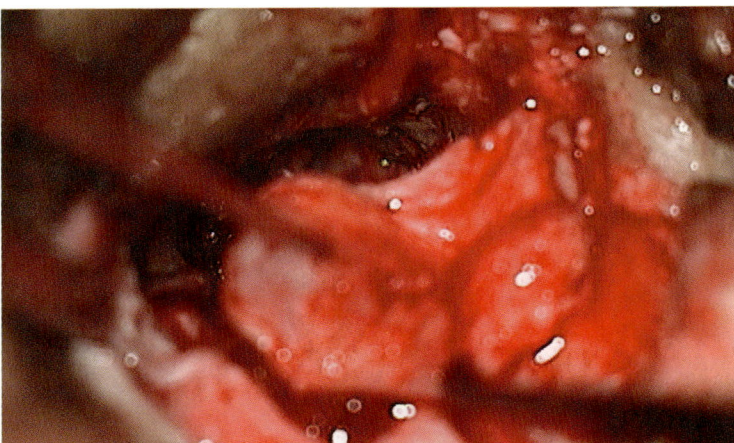

Fig. 10.110 Complete tympanomeatal flap is taken out as free graft.

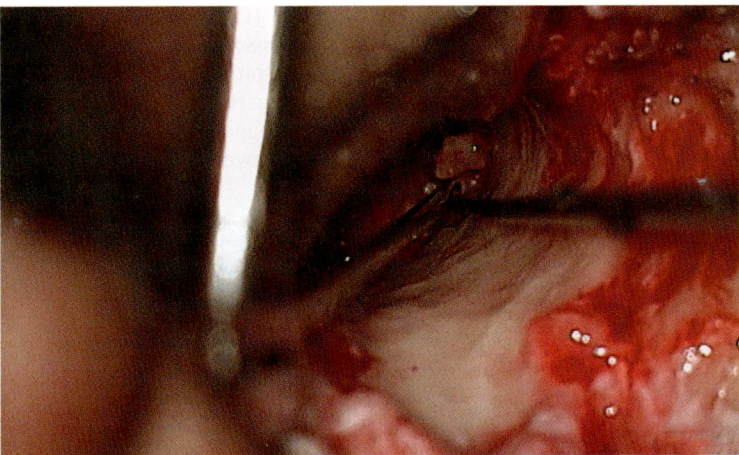

Fig. 10.111 The tip of the handle of the malleus is destroyed. The incus lenticular process is destroyed. The stapes is healthy and mobile.

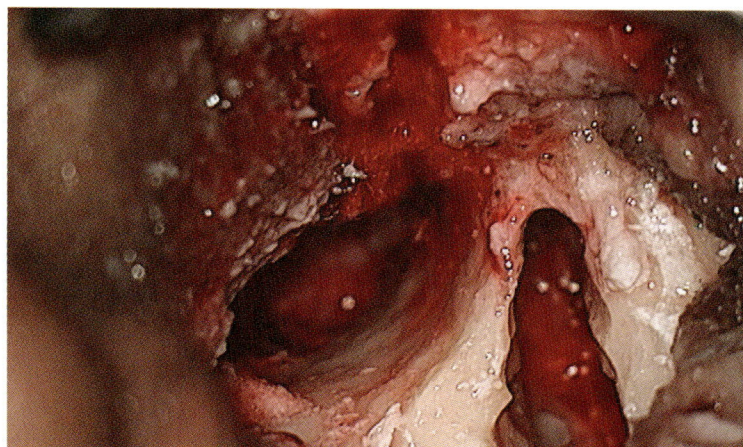

Fig. 10.112 Simple mastoidectomy is done. The attic is cleaned. The water test is positive.

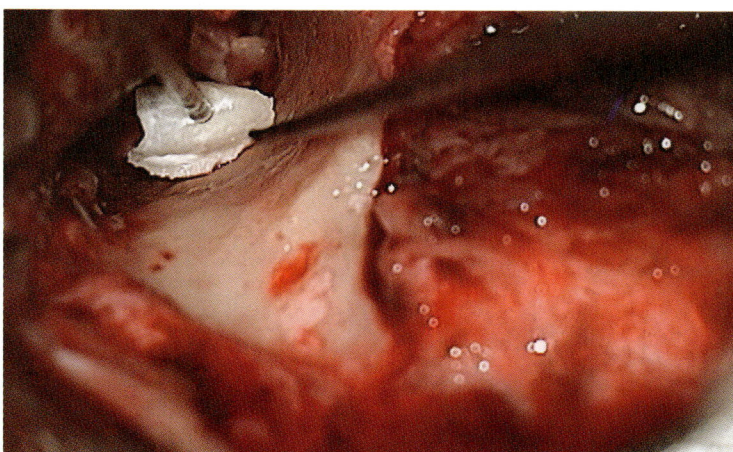

Fig. 10.113 A cartilage piece with the perichondrium is placed in the middle ear. Simple mastoidectomy opening is covered by the pedicled temporalis muscle and periosteal flap.

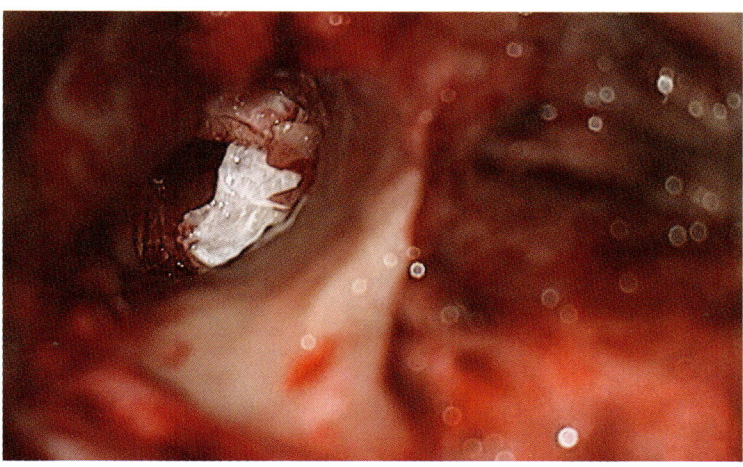

Fig. 10.114 A cartilage with the perichondrium is placed medial to the long process of the incus touching the stapes head lying anteriorly under the malleus remnants. A good contact is maintained between cartilage and the head of the stapes by the pressure of the long process of the incus.

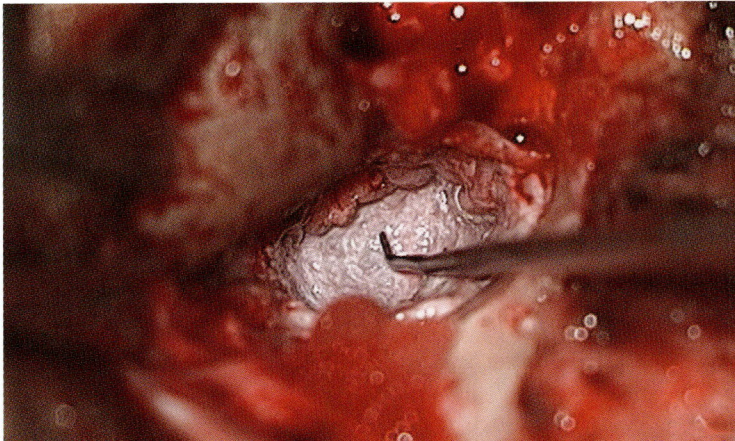

Fig. 10.115 The fascia graft is placed over the middle ear touching the malleus, incus, and cartilage.

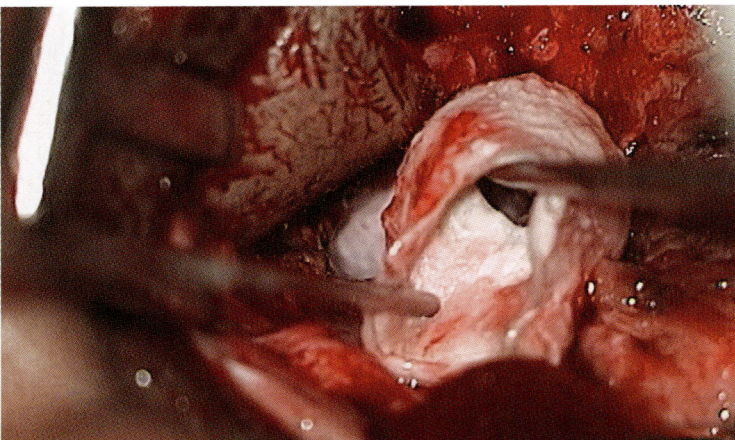

Fig. 10.116 Meatal skin which was taken out as a free graft, is placed in the external auditory canal.

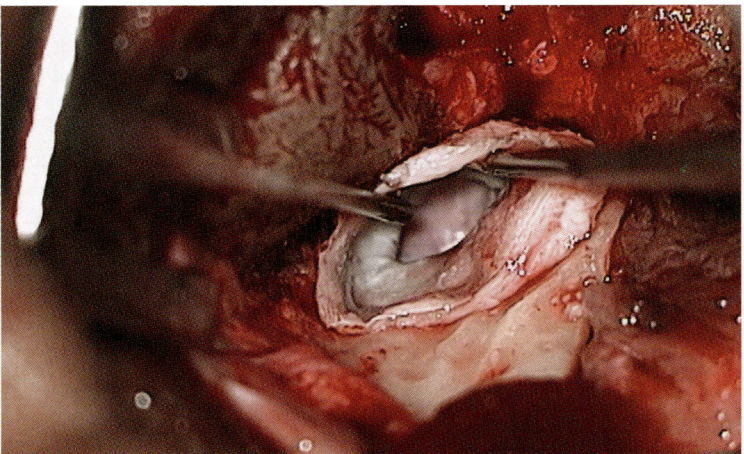

Fig. 10.117 Meatal skin, which was taken out as a free graft, is reposited back into its original position.

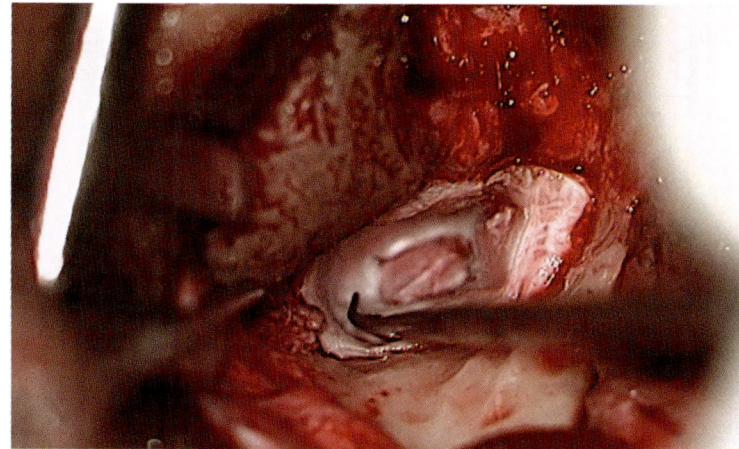

Fig. 10.118 Final position of the meatal skin.

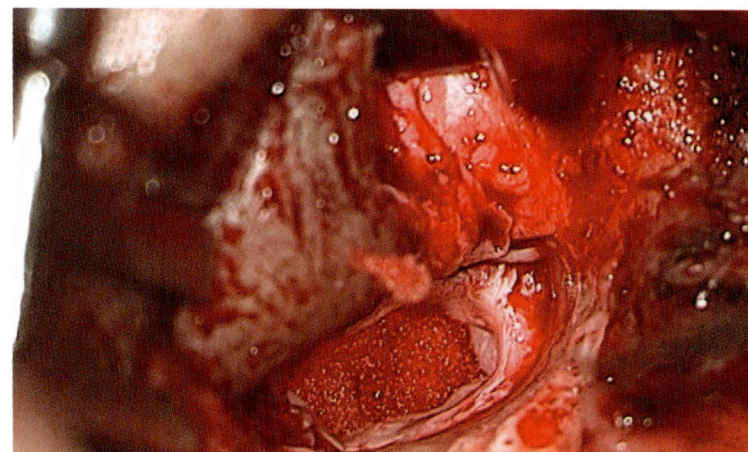

Fig. 10.119 External auditory canal is packed by Gelfoam.

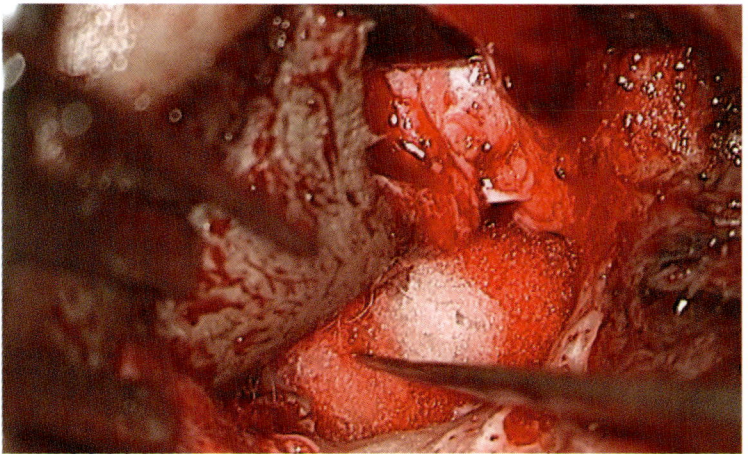

Fig. 10.120 Gelfoam is placed in the canal till its outer end and incision are closed.

11 Canalplasty

Canalplasty

- It is an integral part of tympanoplasty (**Figs. 11.1–11.13**).

- The narrow or bulging bony canal wall is to be widened to the point at which the entire tympanic sulcus can be seen with one position of the microscope.

- The wide external auditory canal makes the postoperative care easy. The self-cleansing of the external canal will be problem free.

- The time spent in performing an adequate canalplasty is compensated by the time saved during placement of graft, due to improved exposure.

- An adequate canalplasty is important for the exposure that is required for doing proper ossiculoplasty.

- Canalplasty facilitates healing and possible second stage surgery.

- When the meatus is narrow or the anterior bony meatal wall is bulging, the anterior part of the tympanic membrane is not seen. It is difficult to work at the anterior sulcus or at the anterior part of the tympanic membrane.

This difficulty can be overcome by canalplasty.

Care to be Taken during Canalplasty

- Canalplasty should be done slowly, gently, without any hurry taking full care of the elevated meatal skin, tympanic membrane, and ossicular chain.

- While drilling, the meatal skin is protected by a thick sheet of silastic or thin aluminum sheet. Small-size cutting burr should be used. In a very narrow space, diamond burr will be safer.

- Anteroinferior bony meatal wall bulge is very common. Full care should be taken not to open the temporomandibular (TM) joint, which can be recognized by bluish or dark discoloration of the bone while drilling. Opening the TM joint by mistake may cause postoperative pain while opening the mouth and some trismus, which persist for a long time. If the bony partition between the external auditory canal and the TM joint is drilled, the head of the mandible bulges into the external auditory canal when the mouth is closed and the head moves forward when the mouth is opened. The patient gets some clicking sound in the ear while chewing. This may disturb the hearing of the patient.

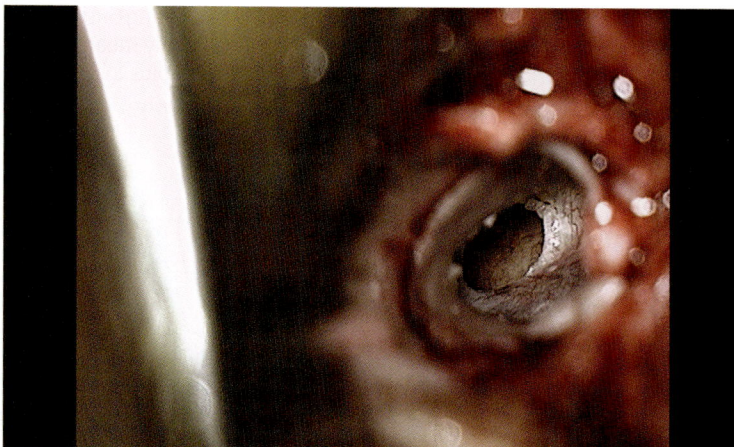

Fig. 11.1 Central perforation. Bulging anterior bony meatal wall hiding the anterior margins of the perforation.

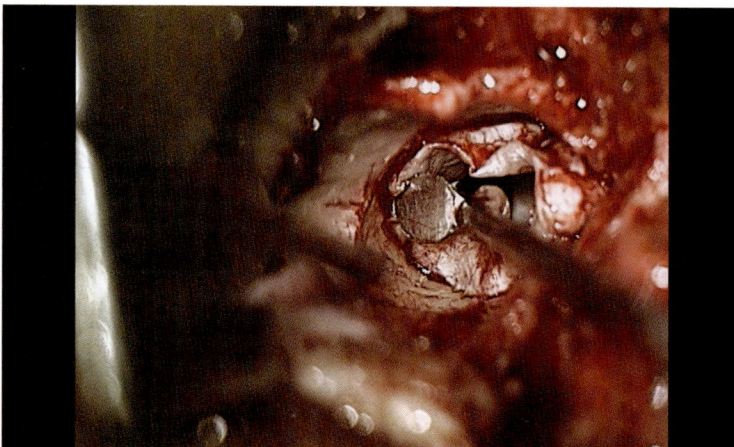

Fig. 11.2 The tympanomeatal flap is elevated.

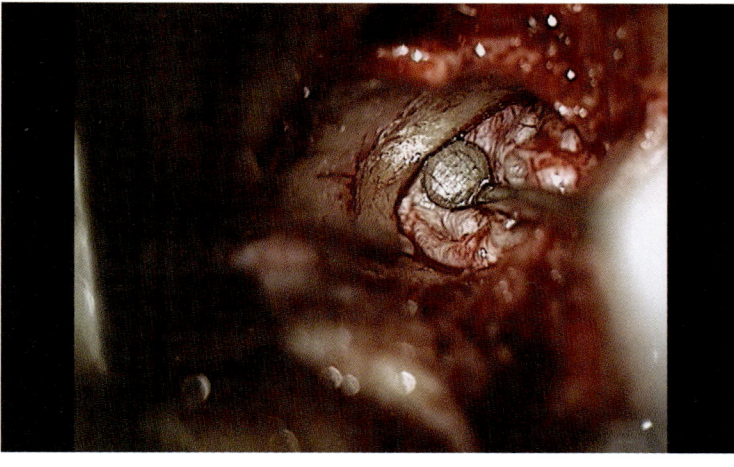

Fig. 11.3 The tympanomeatal flap is elevated all around the canal (360 degrees). Bulging anterior bony meatal wall is exposed.

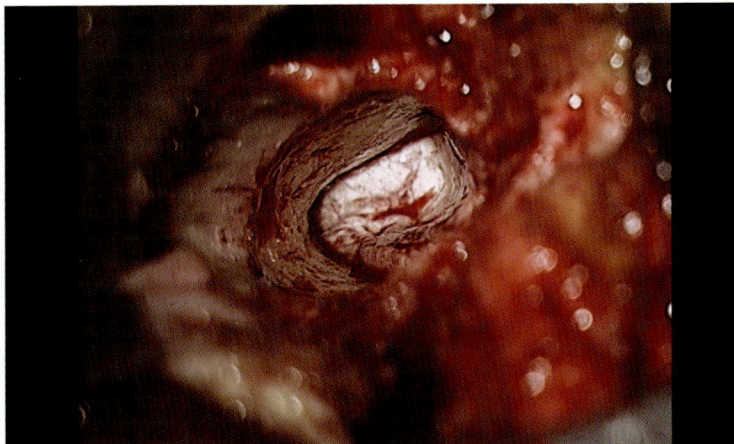

Fig. 11.4 Bulging anterior and inferior bony meatal wall is hiding the annulus.

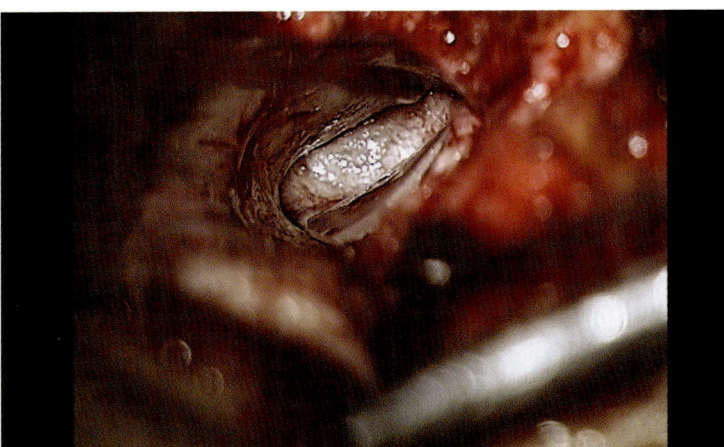

Fig. 11.5 The tympanomeatal flap is covered by a thick silastic sheet to protect it while drilling.

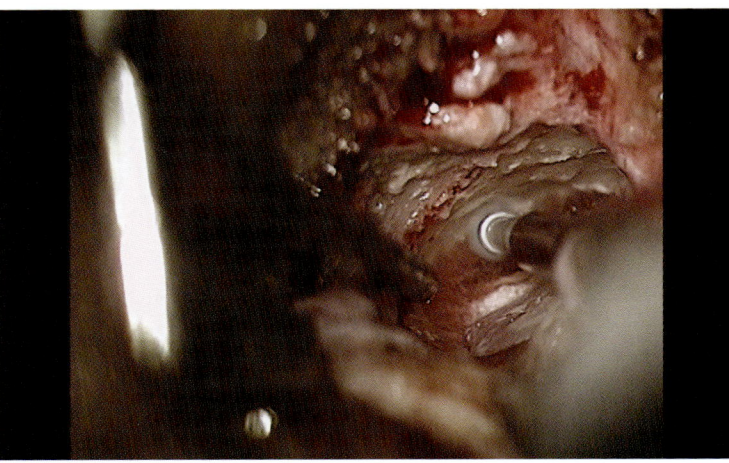

Fig. 11.6 Bulging anterior bony meatal wall is drilled, starting laterally and proceeding medially.

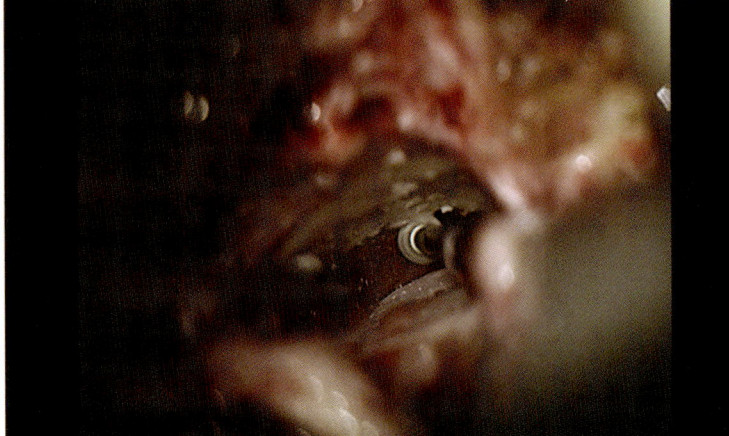

Fig. 11.7 Bulging anterior bony meatal wall is drilled, starting laterally and proceeding medially protecting the tympanomeatal flap by a piece of silastic sheet.

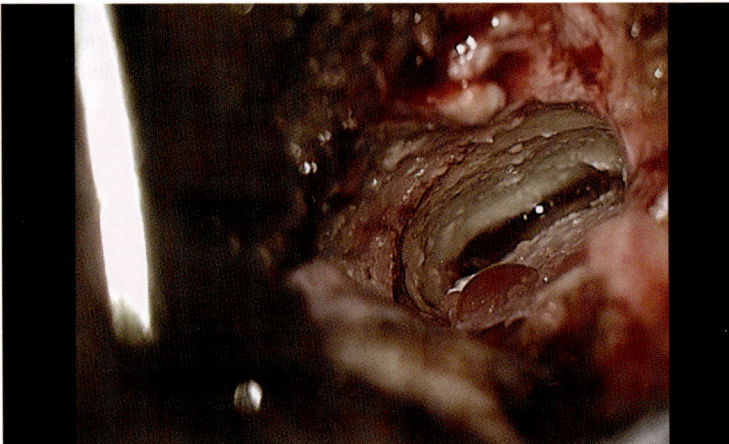

Fig. 11.8 Lateral part of the bulging anterior bony meatal wall is drilled; the medial part is still bulging.

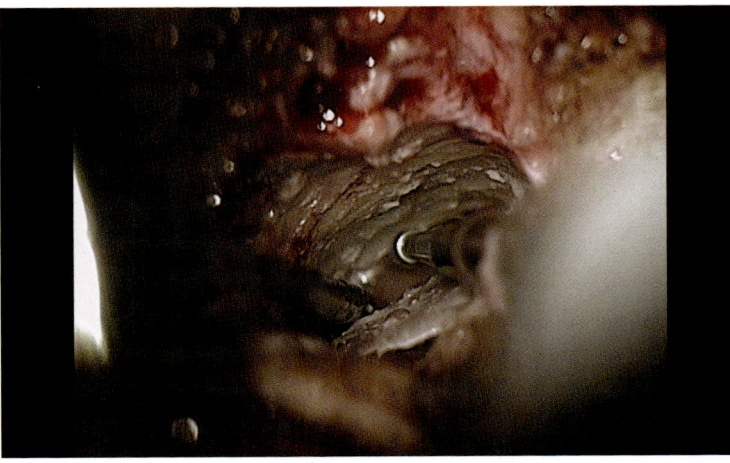

Fig. 11.9 Medial part of the bulging anterior bony meatal wall is drilled by a smaller burr to expose the annulus.

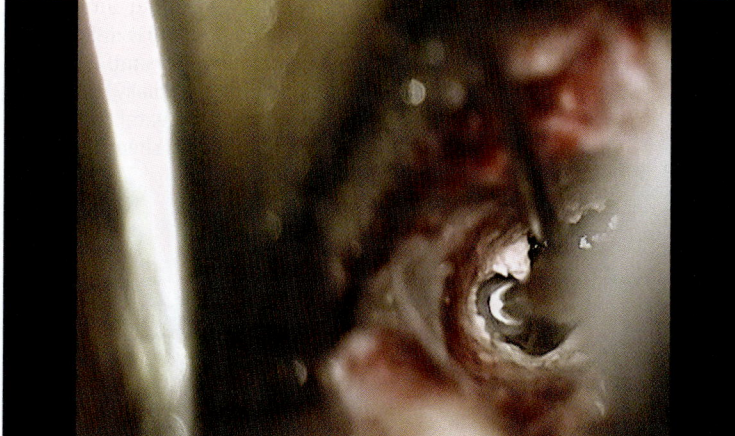

Fig. 11.10   Inferior bony meatal wall close to the annulus is drilled by a diamond burr. It is safe for both the tympanomeatal (TM) flap and joint.

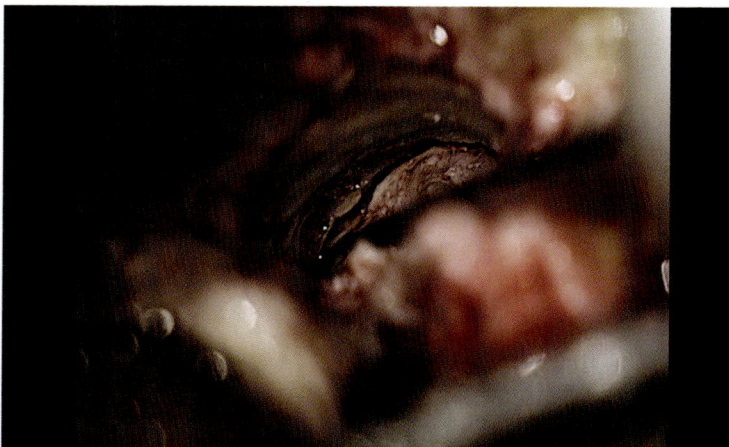

Fig. 11.11   Anterior annulus is seen, separated from the sulcus, and the middle ear is entered.

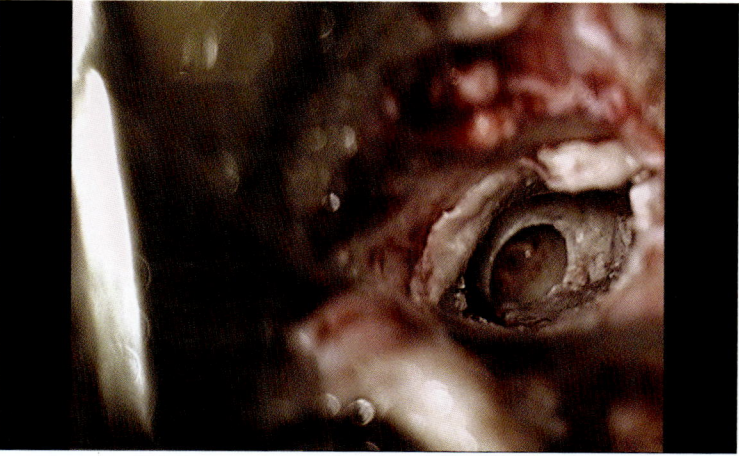

Fig. 11.12   Bulging anterior bony meatal wall is reduced, and the tympanomeatal flap is reposited back. Hidden anterior part of the tympanic membrane, which was not seen earlier, is now completely exposed.

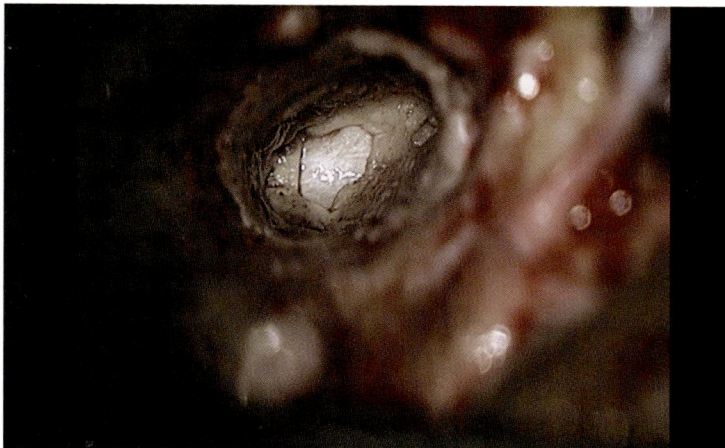

Fig. 11.13 Underlay graft is placed supported by the anterior, inferior, posterior, and superior bony meatal wall. The anterior tympanomeatal angle is well maintained and is skin lined to prevent blunting. Gelfoam is packed in the external auditory canal and incision is closed.

- The bony posterior canal wall bulge is not uncommon, Care should be taken while drilling the posteroinferior bony canal wall bulge, especially near the annulus as the facial nerve is around 2 to 3 mm behind the tympanic sulcus.

- Even if the TM joint is exposed, the capsule of the joint should not be open. Then the problems will be less.

- While drilling the bony canal wall, adequate irrigation of bone by saline should be done so that there should not be any heating of the canal wall bone. All the bone dust should be removed by saline irrigation and suction.

- When there is generalized bony bulge in the canal, space must be created by drilling the posterior bony canal wall first, followed by the remaining canal wall like the inferior, superior, and, at last, the anterior bony canal wall.

12 Mastoidectomy in Safe Otitis Media

In chronic otitis media, the entire middle ear cleft including the mucosa of the mastoid antrum and air cells is edematous, highly vascular, and full of granulations. Simple closure of the perforation without surgical removal of the disease from the mastoid may fail in the long term. Hence, mastoidectomy is essential for long-term results. It is found that more than 50% of patients with safe otitis media have irreversible mastoid pathology.

This includes markedly edematous mastoid mucosa, granulations, cholesterol granuloma, tympanosclerosis, and Koch's disease, even if the ear is dry for a long time.

Hence, simple mastoidectomy with intact posterior canal wall is "MUST," except in patients with traumatic perforation and patients with a radiologically normal (cellular) mastoid.

Success rate is high in patients when the mastoid is opened.

Recently, certain studies showed that mastoidectomy is a must in patients with active mucosal disease with persistent otorrhea and in patients of revision surgery.

Some leading surgeons claim that the results of tympanoplasty or myringoplasty performed without opening the mastoid and with opening the mastoid has no difference. Results are equally good with both techniques, but the mastoid should always be opened to see for any irreversible mucosal disease, granulations, cholesterol granuloma, and tympanosclerosis. It is already mentioned that the primary Koch disease is not uncommon in the middle ear.

Simple Mastoidectomy

Surgical Steps

- Mastoid antrum is opened (**Fig. 12.1a–f**).

- Edematous mucosa, granulations, or cholesterol granuloma may be present in the mastoid.

- A simple mastoidectomy is done. The granulations and bulky diseased mucosa in the mastoid are removed. All the mucosa in the mastoid should not to be removed, so that too much of raw areas in the mastoid air cells are not created.

- The antrum and the attic should be cleaned. Ventilation of the atti-coantral area and mastoid air cells should be established. (Congestion in the mastoid air cells should be released.) The water test should be positive.

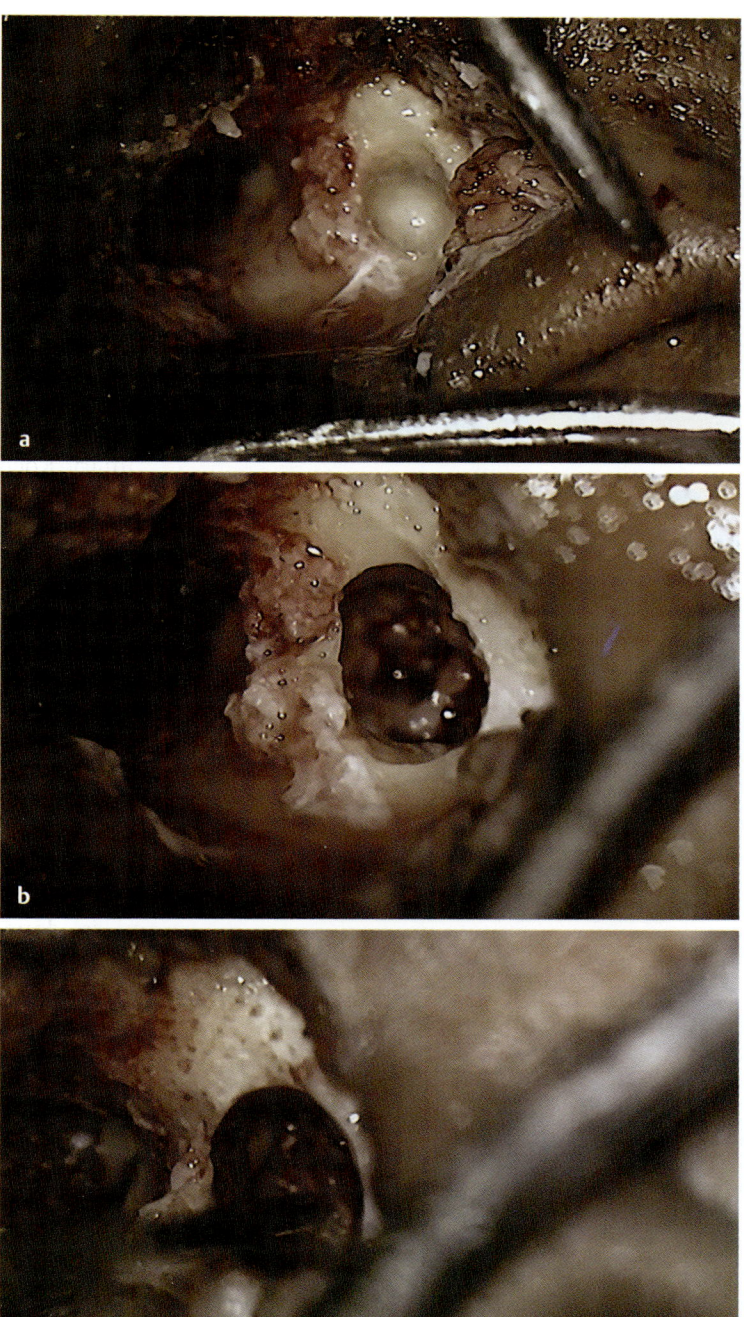

Fig. 12.1 **(a)** This is an endaural incision. A simple mastoidectomy is performed. **(b)** The antrum is opened. Full of markedly edematous, hypertrophied mucosa. The attic is blocked. **(c)** The hypertrophied mucosa in the mastoid is cleared. A simple mastoidectomy is done. The attic is cleared. *(Continued)*

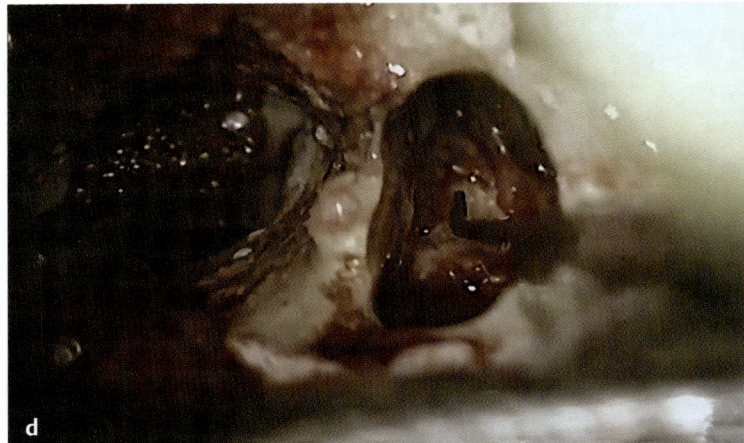

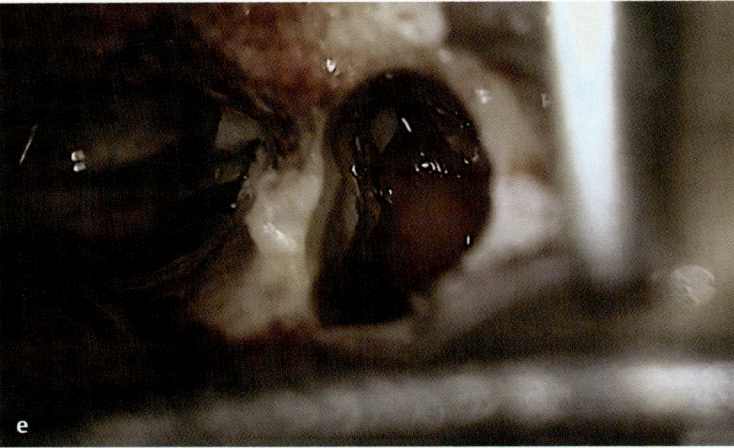

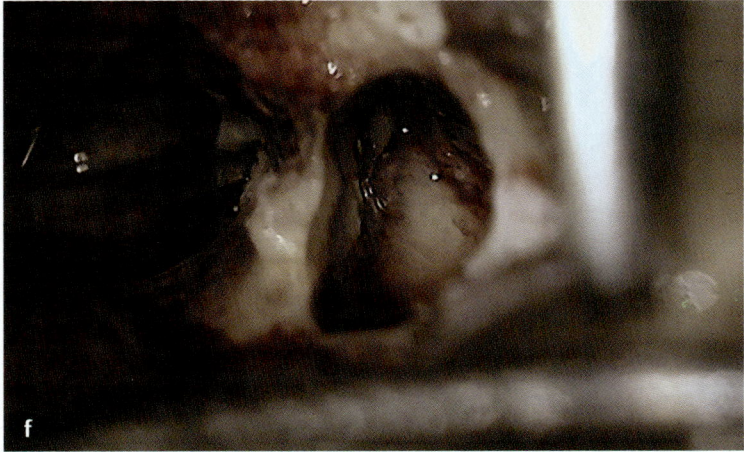

Fig. 12.1 *(Continued)* **(d)** A simple mastoidectomy is completed. Air cells are opened. Air cell congestion is cleared. Good aeration of the mastoid air cells is established. **(e)** The attic is cleaned, the short process of the incus is seen, and the water test is performed by irrigation of the mastoid by a saline solution. **(f)** The water test is positive.

- As per my experience, the mastoid should always be opened to deal with the granulations, bulky edematous mucosa, and cholesterol granuloma in the mastoid air cells to reduce congestion in that area. Good aeration of mastoid air cells should be established.

- If the attic is blocked and water test is negative, the edematous mucosa in the attic should not be disturbed, as the removal of this edematous mucosa around the ossicular chain in the attic is followed by the restricted mobility of the ossicular chain due to healing with fibrosis. It is found that once the middle ear heals up and the graft is taken up well, the edema of the attic mucosa subsides and the attic block clears up automatically, causing good ventilation of mastoid air cells with normal healing.

Rules Should be Followed during Drilling

- Start with the bigger burr, then gradually shift to the smaller burr, so that the edges of the mastoidectomy opening are beveled for better visibility in the depth. Drilling deep in a narrow tunnel may damage important structures.

- While drilling, hold the hand piece like a pen for better control and better stability with the little finger resting over the patient face.

- Drilling should only be started once the drill has been placed at the target. While removing the drill, it should be ensured that the drill is not moving. First stop the drill and then take it out.

- Continuous irrigation while drilling by a normal saline solution should be done. It removes the bone dust generated while drilling and keeps the bone cool. Excessive heat generated while drilling may cause excessive granulation formation postoperatively, especially when the bone is not cooled by proper saline irrigation during drilling.

- While drilling, excessive pressure should not be exerted over the bone. This only happens when the burrs have become blunt. These blunt burrs should be changed to new burrs.

- When close to the important structure, drilling is done by a diamond burr, which is also hemostatic. Drilling near the important structure should be done along the length of the structure to prevent its damage.

13 Treatment of Small Perforations

Small-sized perforation can be treated by repeated chemical cauterization of the edges of the perforation either by 30% silver nitrate or by 50% trichloroacetic acid (TCA).

After chemical cauterization, the edges of the perforation are splinted by a piece of filter paper soaked in betadine solution, which helps in faster healing. This chemical cauterization removes the squamous epithelium at the edges of the perforation and stimulates the middle fibrous layer to grow and promotes the healing of the perforation. This process of chemical cauterization is to be repeated after every 3 weeks till perforation heals up. The speed of closure of the perforation depends upon the healing power of the patient.

Another technique to promote the healing of the perforation is to put a small piece of fat in the perforation after chemical cauterization, which helps in closure of the perforation (fat grafting). Myringoplasty is to be done when all these measures fail.

Tympanoplasty for Small Perforation

Small perforation does not require 360-degree elevation of the tympanomeatal flap. These perforations can be managed by just elevation of the posterior and anterior tympanomeatal flap as sufficient tympanic membrane is there to overlap the fascia graft with high degree of success.Details of the tympanoplasty for small perforation are presented in **Figs. 13.1–13.18**.

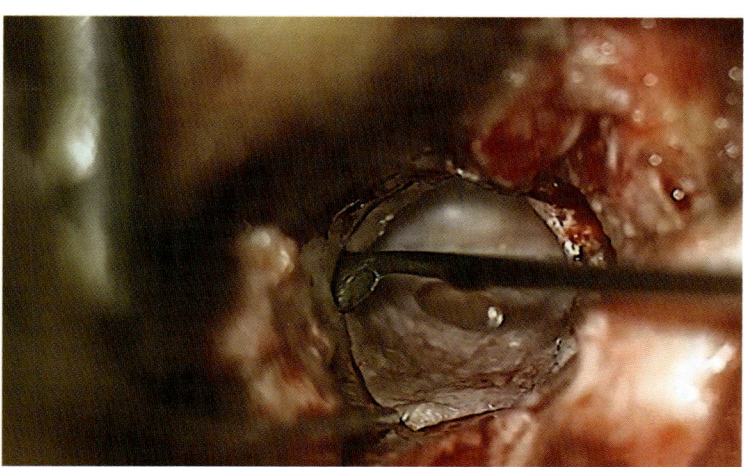

Fig. 13.1 Small perforation can be managed, by just elevation of the posterior and anterior tympanomeatal flap and not the 360-degree elevation of the tympanomeatal flap.

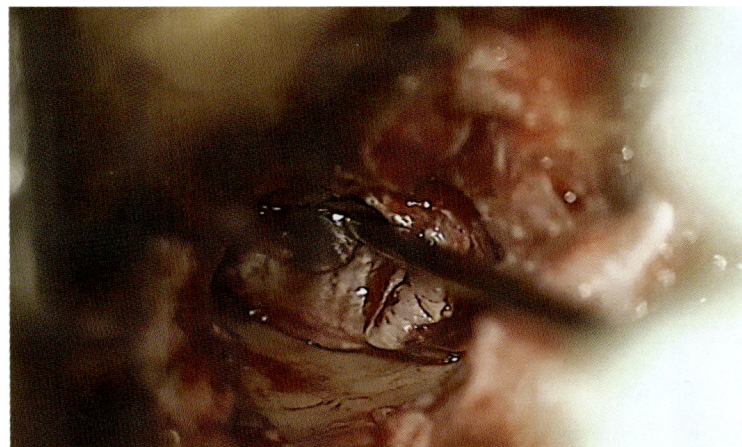

Fig. 13.2 The posterior tympanomeatal flap is elevated.

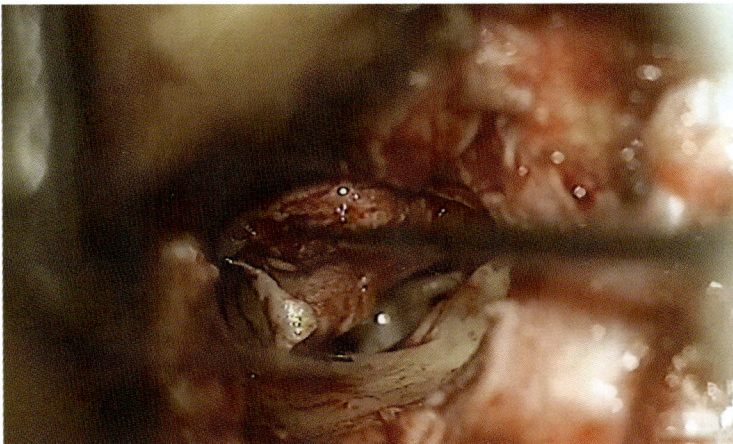

Fig. 13.3 The posterior tympanomeatal flap is elevated. The annulus is lifted from the sulcus and the middle ear is entered.

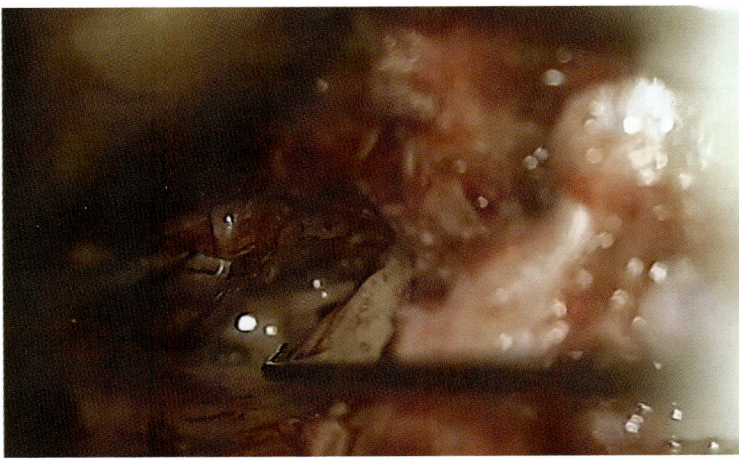

Fig. 13.4 The posterior tympanomeatal flap is elevated. The ossicular chain is examined and it is found to be normal. There is no need for 360-degree elevation of tympanomeatal flap in small perforation. Only anterior and posterior tympanomeatal flap elevation is sufficient to have good overlapping of the tympanic membrane and graft.

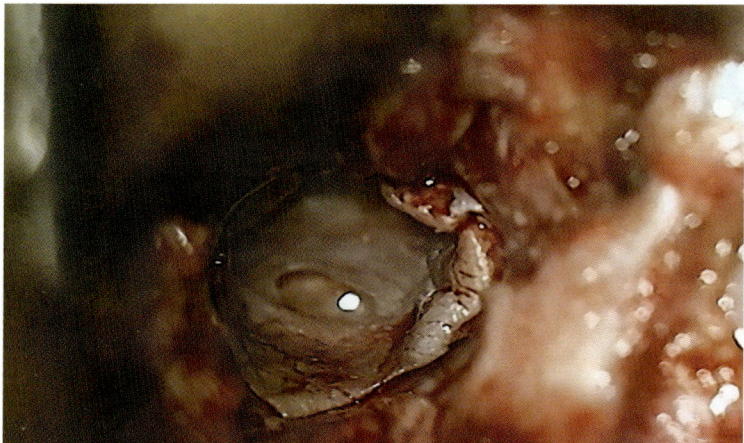

Fig. 13.5 The posterior tympanomeatal flap is reposited back.

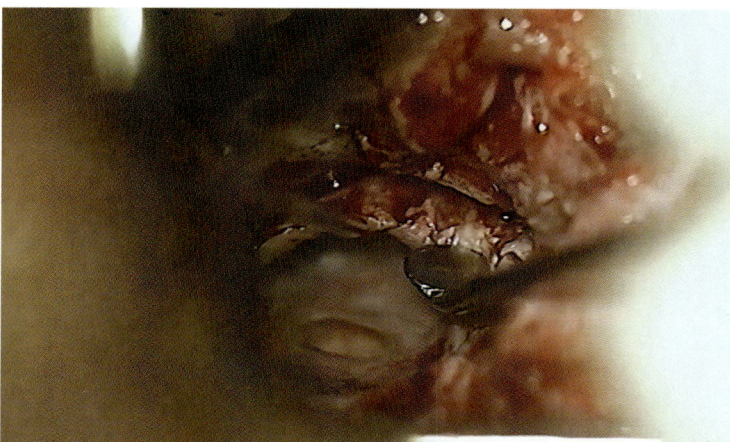

Fig. 13.6 The tympanomeatal flap is elevated anteriorly and superiorly.

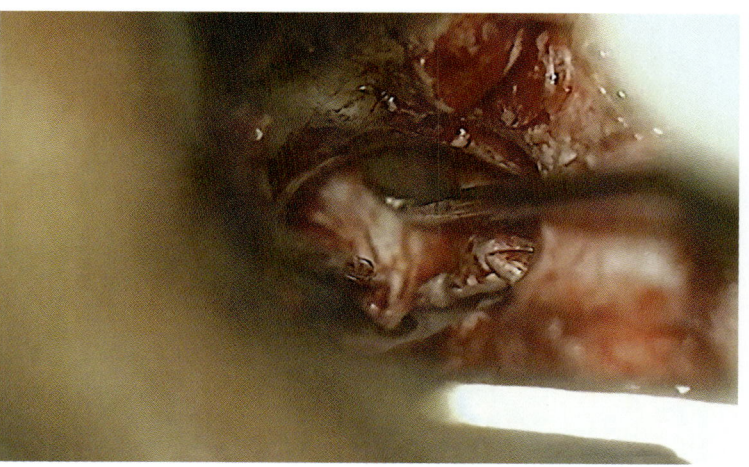

Fig. 13.7 The tympanomeatal flap is elevated anteriorly and superiorly up to the anulus.

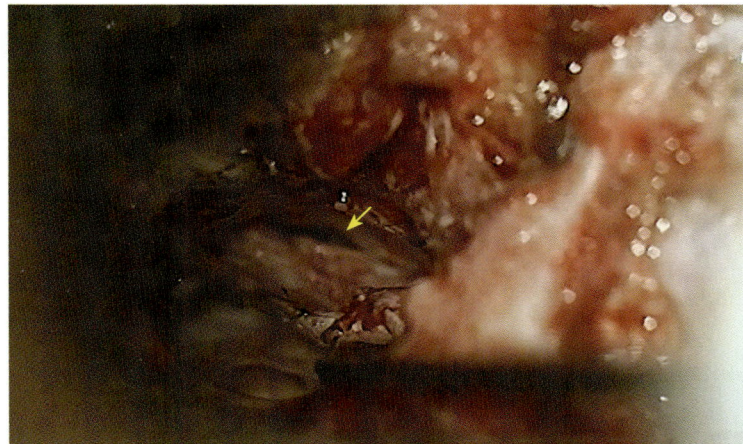

Fig. 13.8 The tympanomeatal flap is elevated anteriorly and superiorly, the annulus is elevated from the sulcus, and the middle ear is entered anterior to the neck of the malleus.

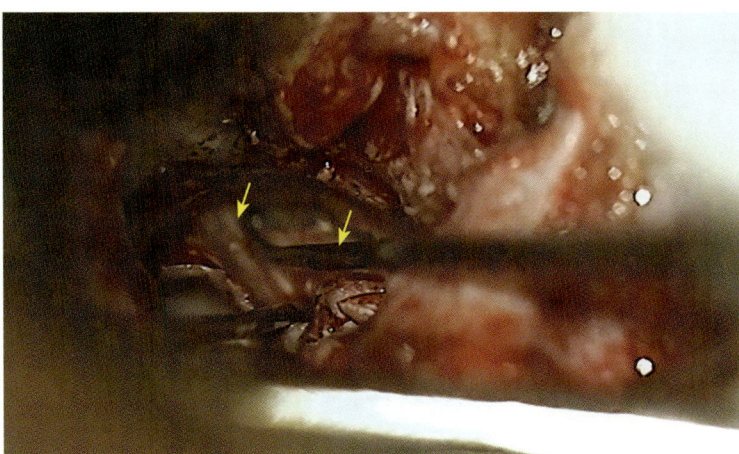

Fig. 13.9 Tympanomeatal flap elevation is continued anteriorly up to the 9 o'clock position and superiorly up to the neck of the malleus.

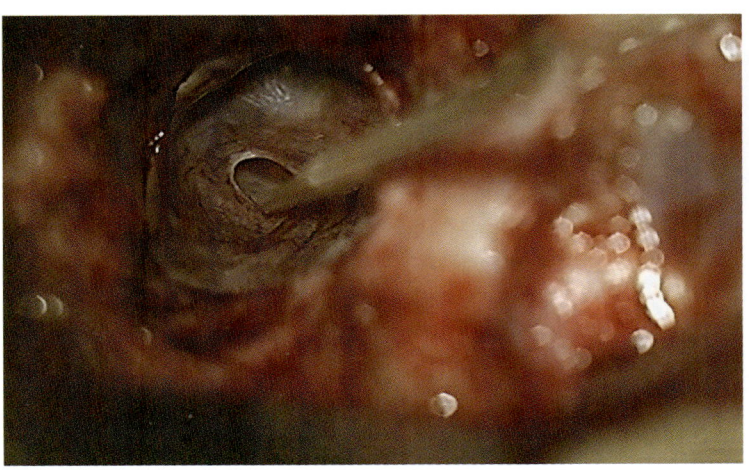

Fig. 13.10 Margins of the perforation is cauterized by 50% trichloroacetic acid (TCA) so that the epithelium at the edges of the perforation is destroyed making the margins of the perforation raw.

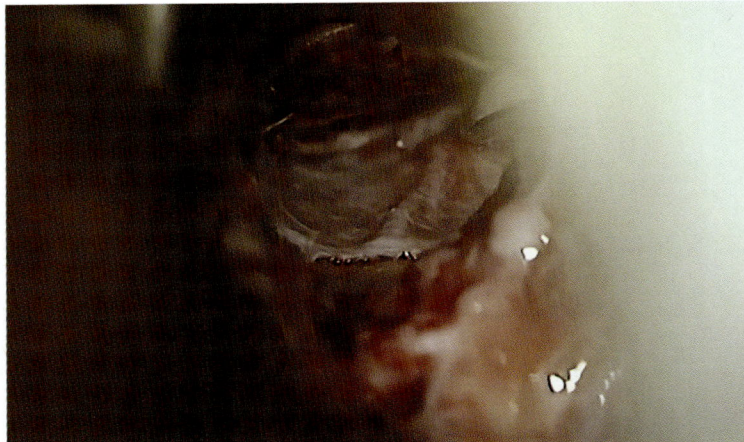

Fig. 13.11 The underlay graft is placed under the posterior tympanomeatal flap, medial to the handle of the malleus.

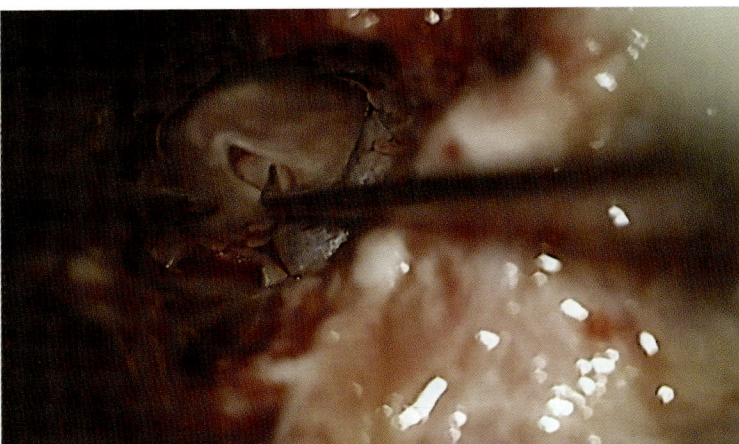

Fig. 13.12 The underlay graft is placed medial to the handle of the malleus. The posterior tympanomeatal flap is reposited back.

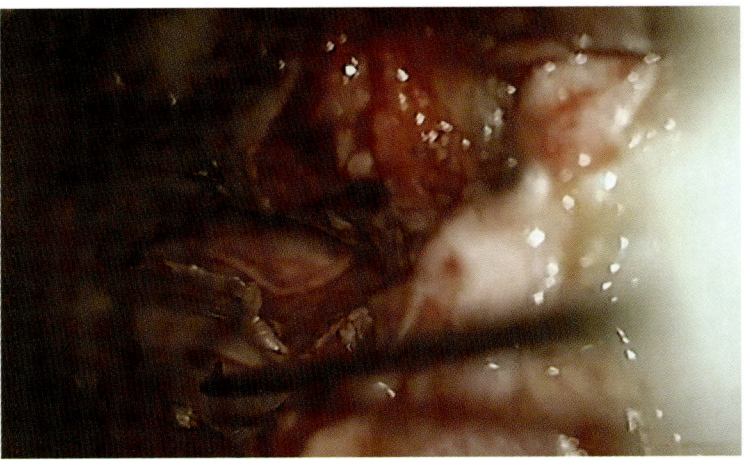

Fig. 13.13 The graft is pulled anterosuperiorly, under the anterior tympanomeatal flap.

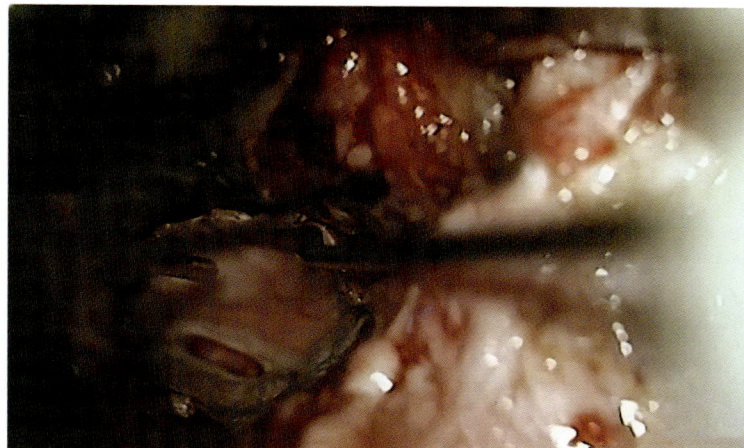

Fig. 13.14 The anterior tympanomeatal flap is reposited back. Now the graft is well supported on the anterior and posterior bony meatal wall lying medial to the tympanic membrane.

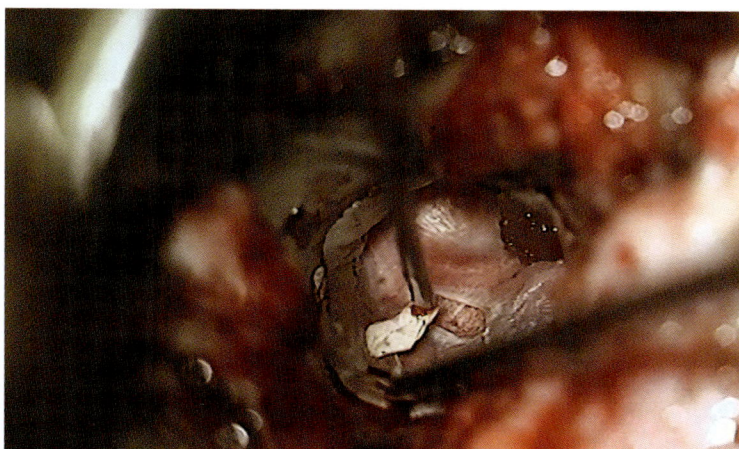

Fig. 13.15 A small piece of meatal skin is taken out to cover the graft.

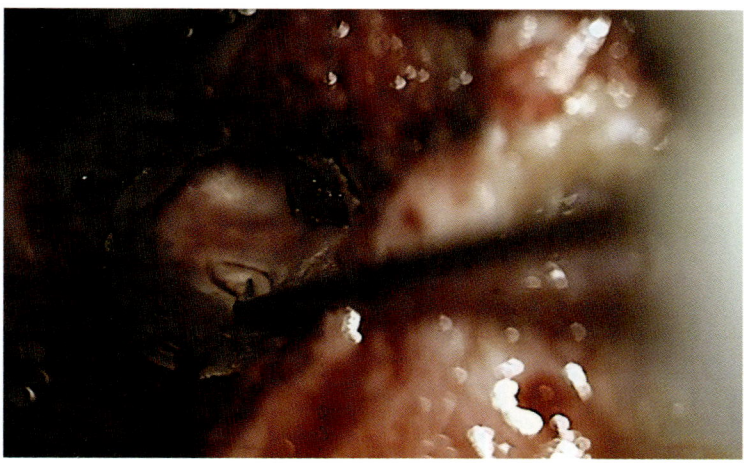

Fig. 13.16 A small piece of meatal skin is placed to cover the graft for faster epithelialization.

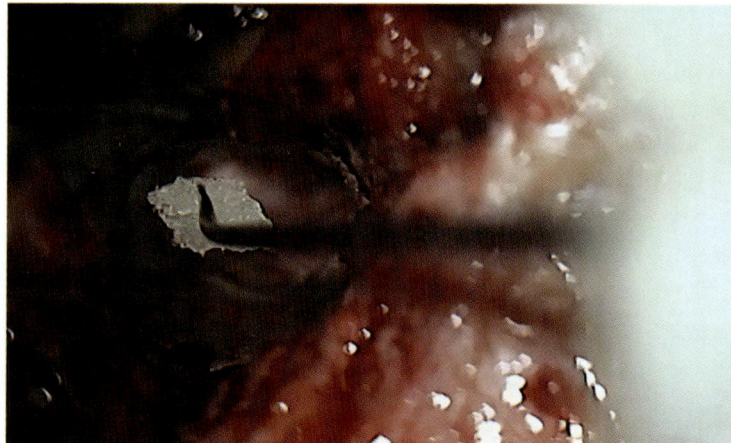

Fig. 13.17   After repositing the tympanomeatal flap, small pieces of Gelfoam are placed in the external auditory canal. Care is taken to maintain the angle between the anterior meatal wall and tympanic membrane less than 90 degrees for complete closure of the air–bone gap.

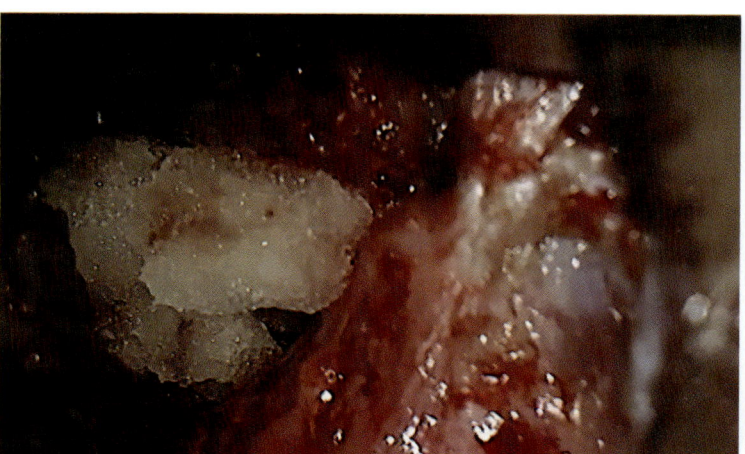

Fig. 13.18   The external auditory canal is packed by Gelfoam and the incision is closed.

14 Surgery in the Wet Ear and in Patients with Granular Myringitis

- Ideally the ear should be dry before grafting.

- If it remains wet, the discharge may be either purulent or mucoid.

- If the discharge is purulent, culture and sensitivity of the pus should be done and a good course of injectable antibiotics should be given as per the culture report. Once the ear becomes dry or less moist, then surgery can be performed.

- Suitable injectable antibiotics should be continued postoperatively for 7 days.

- In these cases, the mastoid should be nicely explored. Simple mastoidectomy should be done. All the bulky edematous mucosa from the mastoid air cells and attic should be removed. Nice ventilation of the mastoid air cells should be established. Any doubtful mucosa or granulations of the middle ear should be sent for histopathology examination to rule out Koch's infection of the middle ear.

- Postoperatively, these patients require antibiotics for longer duration (almost 3 weeks).

- Antibiotics should be changed every week depending upon the culture reports. In general, the chances of failure of surgery are high in the presence of active infection.

- If the discharge is mucoid, mostly it is due to the allergic process in the nose and sinuses. Surgery can be done in these patients without any hesitation.

- This mucoid discharge is associated with edematous, hypertrophied mucosa of the middle ear, and postoperatively antihistamines should be given to these patients for longer duration.

Granular Myringitis

- This is the most common cause of persistent otorrhea. It is a condition in which the tympanic membrane is covered by thick granulation tissue, which keeps the ear wet.

- The epithelial layer is replaced by thick granulations with a healthy middle ear mucosa. The cause of these granulations is not known. It is said to be a growth of the endothelial layer over the epithelium.

- Histopathological examination of these granulations shows nonspecific chronic inflammation.

- The exact cause of granular myringitis is not known.

- In patients with granular myringitis, the ear remains wet in spite of good antibiotic treatment.

- The ear becomes dry temporarily with the local antibiotic and steroid drops.

- X-ray of the mastoid and computed tomography (CT) of the temporal bone is normal in these patients.

- Surgery is the only final solution for granular myringitis.

- Before surgery is planned, superficial curettage of the granulations over the tympanic membrane is tried under the microscope, with chemical cauterization of the raw tympanic membrane so created is helpful in few cases. This cauterization is to be repeated in some cases. The tympanic membrane gradually heals up and gets epithelialized.

- If the surgery is planned for the granular myringitis patients, the myringitis part of the tympanic membrane is to be excised and the edges of the perforation so created is to be cauterized. Then tympanoplasty is performed.

- When the mastoid is explored in these patients, it is found to be normal in most of the cases. Many a time, the granular myringitis is associated with tympanosclerosis.

- In few patients with extensive granular myringitis involving complete tympanic membrane and adjacent meatal wall, skin requires complete excision of the tympanic membrane with the annulus and adjacent meatal wall skin followed by reconstruction (**Figs. 14.1–14.8**).

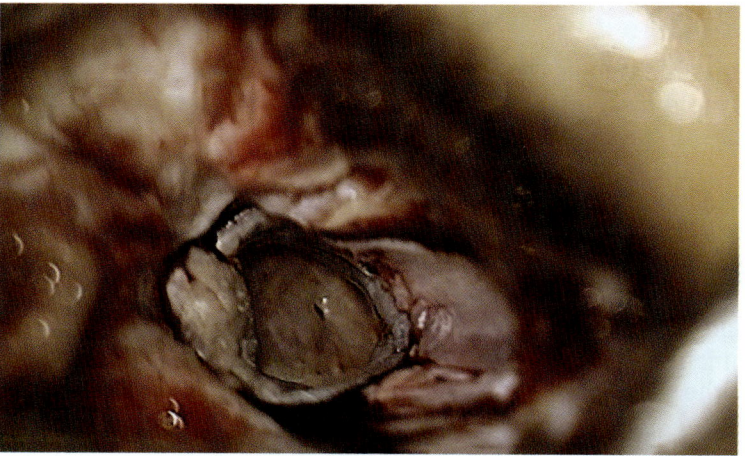

Fig. 14.1 Complete drum myringitis. There is a small central perforation.

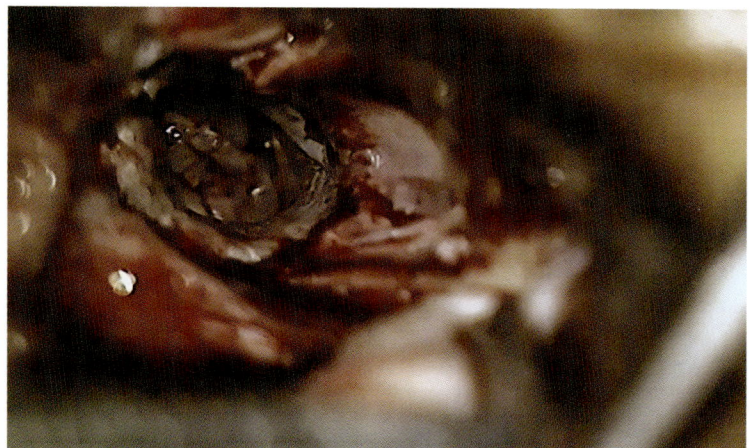

Fig. 14.2 Complete tympanic membrane myringitis is excised by a sickle knife.

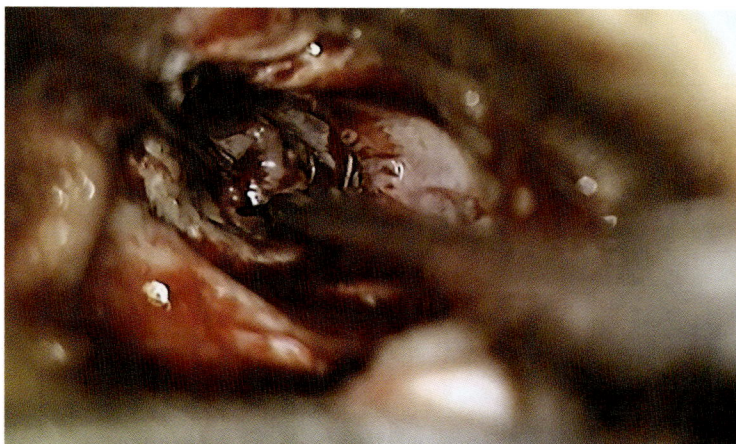

Fig. 14.3 Microscissors are required at times to excise the tympanic membrane with myringitis.

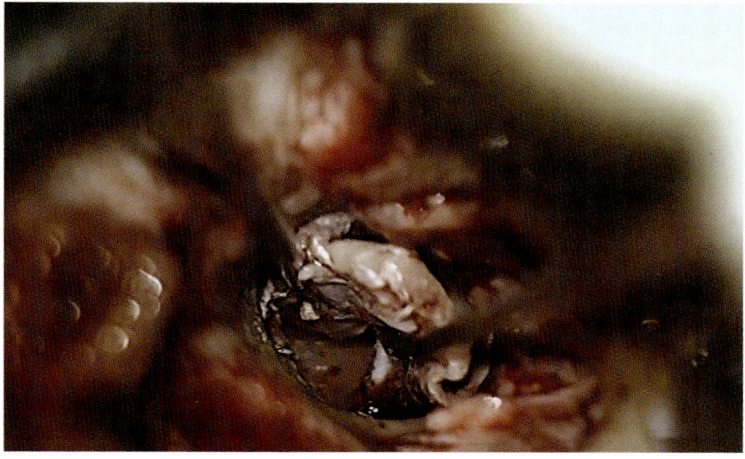

Fig. 14.4 The excised tympanic membrane with myringitis is removed.

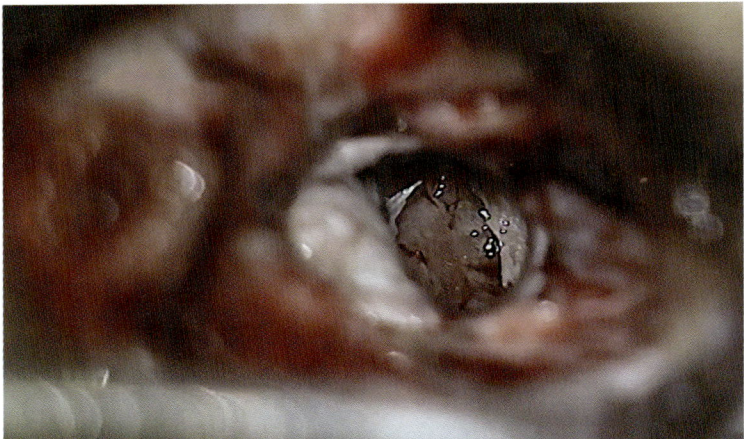

Fig. 14.5 Complete drum with myringitis has been excised leaving the healthy part. A large perforation is created after excising the diseased part.

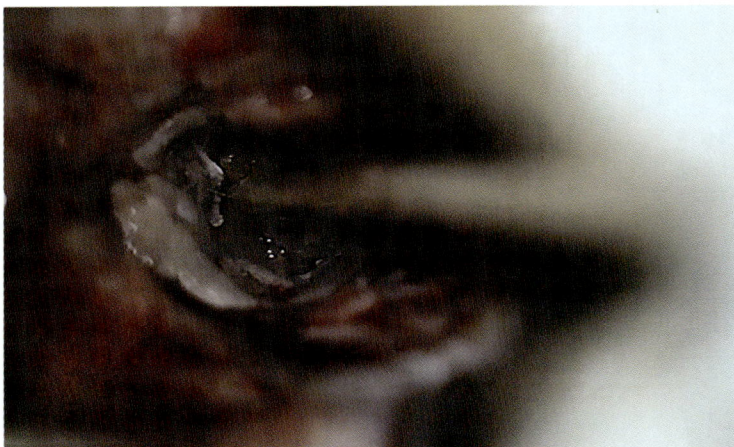

Fig. 14.6 Margins of the perforation so created are cauterized by 50% trichloroacetic acid (TCA).

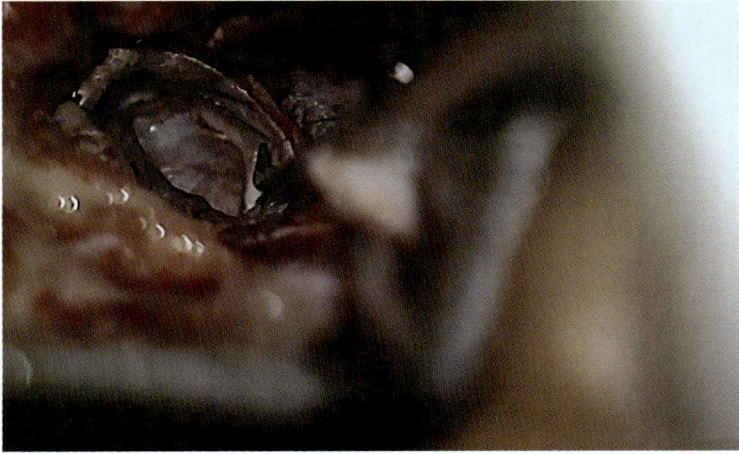

Fig. 14.7 An underlay graft is placed.

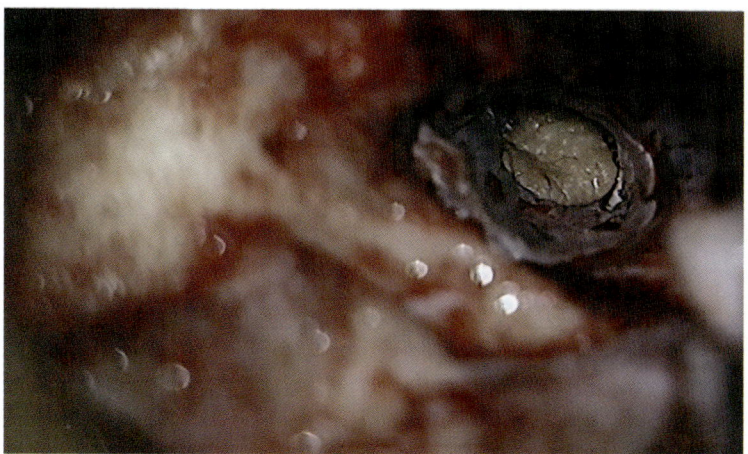

Fig. 14.8   The graft is covered by a piece of full-thickness postaural skin graft.

15 Patient's Age for Tympanoplasty

Tympanoplasty in Children

Normally, tympanoplasty in children should only be done after 12 years of age, as it is difficult to take postoperative care of the operated ear in a very young child.

Before 12 years of the age, the children are more vulnerable to recurrent upper respiratory infection (URI).

Whatever is the age of the child, the nose and throat should be free from any infection (septic focus). Adenoids should not block the eustachian tube (ET); hence, adenoidectomy should always be done before or during tympanoplasty.

A very young child can be operated on, if required, especially if the deafness is affecting his education and social development. This usually happens when the disease is bilateral. Cartilage tympanoplasty in these patients is very much suitable because cartilage is very much resistant to ET dysfunction.

Tympanoplasty in the Older Age Group

Tympanoplasty is not contraindicated in the older age group if the patient is medically fit. An old person of any age can be operated on if he or she is medically fit.

16 Tympanosclerosis

Tympanosclerosis is nothing but hyaline deposits composed of collagen fibers, with calcium phosphate deposits looking like chalks. It gets deposited in the tympanic membrane in the lamina propria between the epithelium and the endothelium or in the subendothelial plane. The formation of tympanosclerotic plaques is due to an abnormal healing process in response to an inflammatory process, especially otitis media. The tympanosclerotic plaque involving the tympanic membrane is known as myringosclerosis.

During tympanoplasty, these myringosclerotic plaques from the tympanic membrane should be removed keeping the epithelium intact, before placing the fascia graft, as these plaques are avascular and may affect the vascularization of the fascia graft. Success rate is high, if the myringosclerotic or tympanosclerotic plaques are removed.

Similarly, tympanosclerotic plaques in the middle ear should be removed, especially if they are affecting the mobility of the ossicular chain. The malleus and incus are mostly fixed in the attic due to tympanosclerotic plaques requiring simple mastoidectomy with posterior atticotomy with removal of tympanosclerotic plaques from the attic fixing the malleus and incus, thus mobilizing the malleus and the incus.

Tympanosclerotic plaque may involve he stapes footplate and superstructure causing fixation of the stapes. This fixation of the stapes can be guessed by doing a Gelfoam patch test before surgery.

During tympanoplasty, it may be possible to mobilize the stapes by removing this tympanosclerotic plaques gently from the stapes, but chances of refixation of the stapes are very high due to deposition of this plaque again causing refixation of the stapes.

Fixed stapes due to tympanosclerotic plaques may be difficult to mobilize at times. Hence, a second-stage stapedectomy can be planned in these patients.

Clinical Cases

- Tympanoplasty in a case of central perforation with tympanosclerosis (myringosclerosis) can be critical (**Fig. 16.1a–g**).

- *A case of tympanosclerosis*: Large central perforation with a myringosclerotic plaque in the anterior part of the tympanic membrane, anterior to the handle of the malleus (**Fig. 16.2a–i**).

- *A case of tympanosclerosis*: The entire eardrum is myringosclerotic with central perforation (**Fig. 16.3a–d**).

- *A case of tympanosclerosis*: Tympanosclerotic plaques around the stapes, fixing the stapes footplate (**Fig. 16.4a–r**).

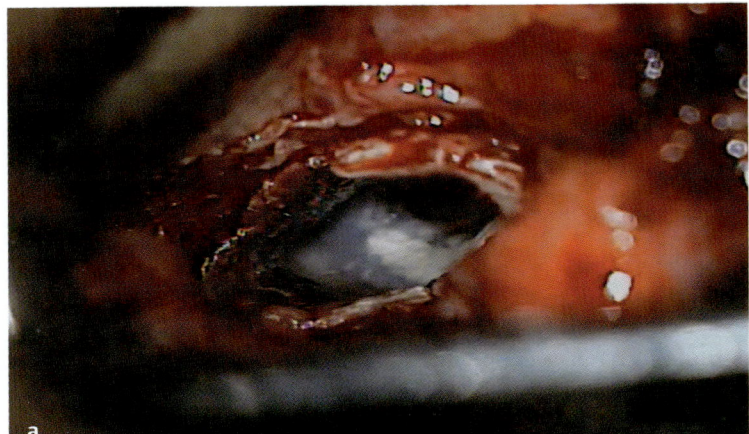

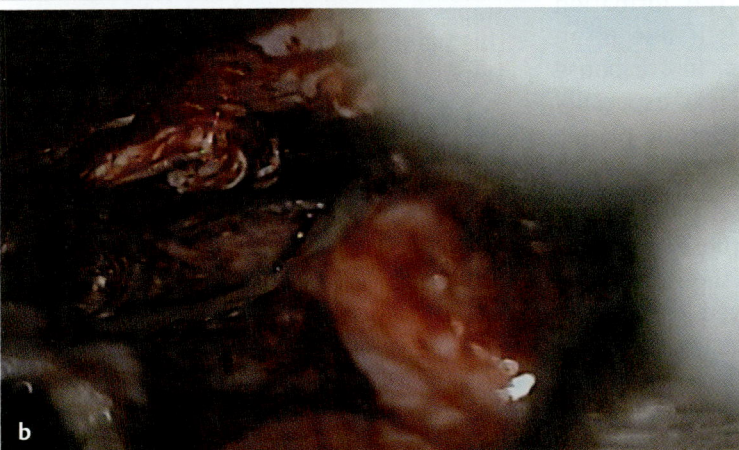

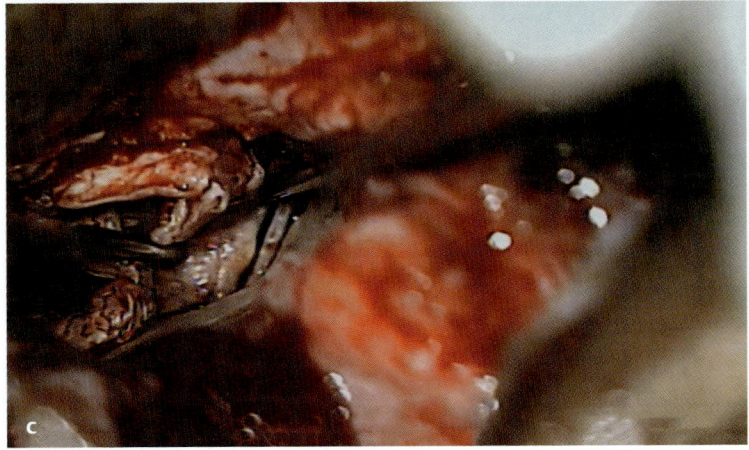

Fig 16.1 **(a)** Plaque of myringosclerosis with central perforation. **(b)** Posterior tympanomeatal flap is elevated. **(c)** Posterior tympanomeatal flap is elevated and the annulus is lifted from the sulcus with limited opening of the tympanic cavity. This limited elevation of the annulus from the sulcus keeps the tympanic membrane stable. *(Continued)*

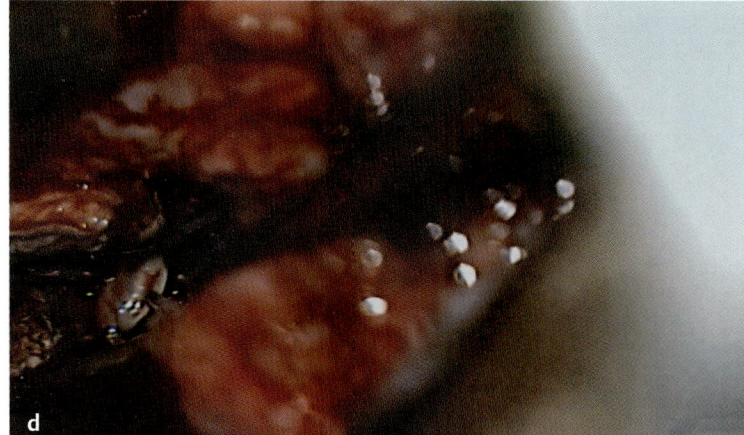

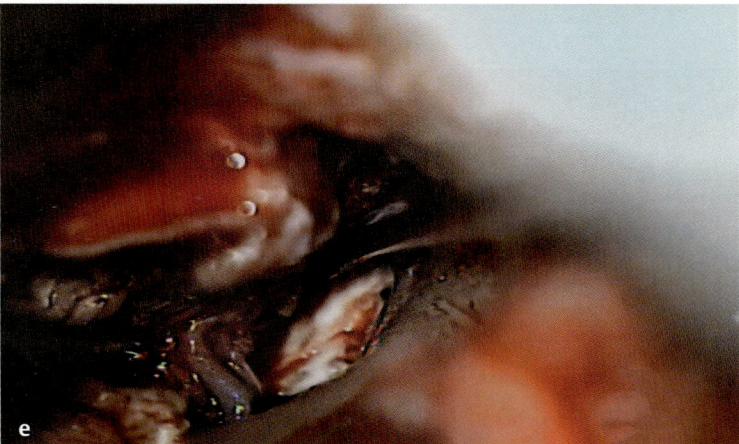

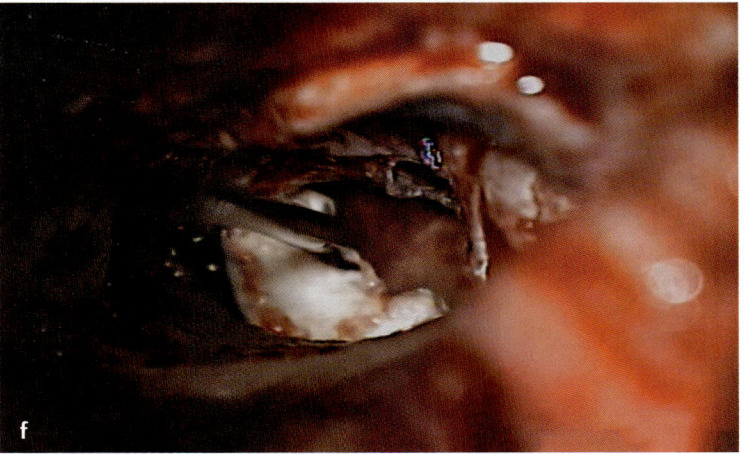

Fig 16.1 *(Continued)*
(d) Myringosclerotic plaque is dissected from the tympanic membrane by a sickle knife. **(e)** Major part of this myringosclerotic plaque is dissected from the tympanic membrane keeping the epithelium intact. **(f)** Complete myringosclerotic plaque is dissected away from the tympanic membrane with intact epithelial layer. This myringosclerotic plaque is removed. *(Continued)*

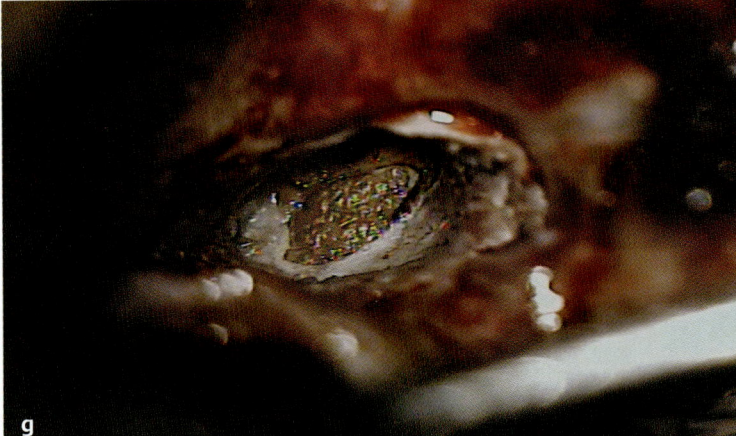

Fig 16.1 *(Continued)* **(g)** An underlay graft is placed. The tympanomeatal flap is reposited back and the graft is covered by postaural skin (full-thickness skin graft).

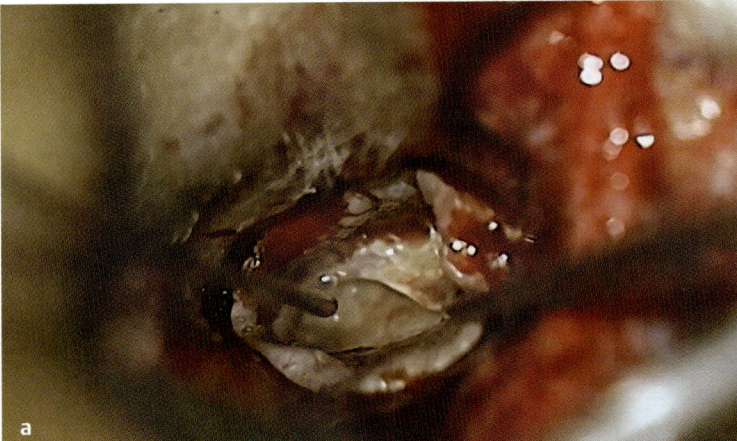

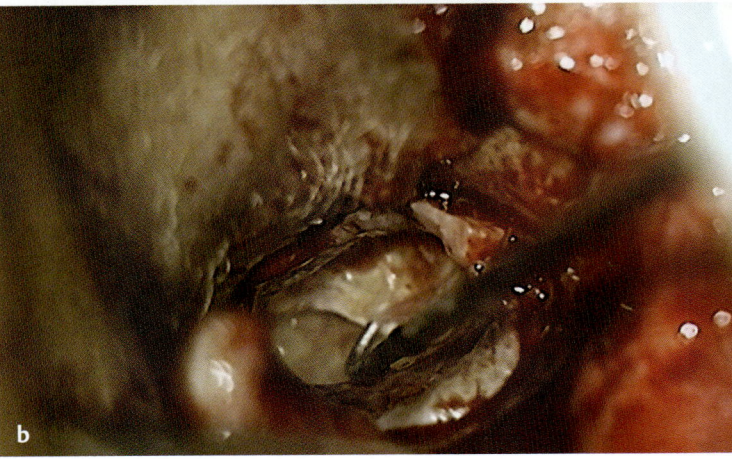

Fig. 16.2 **(a)** Big myringosclerotic plaque in the anterior part of the tympanic membrane. **(b)** The epithelial layer of the tympanic membrane is to be separated from the myringosclerotic plaque by the right-angle hook. *(Continued)*

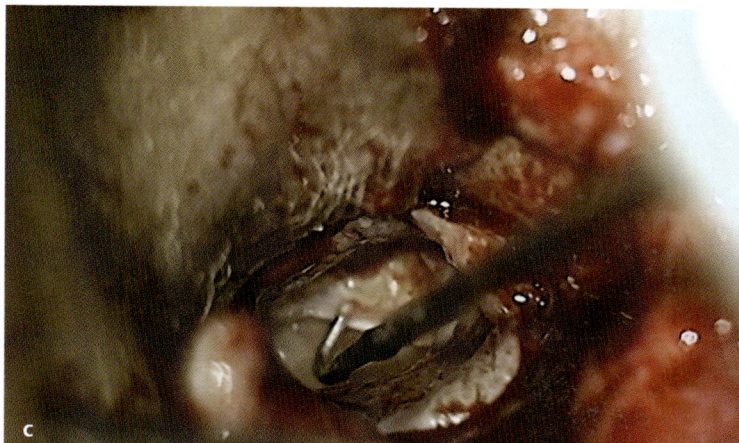

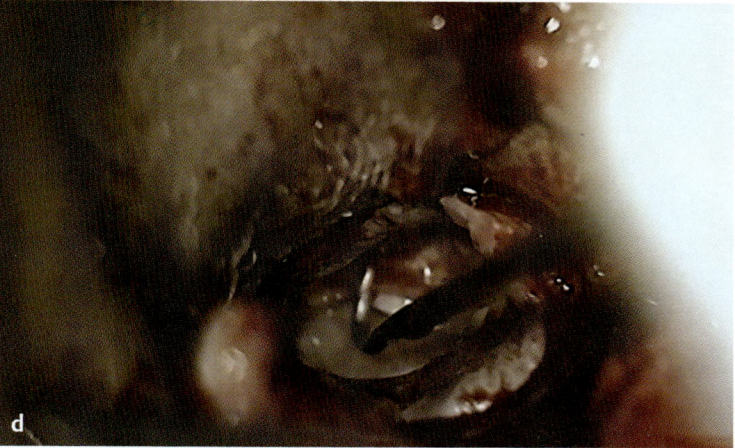

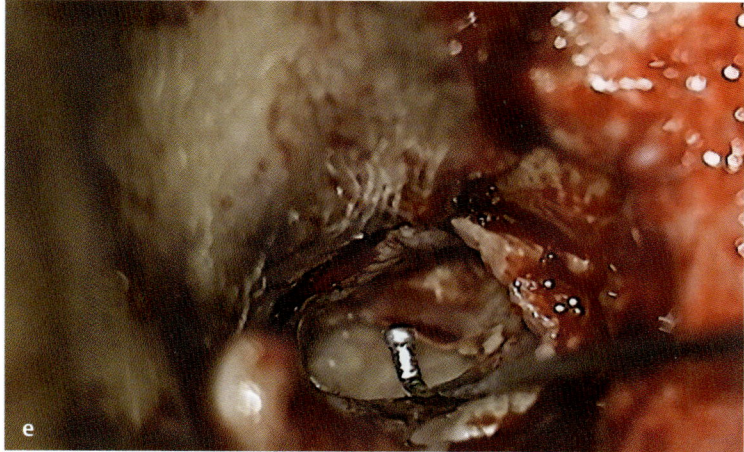

Fig. 16.2 *(Continued)*
(c) Right-angle hook is inserted between the epithelial layer and the myringosclerotic plaque. **(d)** The epithelial layer is separated from the myringosclerotic plaque by right-angle hook. **(e)** A ball probe is inserted between the epithelial layer and the myringosclerotic plaque, to separate the epithelial layer from the myringosclerotic plaque with no risk of flap tearing. *(Continued)*

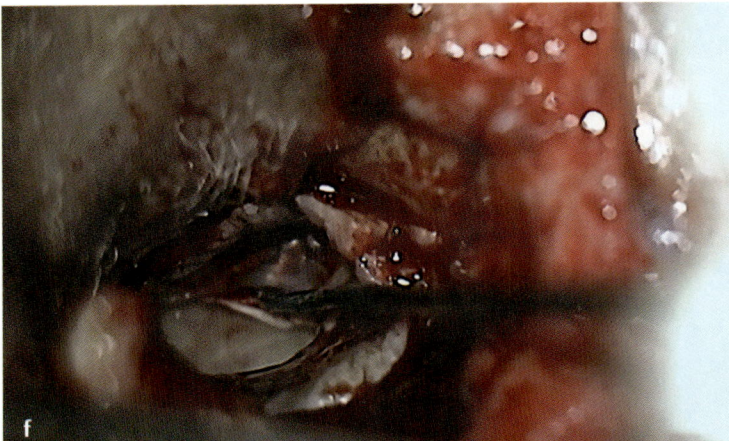

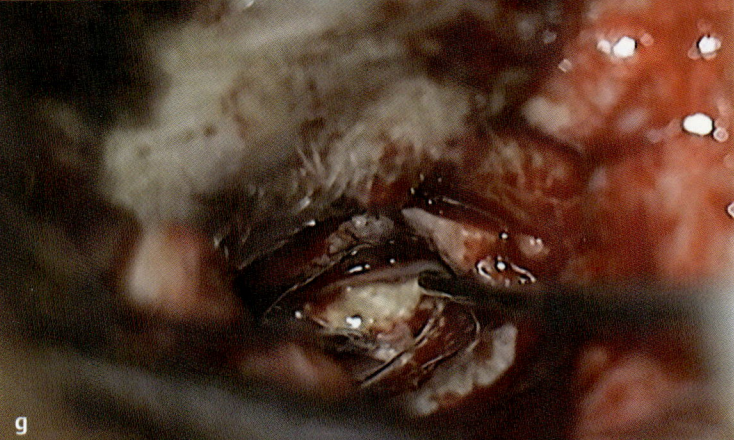

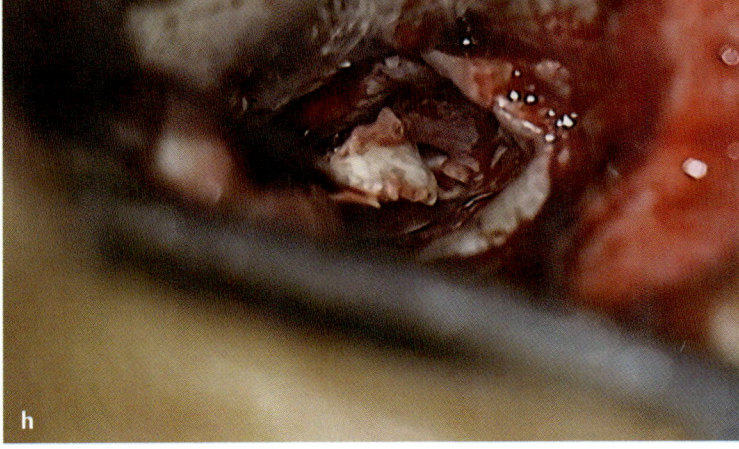

Fig. 16.2 *(Continued)* **(f)** A ball probe is used to separate the epithelial layer from the complete myringosclerotic plaque with no risk of flap tearing. **(g)** The myringosclerotic plaque has been completely dissected out from the tympanic membrane keeping the epithelial layer intact. **(h)** The whole myringosclerotic plaque has been dissected out from the tympanic membrane keeping the epithelial layer intact. *(Continued)*

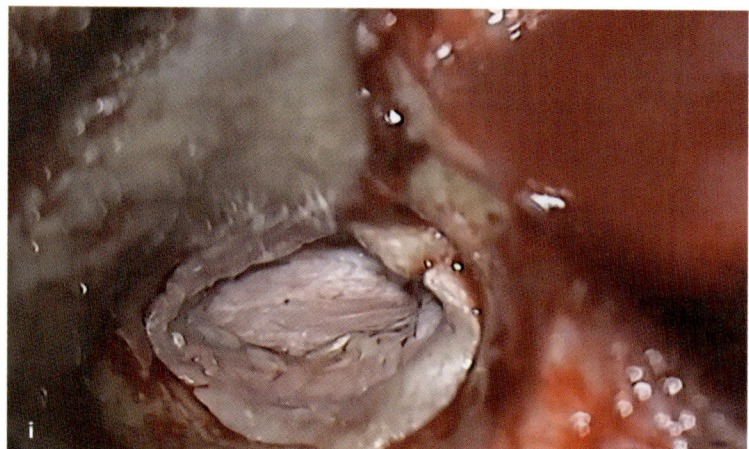

Fig. 16.2 *(Continued)* **(i)** An underlay graft is placed and the tympanomeatal flap is reposited back.

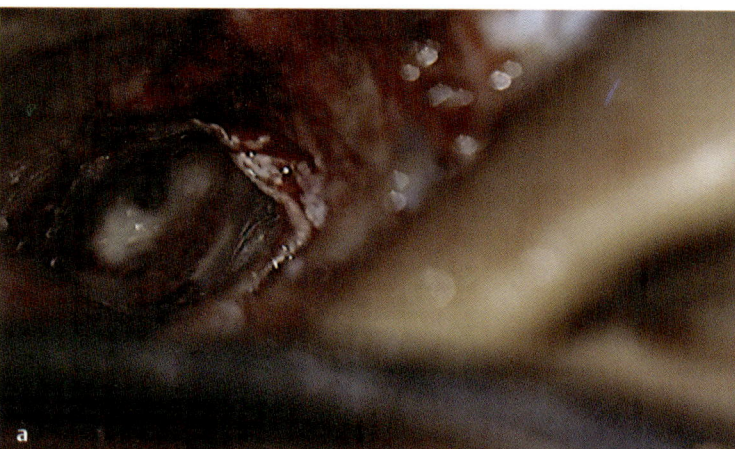

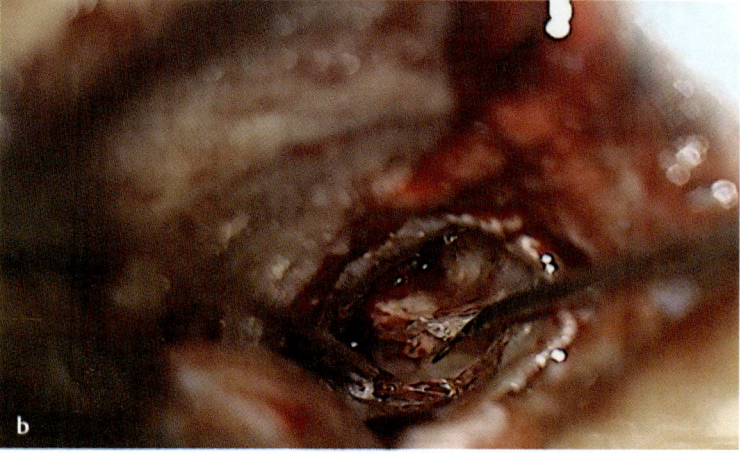

Fig. 16.3 **(a)** The entire eardrum is myringosclerotic with a small central perforation. **(b)** The entire eardrum is myringosclerotic. It is not possible to separate the epithelial layer from the myringosclerotic plaque. Hence, the entire eardrum is excised by a sickle knife. *(Continued)*

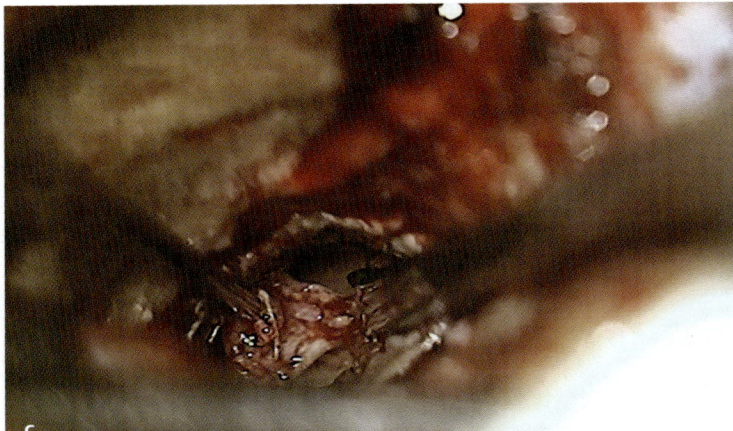

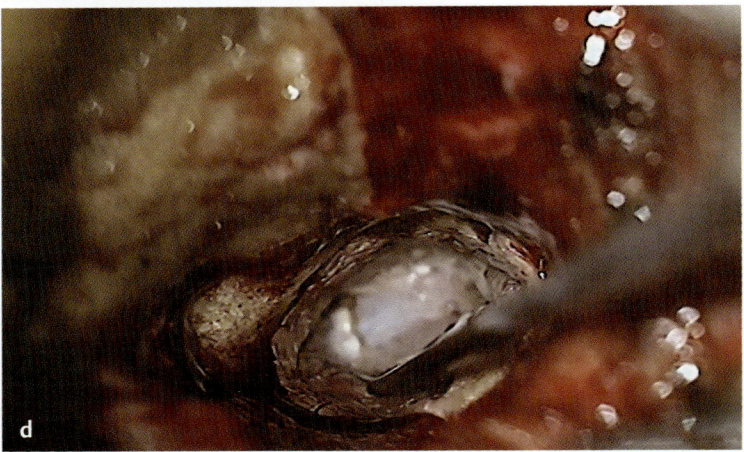

Fig. 16.3 *(Continued)*
(c) Complete myringosclerotic drum is excised by scissors. It is also dissected from the handle of the malleus by scissors. **(d)** After excising the myringosclerotic plaque, the tympanic membrane perforation so created is reconstructed by an underlay graft.

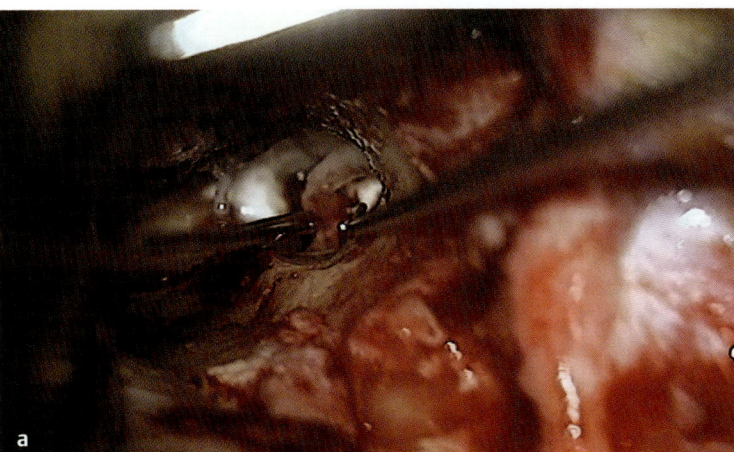

Fig. 16.4
(a) Tympanosclerotic plaques around the stapes. Fixing the stapes footplate. A big tympanosclerotic plaque is seen over the promontory. *(Continued)*

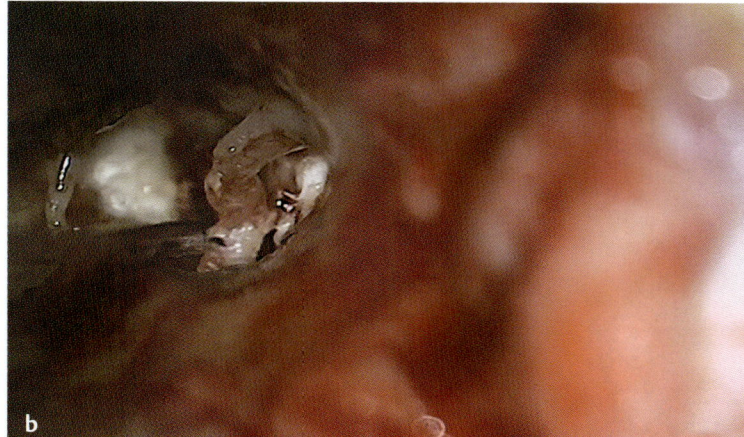

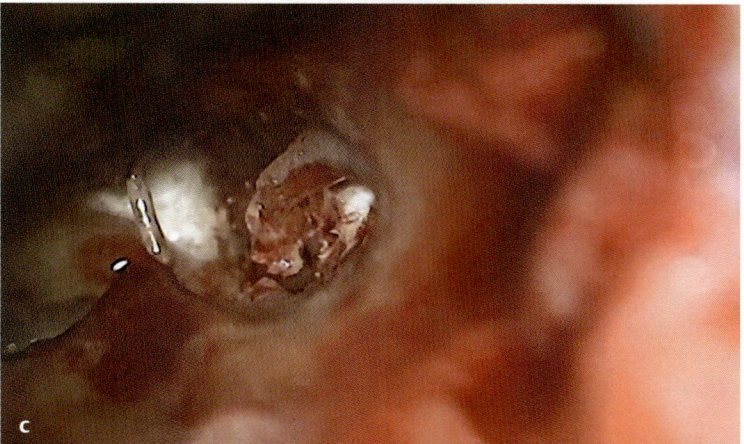

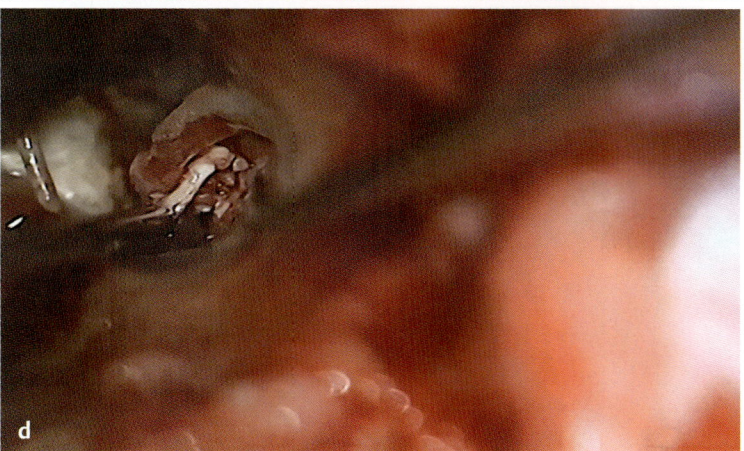

Fig. 16.4 *(Continued)* **(b)** The stapedius muscle is embedded in the tympanosclerotic plaques. **(c)** The stapedius muscle is cut by microscissors. The tympanosclerotic plaque is seen over the superior part of the stapes extending over the fallopian canal. **(d)** The tympanosclerotic plaque at the superior part of the stapes and fallopian canal is removed. *(Continued)*

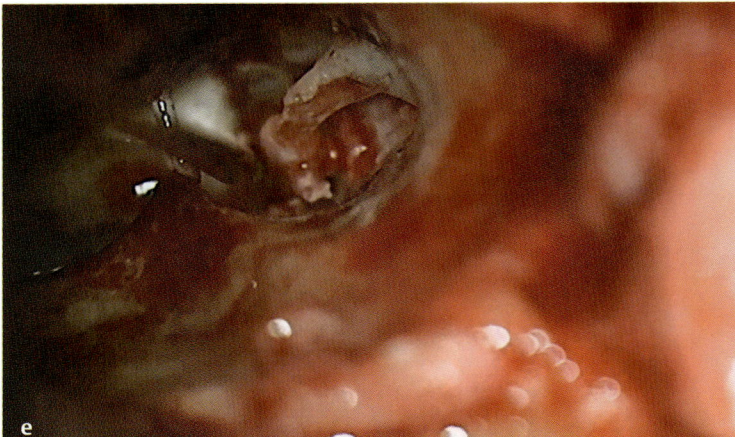

Fig. 16.4 *(Continued)* **(e)** The superior part of the stapes is freed from tympanosclerotic plaques. **(f)** Remnants of the incus is removed. Tympanosclerotic plaques all around the stapes footplate are removed. **(g)** The stapes got mobilized after removal of the tympanosclerotic plaque. *(Continued)*

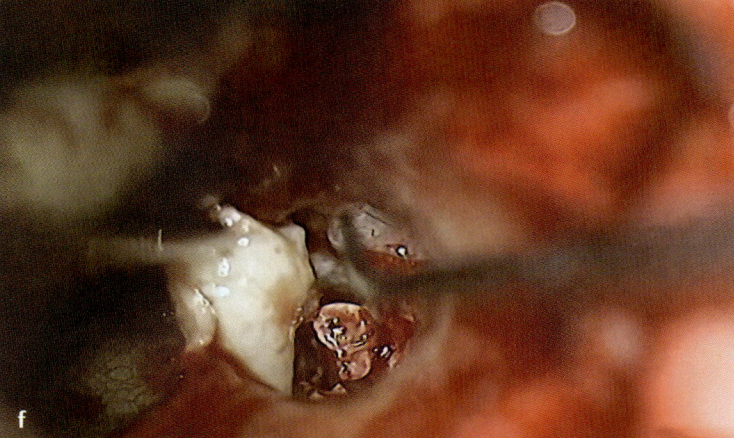

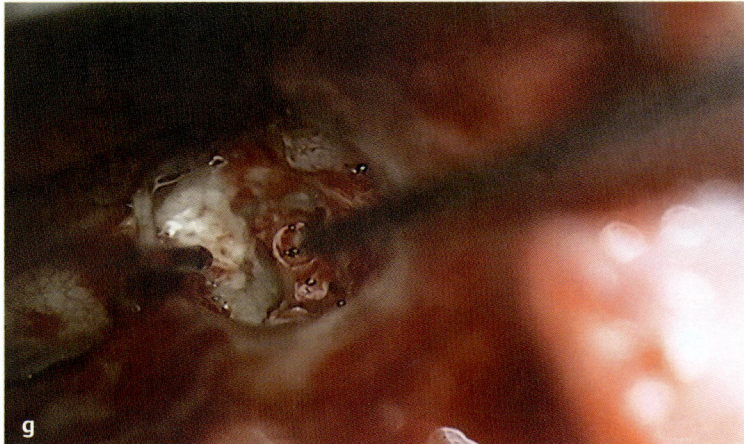

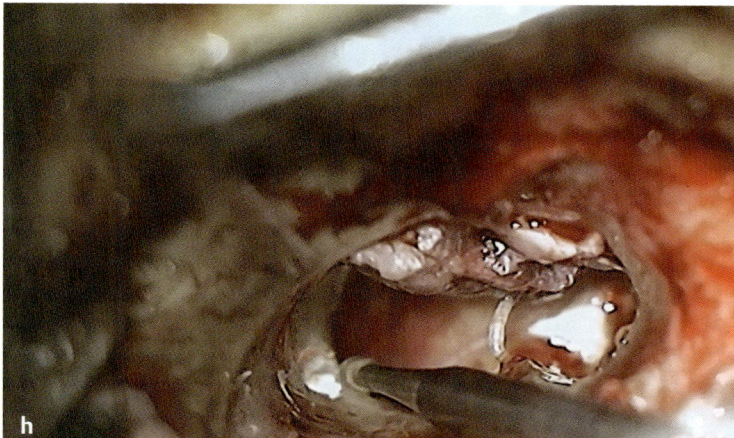

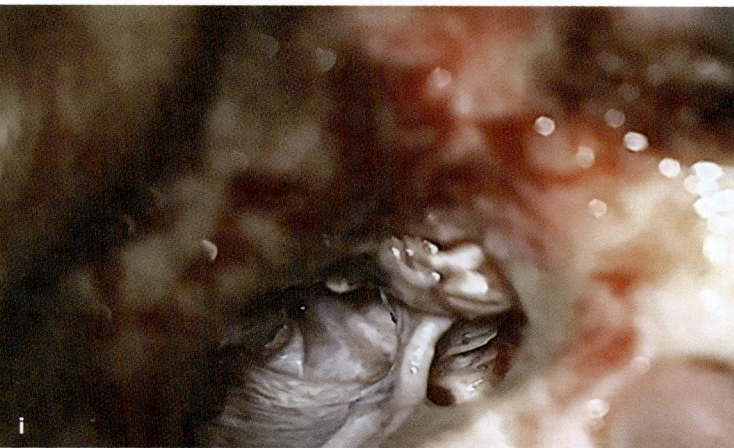

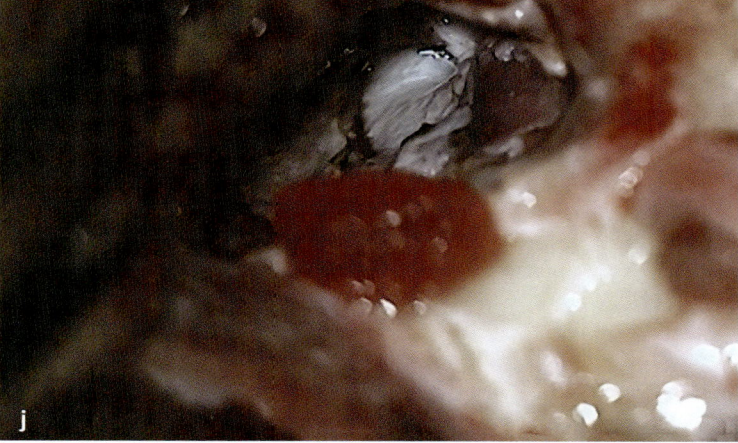

Fig. 16.4 *(Continued)* **(h)** A small depression has been made at the inferior sulcus at the 6 o'clock position, by 1.00-mm cutting burr for placement of the cartilage. **(i)** An underlay graft is placed. **(j)** An underlay graft is placed. The tympanomeatal flap is reposited back. *(Continued)*

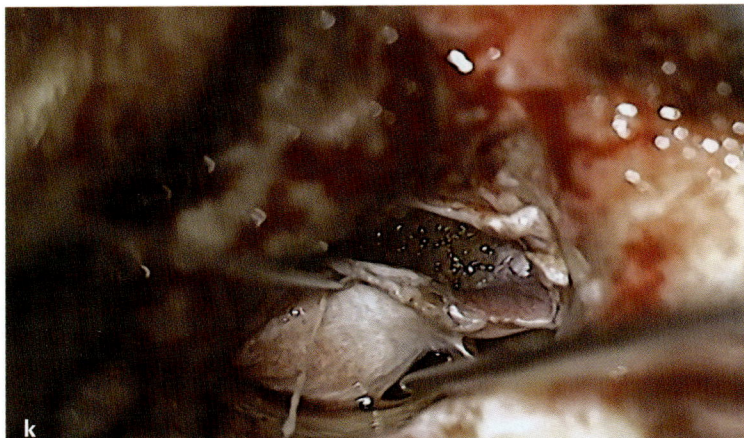

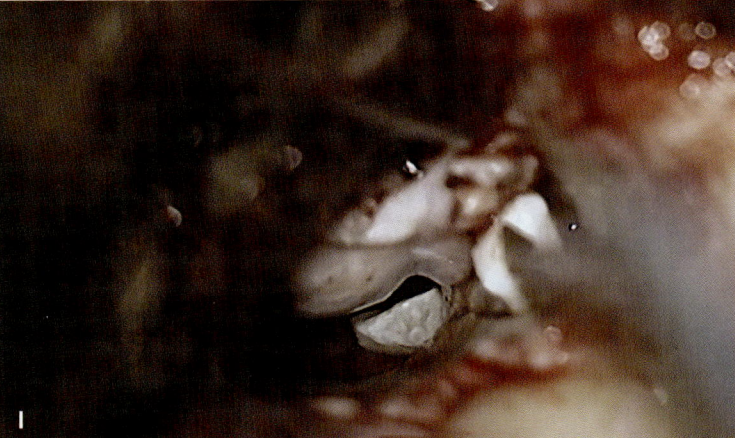

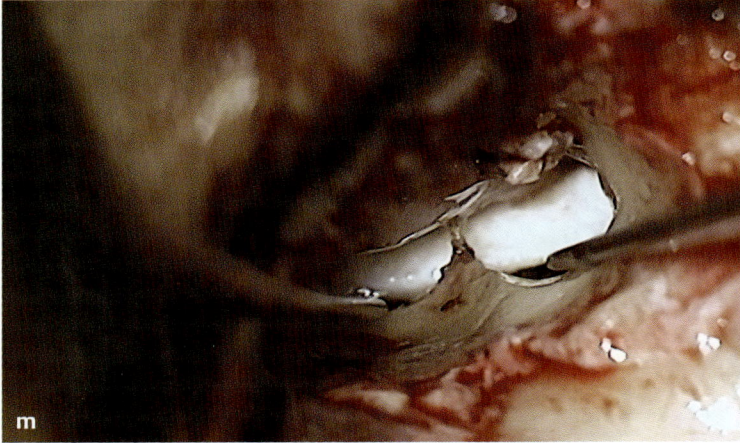

Fig. 16.4 *(Continued)* **(k)** The graft with the tympanomeatal flap is lifted up again, to expose the middle ear, for placement of the cartilage. **(l)** A triangular piece of the cartilage is introduced in the middle ear. **(m)** The cartilage is placed horizontally in the middle ear with its lower end resting on the depression at the inferior sulcus. *(Continued)*

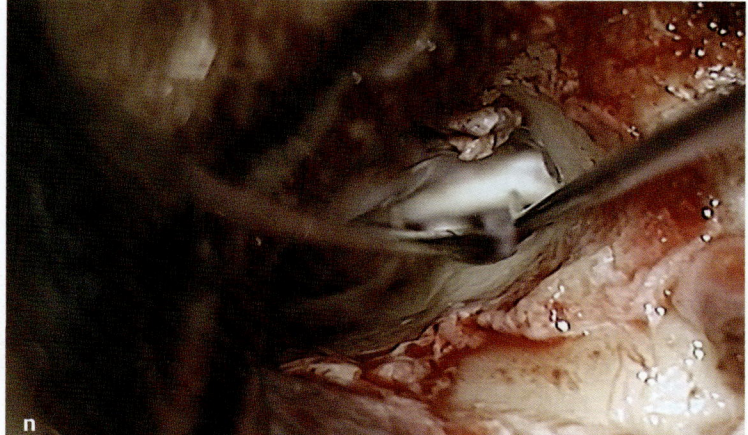

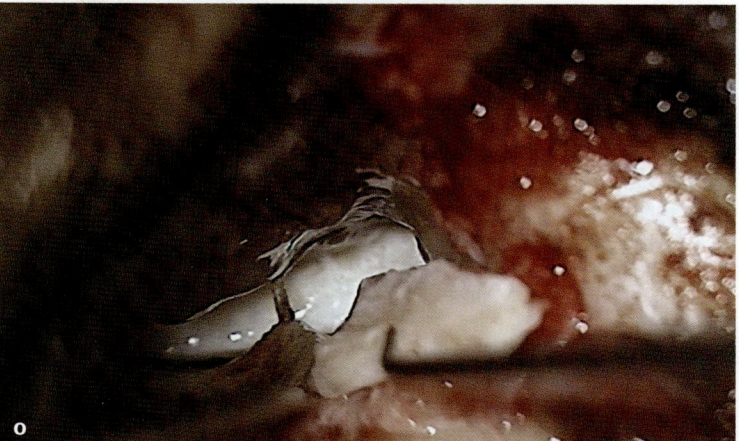

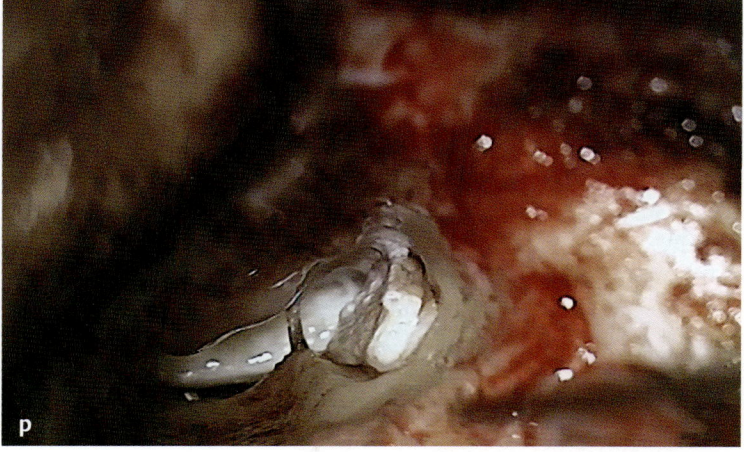

Fig. 16.4 *(Continued)* **(n)** Upper end of the horizontal cartilage is resting over the stapes head, touching the stapes head and supporting the graft. **(o)** A second cartilage is placed to close the defect in the posterosuperior bony meatal wall. **(p)** The second cartilage is placed to close the defect in the posterosuperior bony meatal wall and it exerts some pressure over the first cartilage to maintain good contact between the first cartilage and the stapes. *(Continued)*

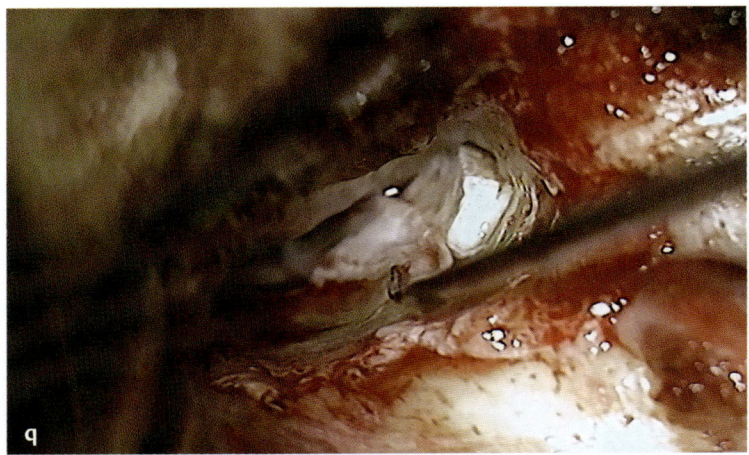

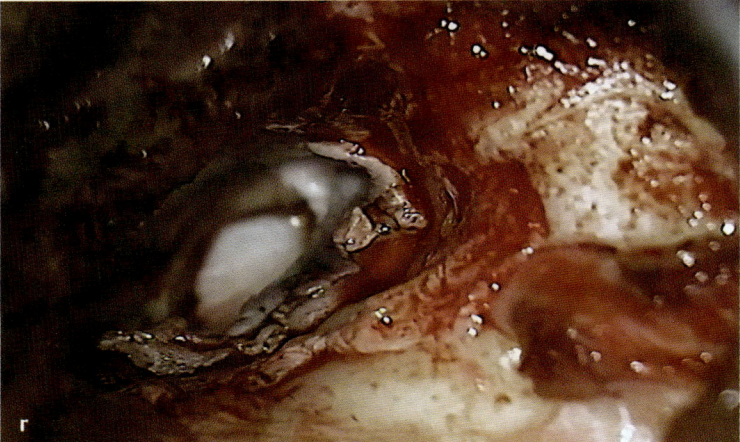

Fig. 16.4 *(Continued)* **(q)** The cartilage is covered by the perichondrium. **(r)** The tympanomeatal flap is reposited.

17 Tuberculous Otitis Media

Tuberculous otitis media is not uncommon in India. Clinically these patients present like nonspecific chronic otitis media with no specific symptoms and signs to indicate tuberculous otitis media.

This infection in the middle ear is either secondary to pulmonary infection or primary infection involving the middle ear only. The secondary infection reaches the middle ear either through tympanic membrane perforation or via the eustachian tube. Infection can also reach the middle ear through the hematogenous route.

Symptoms are the same as nonspecific otitis media, but otorrhea, which is not responding to routine antibiotics, gives some suspicion about Koch's infection. These cases can be distinguished clinically by microscopic examination, which shows markedly pale, edematous middle ear mucosa seen through the perforation with granulations.

Various complications due to associated fast bony destruction in tuberculous otitis media are facial nerve palsy and labyrinthitis leading to sensorineural hearing loss (SNHL).

If tuberculous otitis media is suspected before surgery, diagnosis is confirmed by taking out granulations from the middle ear for histopathological examination before proceeding for tympanoplasty.

If tuberculous otitis media is suspected during tympanoplasty or mastoidectomy, middle ear tissue, especially middle ear granulations, should be sent for histopathological examination.

The histopathological examination shows granulations with caseation necrosis epithelioid cells and Langerhans giant cells. Pus from the ear canal can be sent for culture and sensitivity for tuberculous bacilli, but negative test does not rule out tuberculous otitis media.

Radiologically plain X-ray mastoid is not useful. Computed tomography (CT) scan of the temporal bone in the beginning shows either minimum sclerosis of the mastoid or cellular mastoid with soft tissue in the middle ear without any erosion. Advance disease shows diffuse destruction in the temporal bone. Destruction in the temporal bone without any evidence of cholesteatoma clinically is in favor of tuberculous otitis media, but final diagnosis is by histopathological examination.

Various conditions with similar picture are nonspecific otitis media, cholesteatoma, Wegener's granuloma, and histiocytosis.

Management

- The main therapy is antituberculosis (anti-TB) drugs.

- Surgical management is simple mastoidectomy with tympanoplasty, especially in undiagnosed cases.

- Biopsy is done in the suspected cases from the middle ear mucosa or from the mastoid to confirm the diagnosis.

- If diagnosis is confirmed after surgery by histopathological examination, then a 6-month anti-TB treatment is given. The anti-TB drugs control the infection and the middle ear heals up nicely and tympanoplasty is successful in most of the cases.

- If diagnosis is confirmed before surgery, then anti-TB treatment is given for 6 months followed by tympanoplasty with mastoidectomy.

- In advance cases, surgery is required to remove the middle ear granulations, to drain the pus and to remove the unhealthy bone. Facial nerve decompression is required if the patient develops facial nerve palsy.

TB infection is suspected in the following cases:

- In the cases with persistent otorrhea that is not responding to even broad-spectrum antibiotics.

- In the cases of otitis media with unexpected complications, especially facial nerve palsy.

Suspected tuberculous otitis media. Middle ear biopsy confirmed the diagnosis (**Figs. 17.1–17.24**).

Once the diagnosis is confirmed by histopathological examination of middle ear granulations after surgery, 6 months of anti-TB treatment is given. The anti-TB drugs control the infection and the middle ear heals up nicely and tympanoplasty is successful in most of the cases.

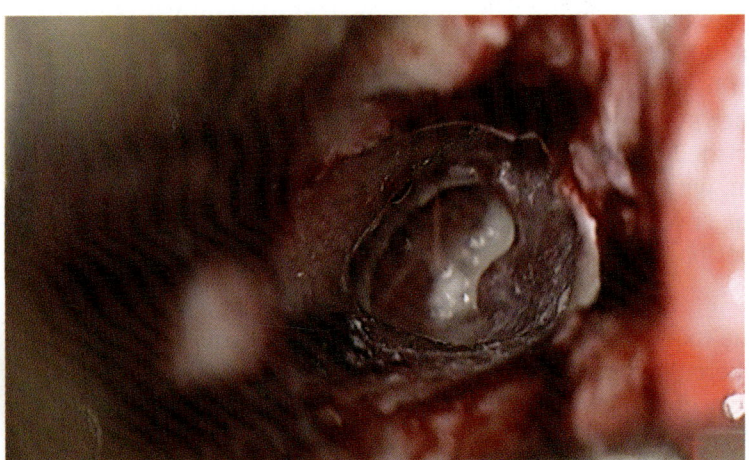

Fig. 17.1 A patient of chronic otitis media with markedly edematous, pale middle ear mucosa with persistent otorrhea not responding to routine antibiotics. Earlier cholesteatoma was suspected.

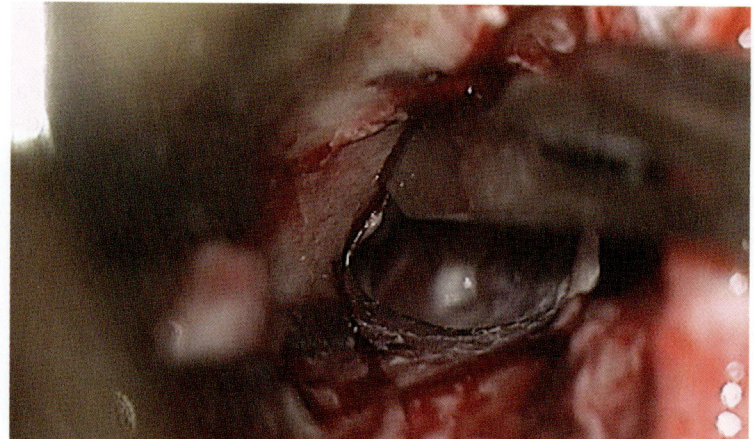

Fig. 17.2 A circumferential meatal wall skin incision is given.

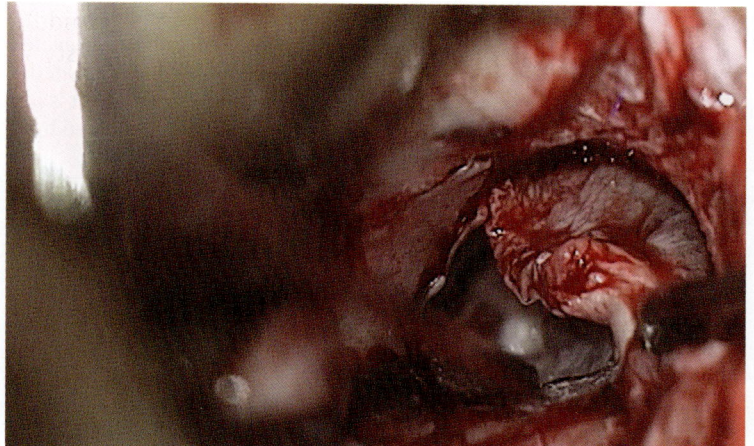

Fig. 17.3 Superior meatal wall skin is elevated.

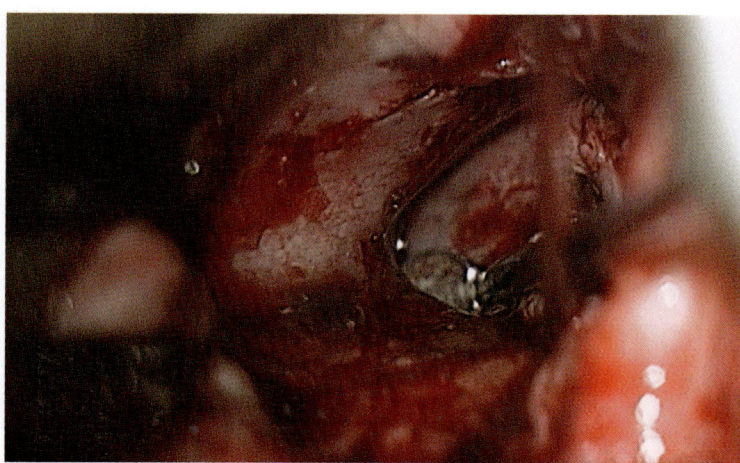

Fig. 17.4 Anterior and inferior meatal wall skin is elevated.

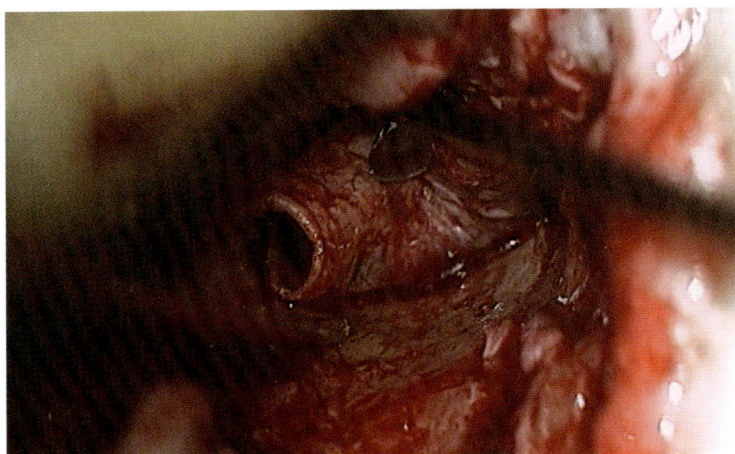

Fig. 17.5 Posterior meatal wall skin is elevated.

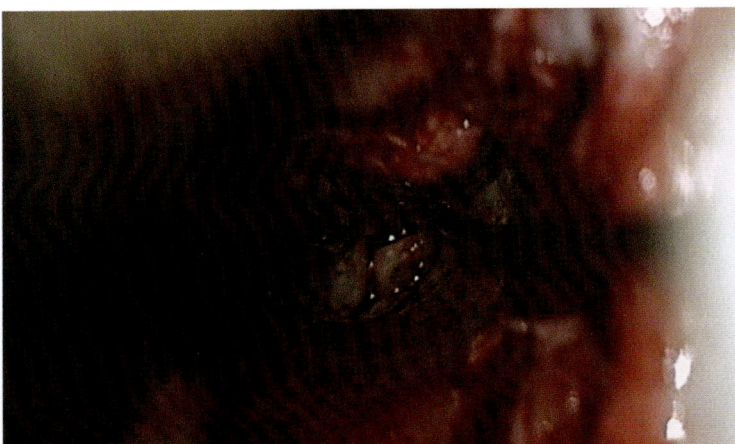

Fig. 17.6 Posterior tympanomeatal flap is elevated and the middle ear is entered. The incudostapedial joint is seen. The incus is covered by the edematous mucosa.

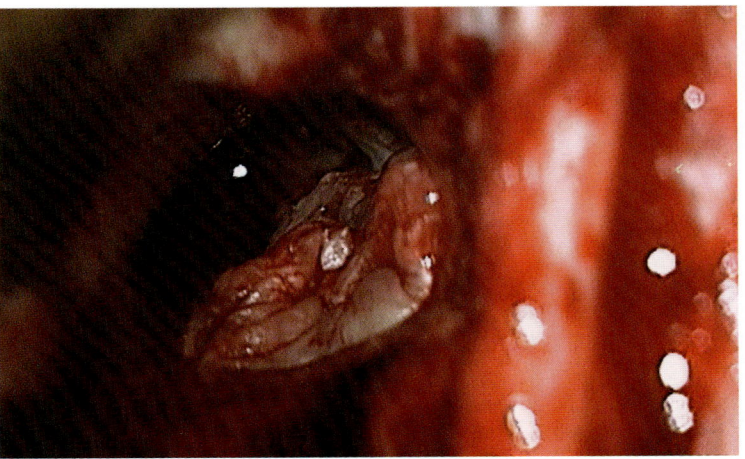

Fig. 17.7 Tympanomeatal flap is elevated anteriorly and inferiorly. The annulus is separated from the sulcus and the middle ear is entered.

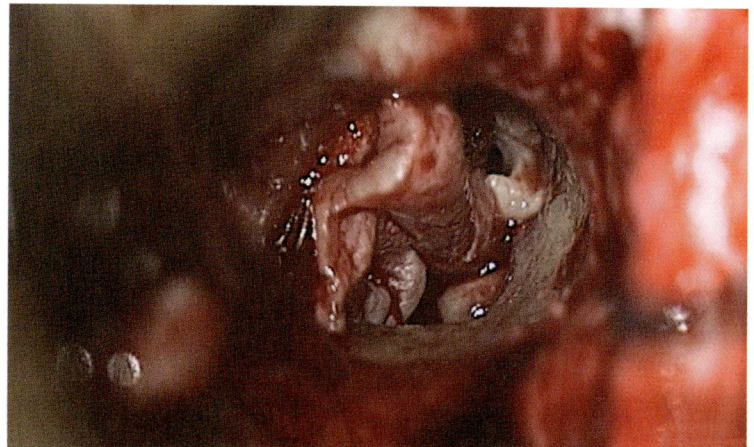

Fig. 17.8 Tympanomeatal flap is elevated superiorly. The lateral process of the malleus is seen.

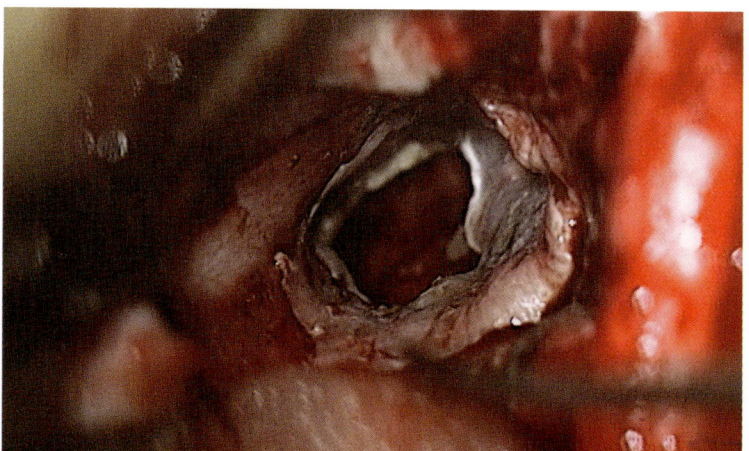

Fig. 17.9 Complete margins of perforation is cauterized by 50% trichloroacetic acid (TCA).

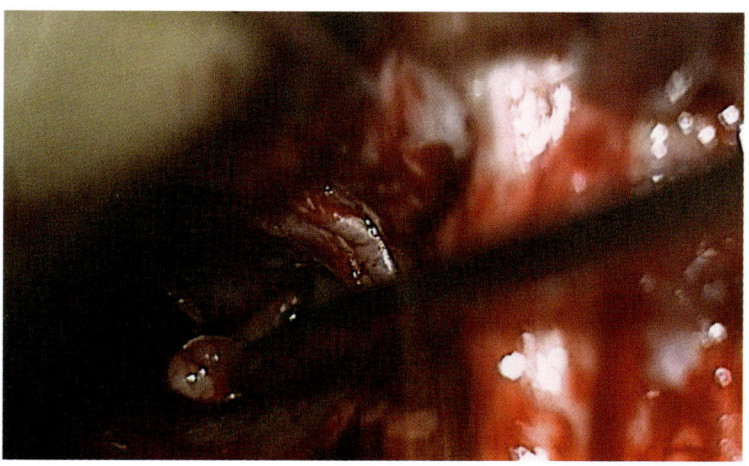

Fig. 17.10 Middle ear granulations were removed for histopathological examination.

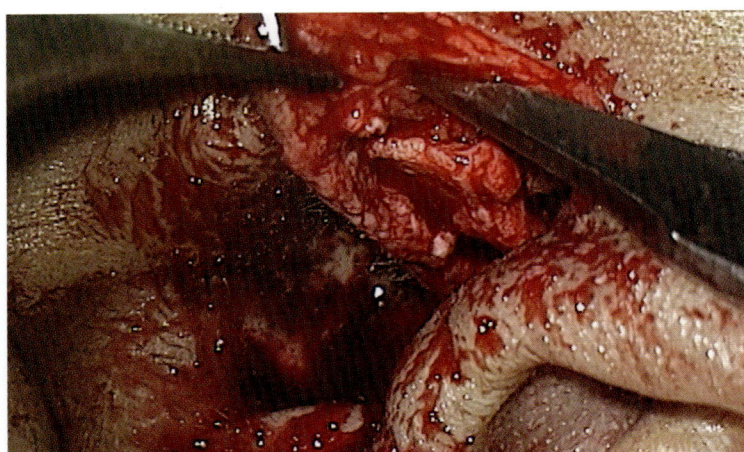

Fig. 17.11 Tragal cartilage is removed.

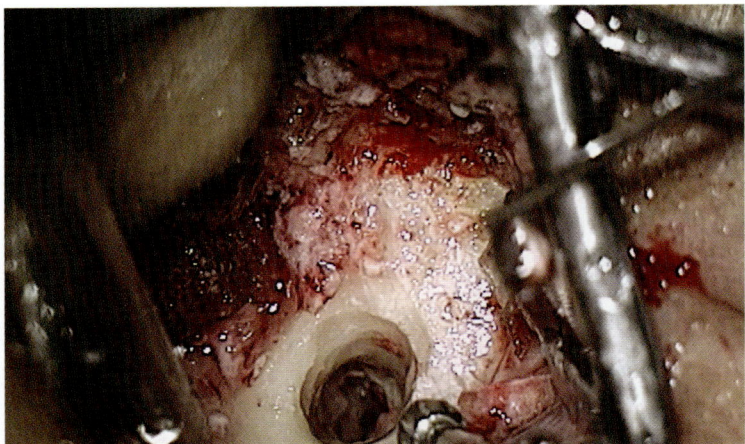

Fig. 17.12 The mastoid is opened. The mastoid is full of edematous mucosa and granulations.

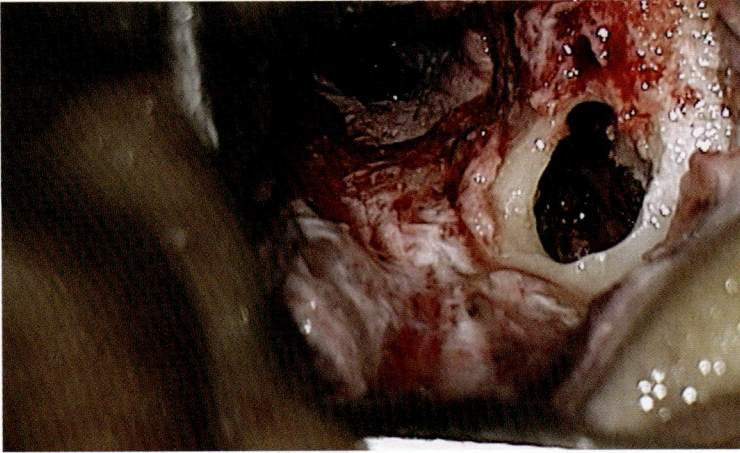

Fig. 17.13 Simple mastoidectomy is done. The mastoid is full of edematous mucosa and granulations. Granulations are removed and have been sent for histopathological examination.

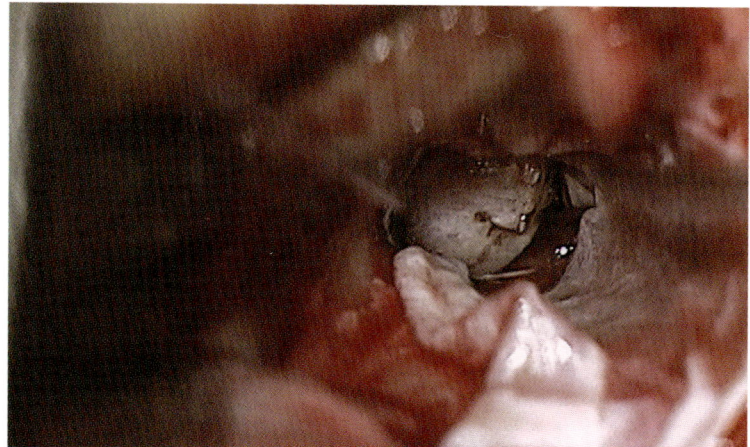

Fig. 17.14   An underlay graft is placed medial to the handle of the malleus.

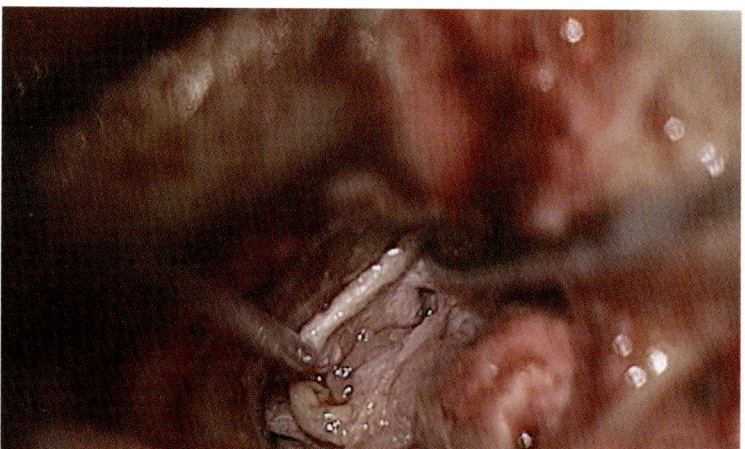

Fig. 17.15   Graft is pulled anteriorly under the anterior tympanomeatal flap.

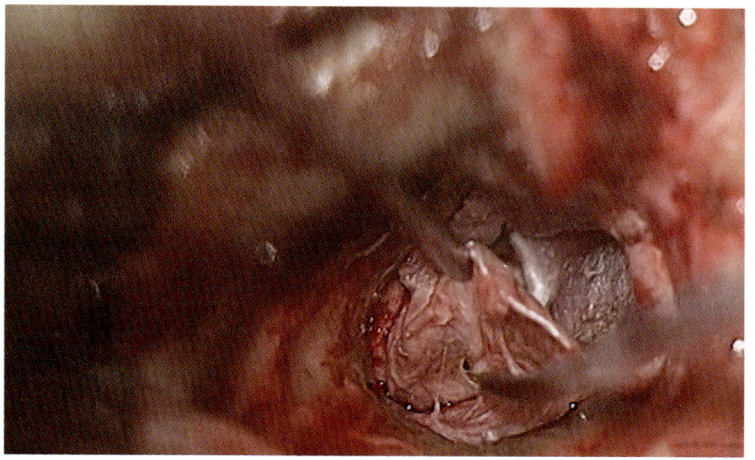

Fig. 17.16   Graft is supported inferiorly by the inferior bony meatal wall.

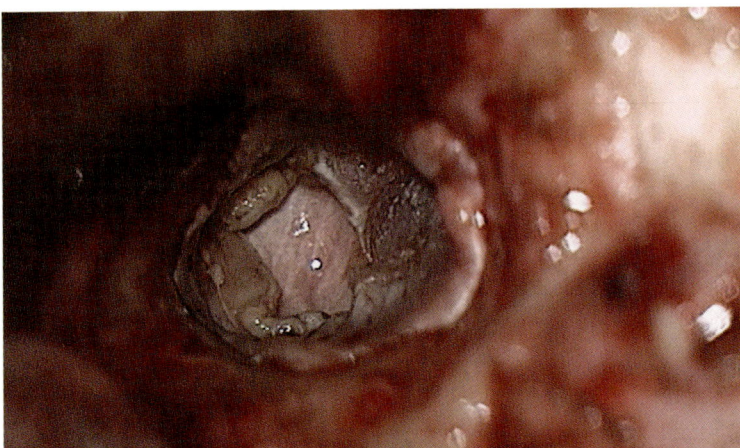

Fig. 17.17 Complete tympanomeatal flap is reposited back.

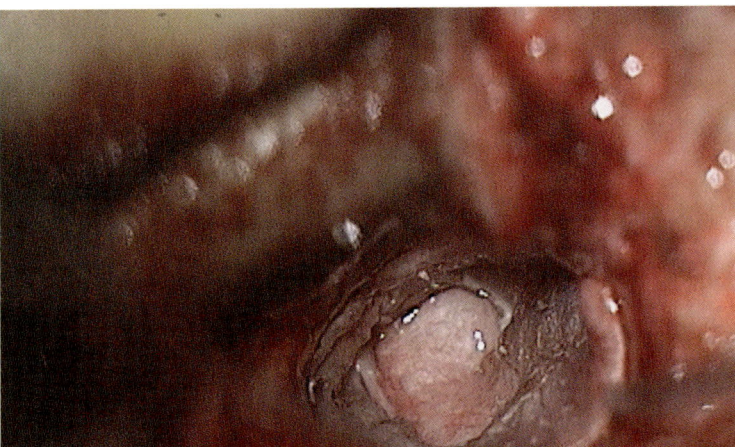

Fig. 17.18 Graft is well supported on all the sides on the meatal wall with final position of the tympanomeatal flap.

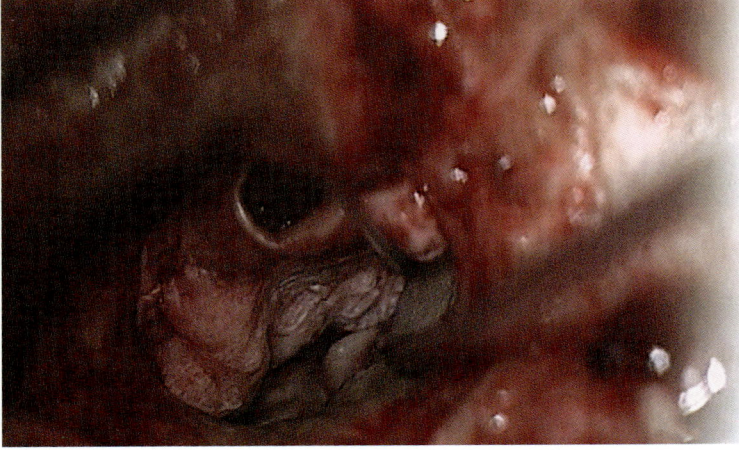

Fig. 17.19 Posterior tympanomeatal flap with the graft is elevated again for placement of the cartilage in the middle ear. Cartilage is placed under the fascia graft to support it and to prevent its contact with the edematous middle ear mucosa, to prevent future adhesions.

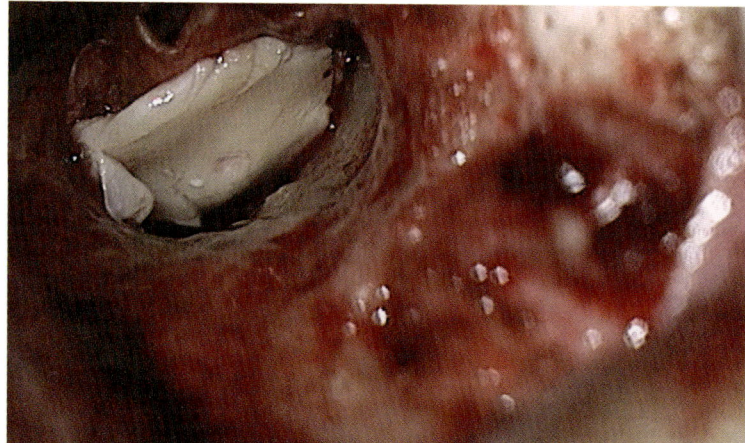

Fig. 17.20 Tragal cartilage with perichondrium on one side (lateral side) is placed in the middle ear medial to the fascia and the handle of the malleus supporting the temporalis fascia graft preventing its contact with the edematous middle ear mucosa.

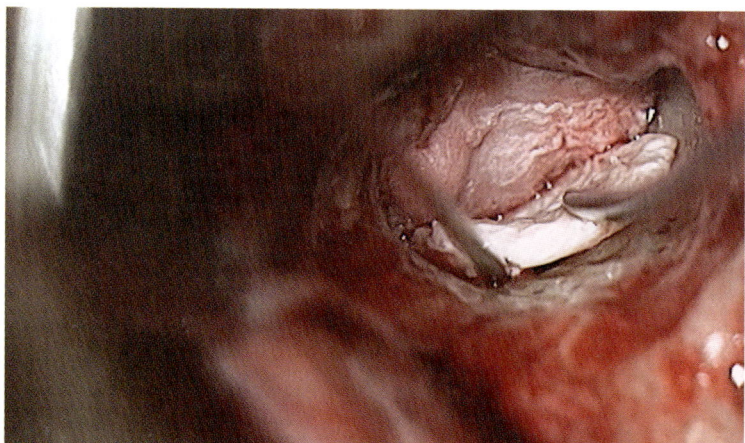

Fig. 17.21 Tragal cartilage with perichondrium on one side (lateral side) is placed in the middle ear, medial to the fascia and the handle of the malleus supporting the temporalis fascia graft, preventing its contact with the edematous middle ear mucosa.

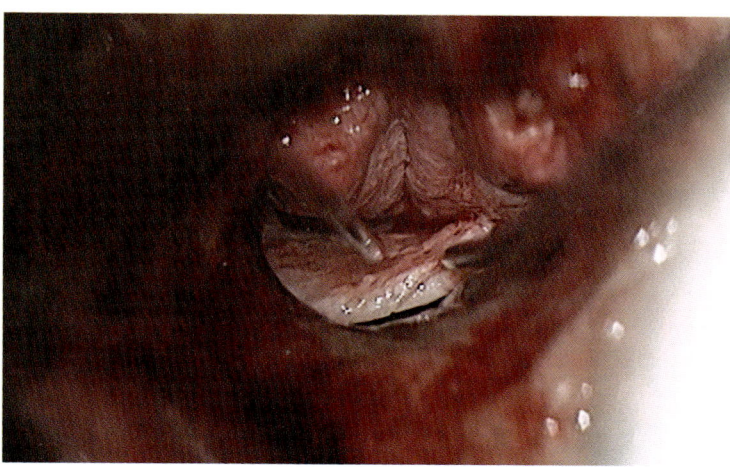

Fig. 17.22 Cartilage is resting on the groove made on the inferior bony meatal wall at the level of the sulcus.

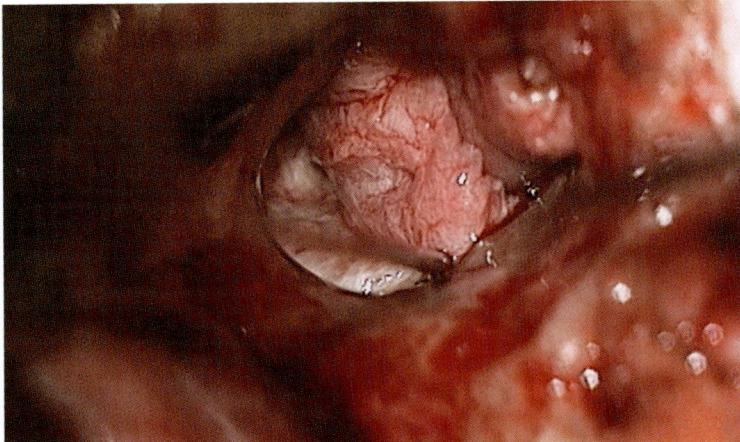

Fig. 17.23 Cartilage is resting on the groove made on the inferior and anterior bony meatal wall, supporting the fascia graft, maintaining middle ear space, preventing contact of the fascia with the edematous promontory mucosa to prevent future adhesions.

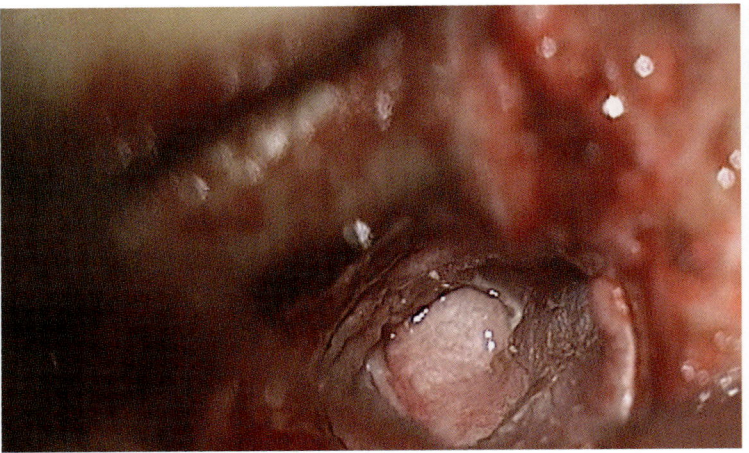

Fig. 17.24 Tympanomeatal flap is reposited back. Gelfoam is placed in the external auditory canal and the incision is closed.

18 Cartilage Tympanoplasty

The most commonly used graft material is the temporalis fascia and perichondrium. Cartilage is another graft material most commonly used for revision surgery and in cases of atelectatic drum.

Cartilage tympanoplasty is very much useful in patients with compromised eustachian tube function, to avoid postoperative retraction of the graft or tympanic membrane (**Figs. 18.1–18.12**).

Cartilage is more successfully used in patients with large perforations as the cartilage is more stable and stronger than the temporalis fascia and success rate is very high, as compared to the fascia and the perichondrium.

The most common source of cartilage is the tragus or concha. It is advisable to use cartilage with the perichondrium. A piece of 1 cm × 1 cm cartilage is removed. The perichondrium from one side is separated and preserved. The cartilage is trimmed to required size. A very small strip of cartilage is removed radially from one side of the cartilage to accommodate the handle of the malleus. The posterior part of the cartilage can also be trimmed to make space for the incus.

This cartilage is placed medial to the temporalis fascia resting over the bony meatus.

The hearing results in tympanoplasty with cartilage are at par with the temporalis fascia or the perichondrium. Initially, immediate postoperatively, hearing results with the fascia are better than cartilage, but later on, after few months to 1 year, hearing results are similar with cartilage and fascia.

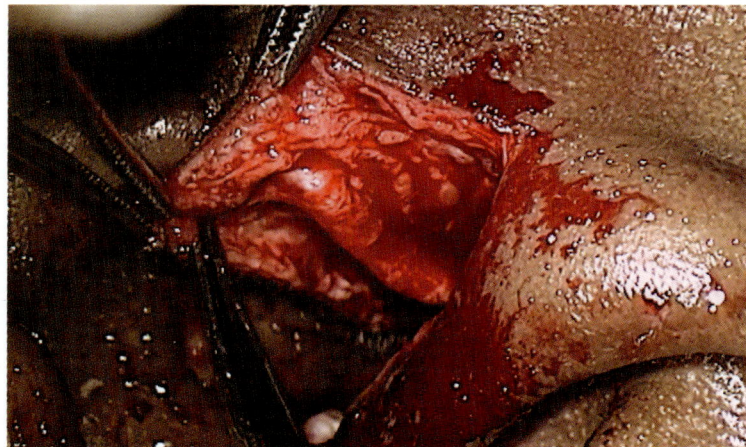

Fig. 18.1 Endaural incision is made. Cartilage is removed from the tragus. When an endaural incision is made, cartilage can be removed from the same incision. No separate incision is required.

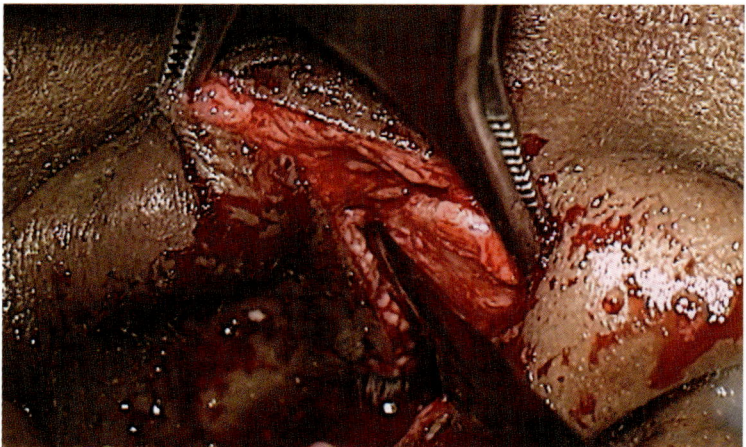

Fig. 18.2 Tragal cartilage is dissected by scissors.

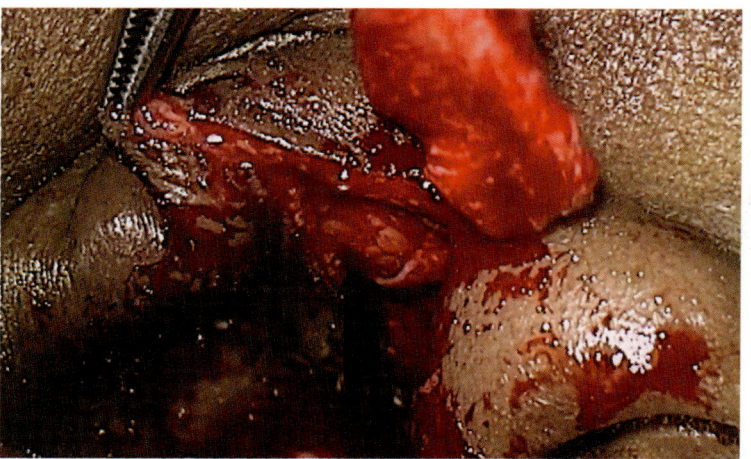

Fig. 18.3 Tragal cartilage piece is removed.

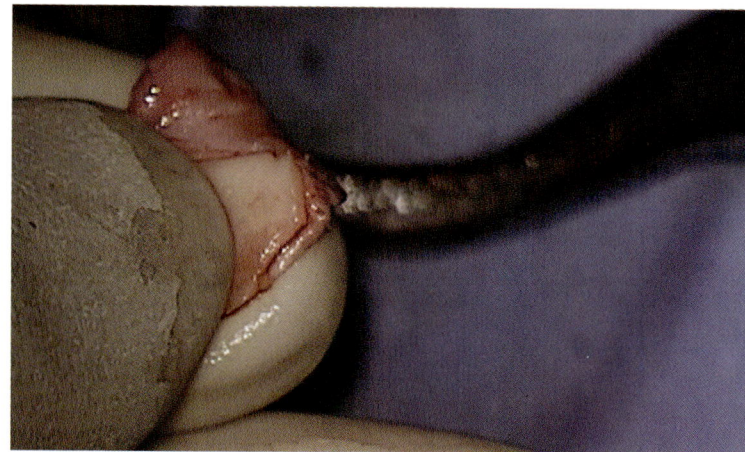

Fig. 18.4 The perichondrium from one side of the cartilage is elevated and excised. It is preserved as free graft.

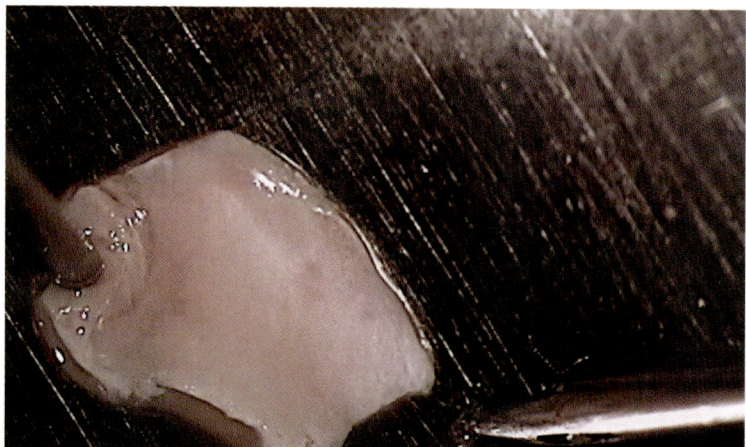

Fig. 18.5 Free perichondrium is removed from the tragal cartilage.

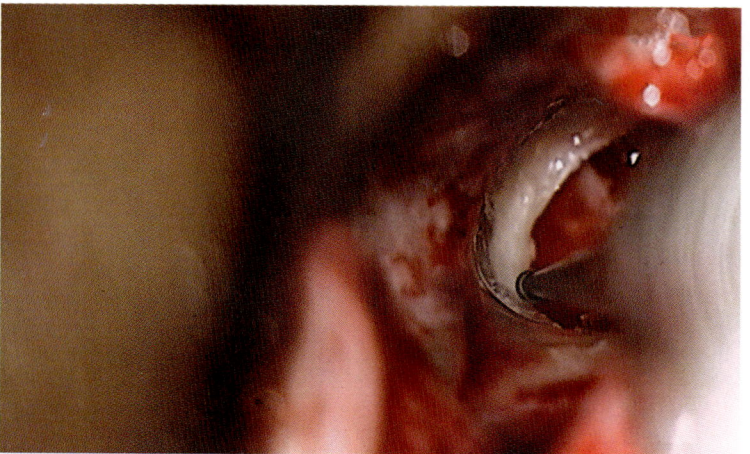

Fig. 18.6 A groove is made at the inferior part of the external auditory canal near the sulcus by a 1.00-mm burr.

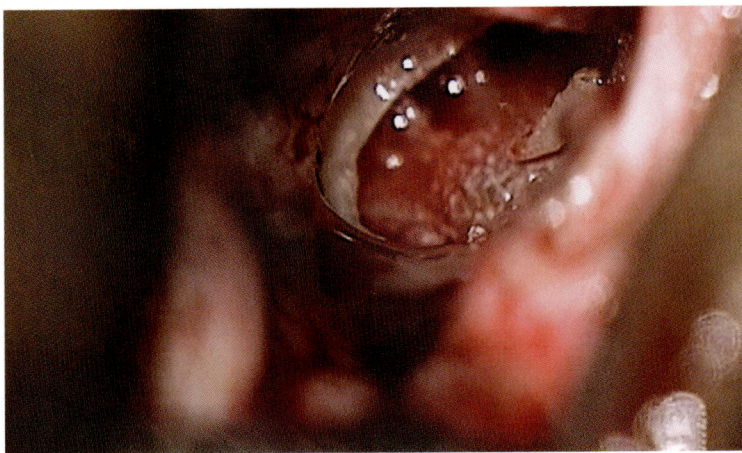

Fig. 18.7 A groove is made at the inferior part of the external auditory canal near the sulcus to accommodate the cartilage.

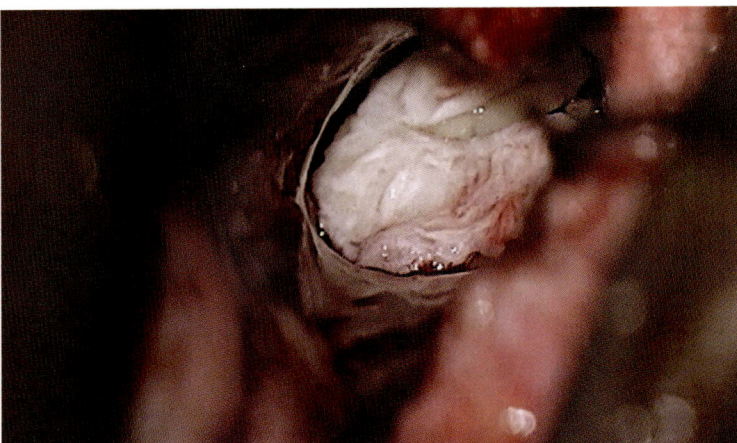

Fig. 18.8 Cartilage of required size is prepared. A radial cut is made in the cartilage to accommodate the handle of the malleus.

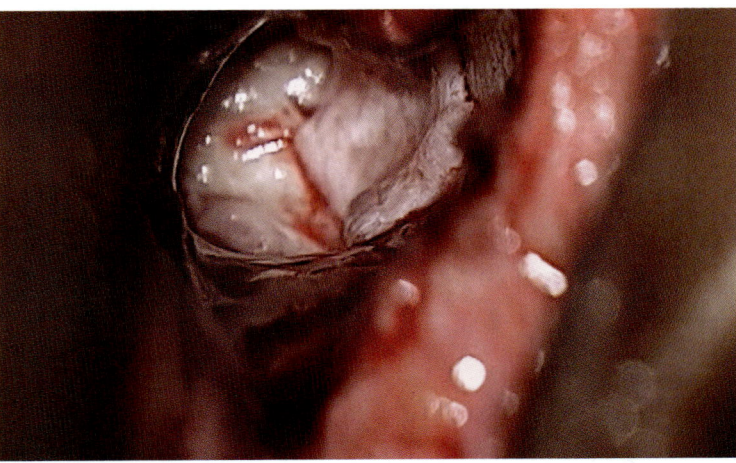

Fig. 18.9 Upper part of the cartilage with radial cut for the handle of the malleus and the adjacent meatal wall is covered by the perichondrium.

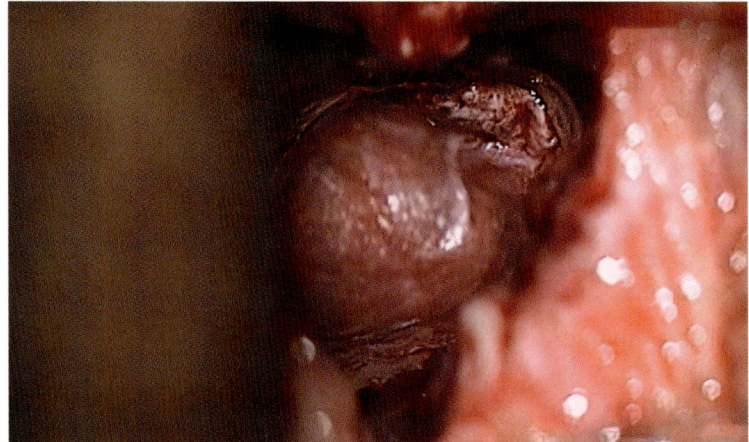

Fig. 18.10 Cartilage is covered by the temporalis fascia graft.

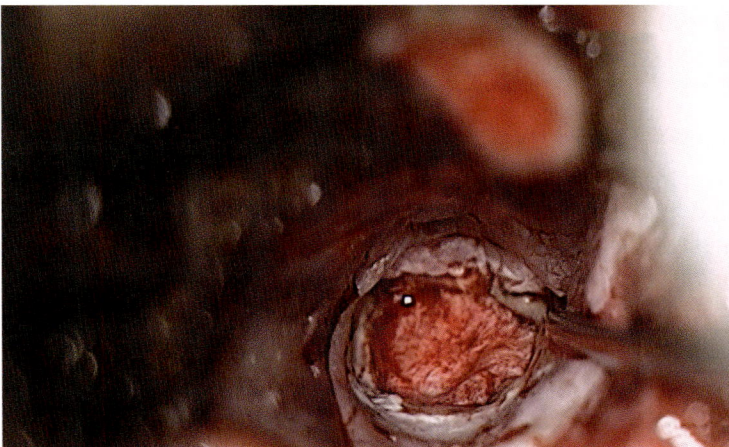

Fig. 18.11 Fascia graft and adjacent meatal wall is covered by free tympanomeatal skin flap, which was elevated and taken out earlier and preserved as free graft.

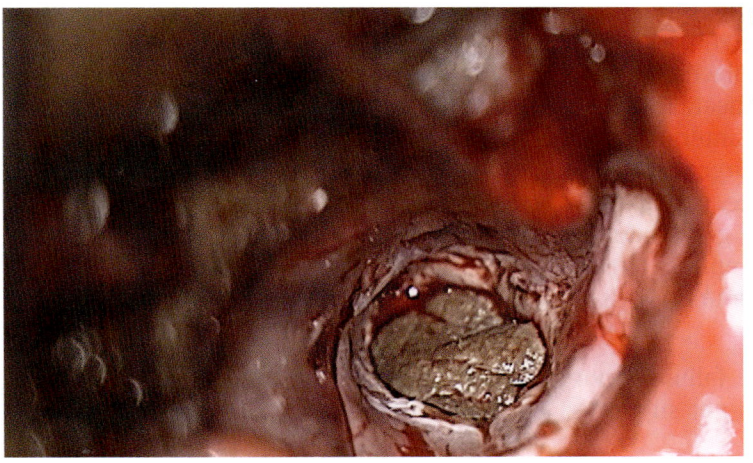

Fig. 18.12 Graft is covered by partial-thickness postaural skin piece. Gelfoam is packed and the incision is closed.

19 Tympanoplasty Failure

Tympanoplasty is considered to be successful under the following conditions:

- When the perforation in the tympanic membrane has closed after surgery and the eardrum has healed up and well epithelialized.

- The angle between the tympanic membrane and anteroinferior bony meatal wall is less than 90 degrees and is well epithelialized without blunting.

- The hearing is normal or near normal.

- As the perforation has closed and the eardrum has healed up, water precautions are not necessary and the patient can swim or take part in various water sports without any problem.

Usually, there is more than 90% success rate in tympanoplasty if the surgery is properly performed and the graft is well supported on the bony meatal wall, especially on the anterior bony meatal wall.

Proper reposition of the tympanomeatal flap and proper Gelfoam placement after repositing the tympanomeatal flap is important to maintain the anterior meatal wall angle. When the surgery is done by the underlay technique, there is no chance of lateralization of graft, blunting of the anterior sulcus, and epithelial pearl formation, which is more common with the overlay technique.

In the underlay technique, failure is more common when the graft is not supported anteriorly by the anterior bony meatal wall so that the graft falls away from the anterior margins of the perforation due to inadequate overlapping of the graft and the eardrum margin especially in patients with subtotal perforation. This failure requires a revision.

Causes of Tympanoplasty Failure

There are various causes of graft failure:

- Postoperative infection is one of the commonest causes of graft failure.

- Lack of support to the graft by the bony meatal wall on all the sides is associated with falling of graft medially in the middle ear and failure.

- Inadequate overlapping of the graft with the tympanic membrane remnant is always associated with graft failure.

- In the pre-antibiotic era, mastoid infections, which were not treated by simple mastoidectomy, were associated with residual perforation or recurrence of perforation especially in patients with mastoid reservoir. These problem are not there in the present scenario due to availability of various broad-spectrum antibiotics

- In addition to this, there are various systemic disorders that are associated with poor surgery results. These are diabetes, cardiac disease, anemia, obesity, smoking, alcohol consumption, and poor nutrition. All these conditions are associated with decreased tissue oxygenation associated with graft failure.

Blunting of the anterior sulcus occurs mainly in the overlay technique resulting in conductive hearing loss. This usually happens when the graft is not covered by the epithelium at the anteroinferior angle. This may require a revision surgery. Revision surgery in these cases should be performed by the underlay technique after excising the thick scar tissue.

Lateralized Tympanic Membrane

Lateralized tympanic membrane is a problem that is common with the overlay technique. The graft moves laterally away from the handle of the malleus. This is associated with conductive hearing loss of severe degree and requires revision surgery.

When the graft is placed lateral to the handle of the malleus, sometimes it falls away from the malleus due to the following:

- Pull from the lateral side, due to healing with fibrosis pulling the graft laterally.

- Lateral push from the medial side could be due to transmitted air pressure from the eustachian tube due to vigorous blowing of nose, pushing the graft laterally away from the handle of the malleus.

The best is to prevent this problem is by performing tympanoplasty by the underlay technique, by placing the graft medial to the handle of the malleus and the tympanic membrane. Thus, there is no chance of graft getting lateralized.

20 Revision Tympanoplasty

Unlike stapedectomy, results of revision tympanoplasty are good. When required, it should be done with all possible precautions. Revision surgery is very much indicated with residual perforations due to failed previous surgery, in patients with lateralized tympanic membrane and blunting of the anterior sulcus with conductive deafness.

There are few challenges with revision surgery. The graft material, especially temporalis fascia graft, is used by the previous surgeon. Hence, adequate fascia graft may not be available during revision surgery. After fascial graft, tragal perichondrium is the next most suitable graft material available for tympanoplasty and it is easily available. Cartilage tympanoplasty also plays a very important role in getting better results in revision cases with equally good closure of the air–bone gap.

Before revising these cases, thorough ear examination including audiogram should be done to assess the condition of the middle ear and the extent of damage done, and patients should be counseled properly. The patient should be told before surgery regarding the possibility of hearing improvement after revision surgery as complete restoration of hearing may not be possible with revision surgery in spite of doing a good job.

The revision surgery is a little difficult compared to the first surgery due to scarring, and there is more bleeding during revision surgery compared to the first surgery. Hence, these surgeries should be done by an experienced surgeon.

Revision tympanoplasty for the lateralized tympanic membrane with severe conductive hearing loss is depicted in **Figs. 20.1–20.33**.

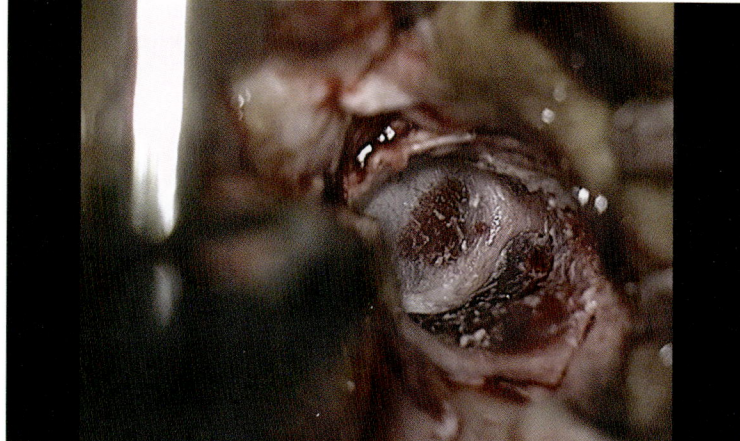

Fig. 20.1   Lateralized tympanic membrane. Revision surgery is done by endaural incision.

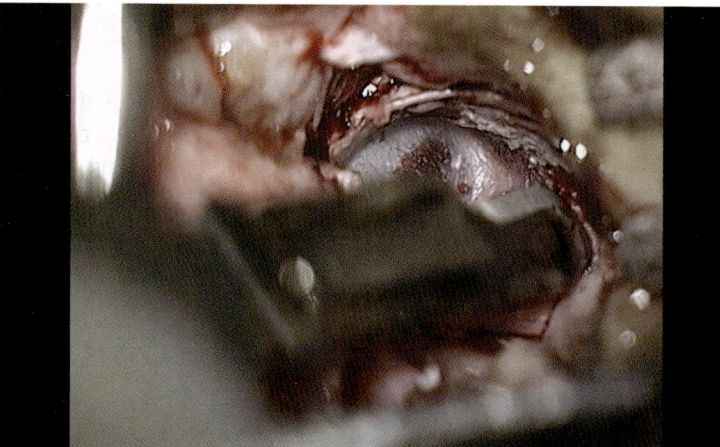

Fig. 20.2   Circumferential meatal wall skin incision is made by a no. 15 blade.

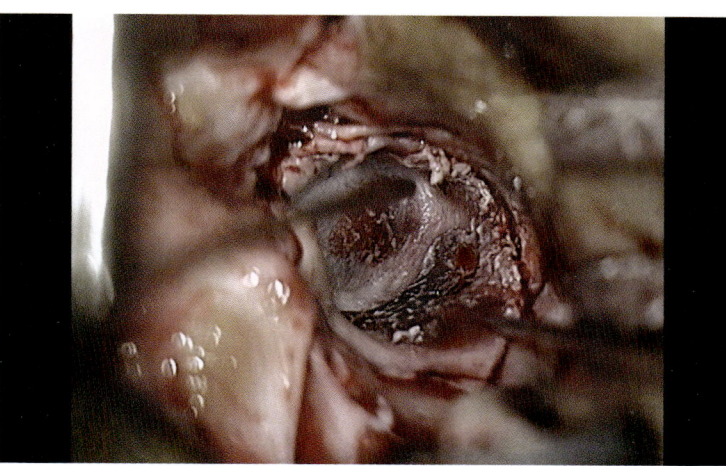

Fig. 20.3   Circumferential meatal wall skin incision is completed.

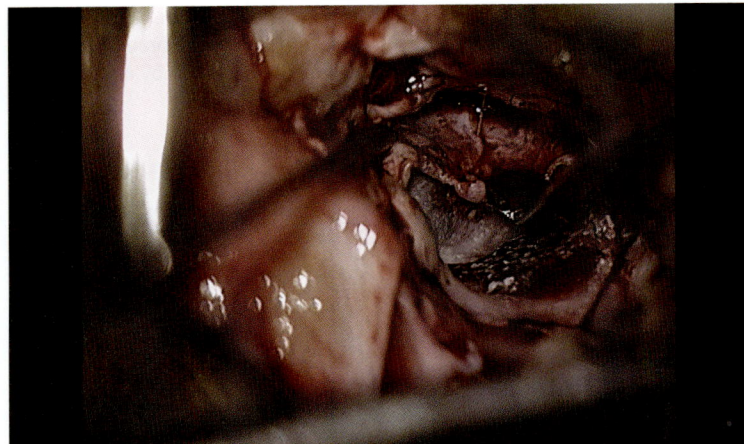

Fig. 20.4 Anterior meatal wall skin is elevated.

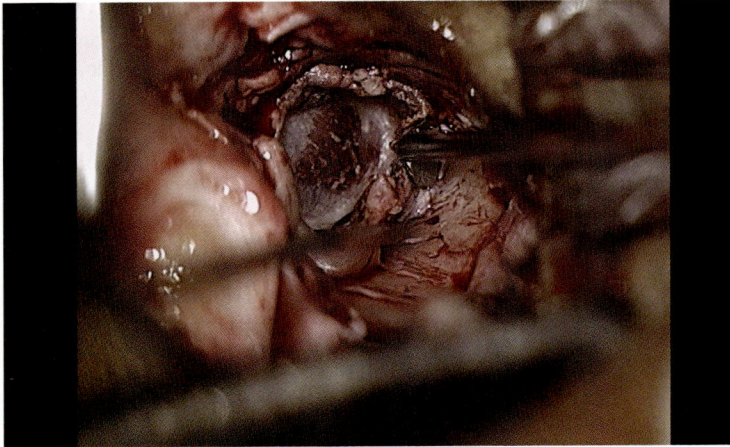

Fig. 20.5 Anteroinferior meatal wall skin is elevated.

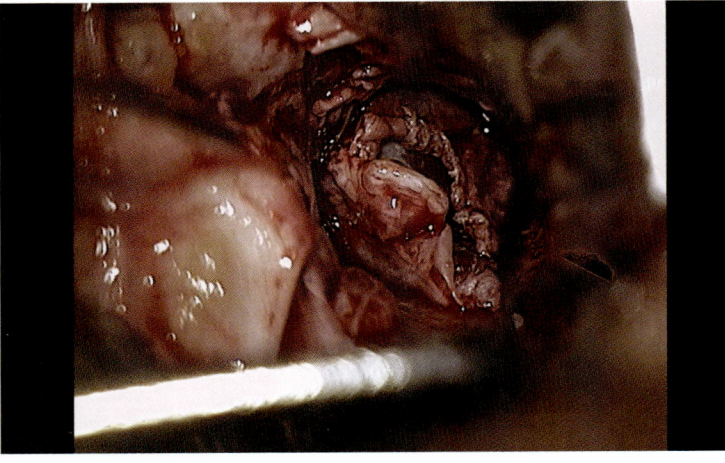

Fig. 20.6 Posterior meatal wall skin is elevated.

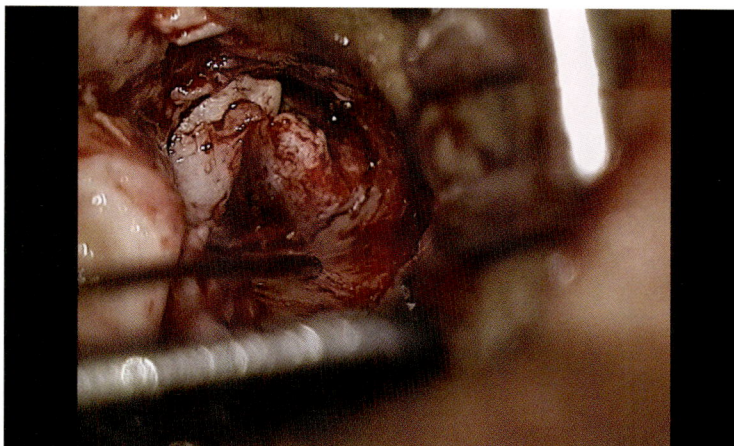

Fig. 20.7 Circumferential meatal wall skin elevation is continued till the annulus.

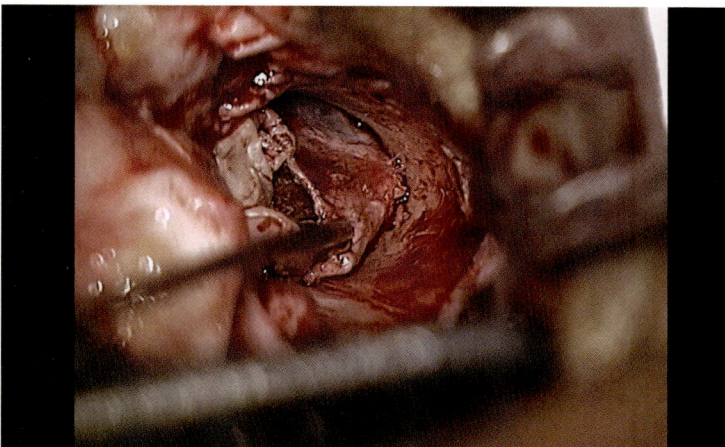

Fig. 20.8 Anterior meatal wall skin is elevated till annulus.

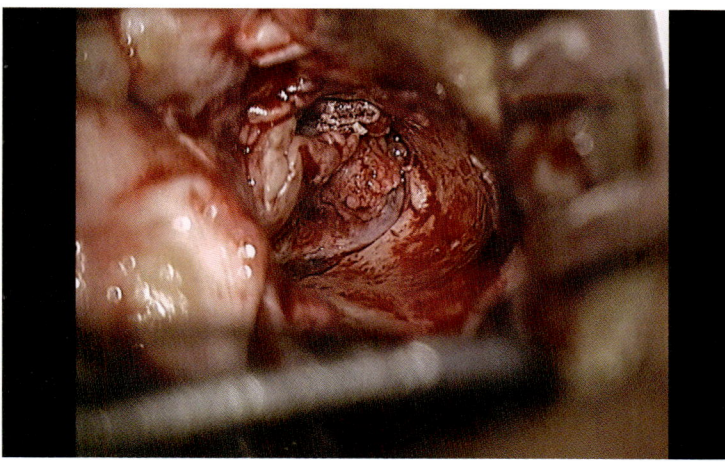

Fig. 20.9 Inferior meatal wall skin is elevated till annulus.

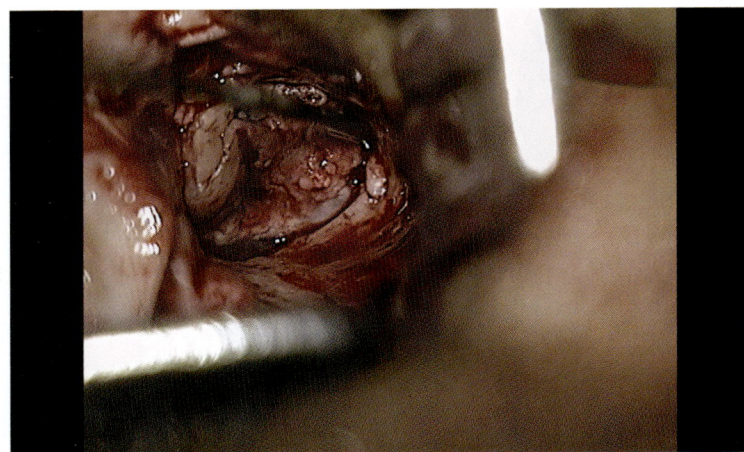

Fig. 20.10 Posterior meatal wall skin is elevated till the annulus.

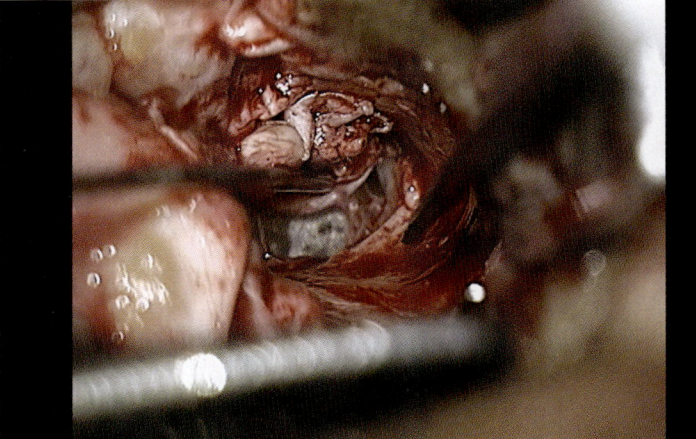

Fig. 20.11 The annulus is lifted from the sulcus and the middle ear is entered. Silastic is seen in the middle ear covering the promontory (kept by the previous surgeon).

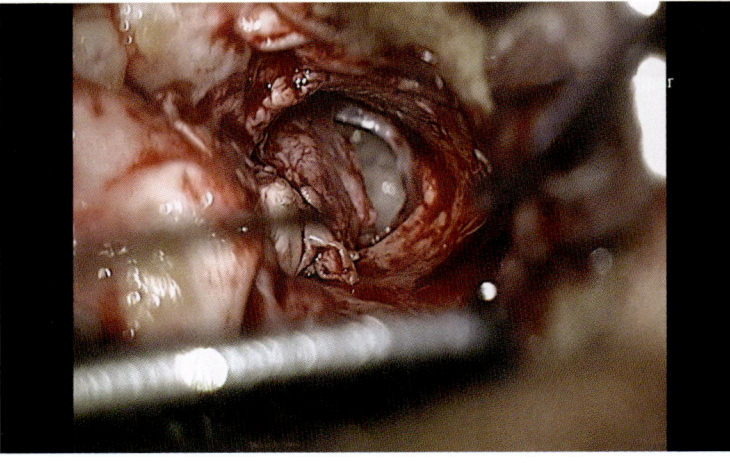

Fig. 20.12 The annulus is lifted anteriorly from the sulcus.

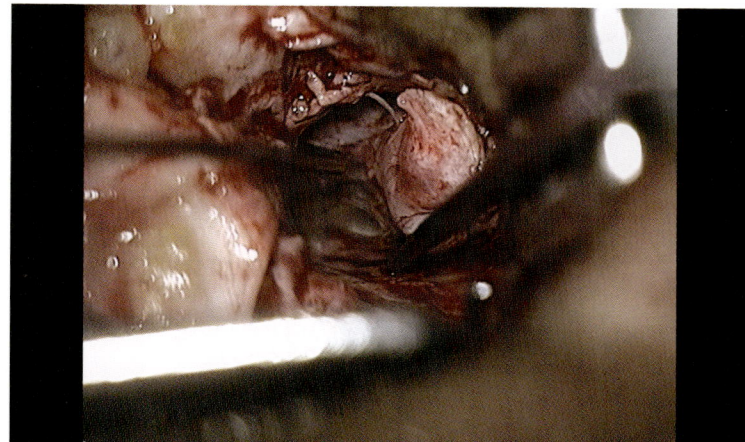

Fig. 20.13 Circumferential complete tympanomeatal flap has been elevated along with the annulus.

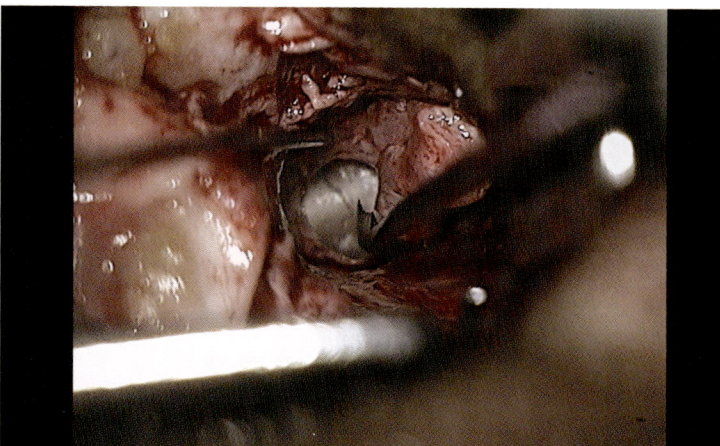

Fig. 20.14 Complete tympanomeatal flap with the tympanic membrane is elevated as one piece.

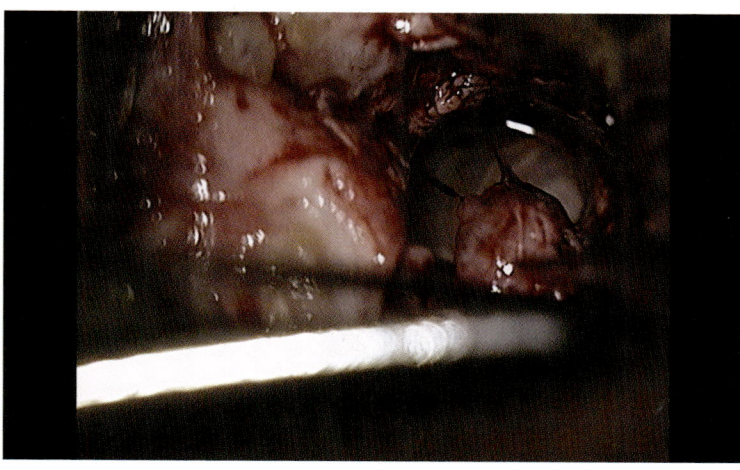

Fig. 20.15 Complete tympanomeatal flap with intact tympanic membrane has been taken out as a free graft.

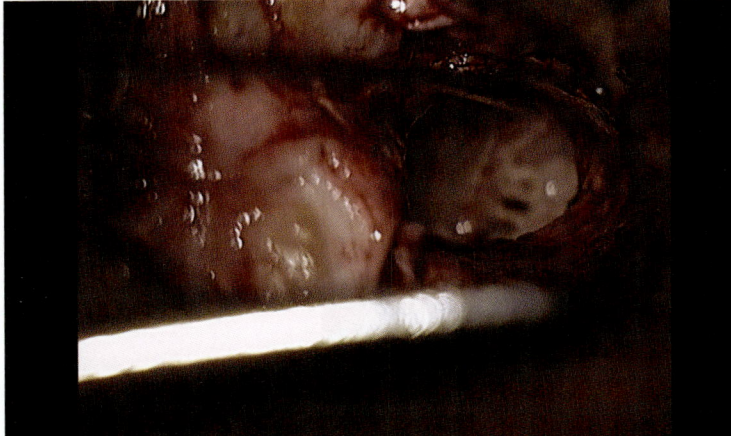

Fig. 20.16 A silastic sheet (kept by the previous surgeon) is found to be covering the tympanic cavity but superiorly lying lateral to the handle of the malleus and is responsible for lateralization of the tympanic membrane (graft) away from the handle of the malleus. (This was the main cause for lateralization of the tympanic membrane in this patient.)

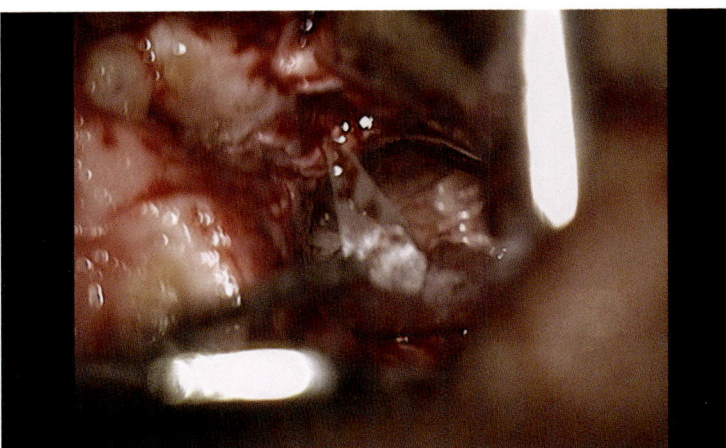

Fig. 20.17 Silastic sheet from the tympanic cavity is removed.

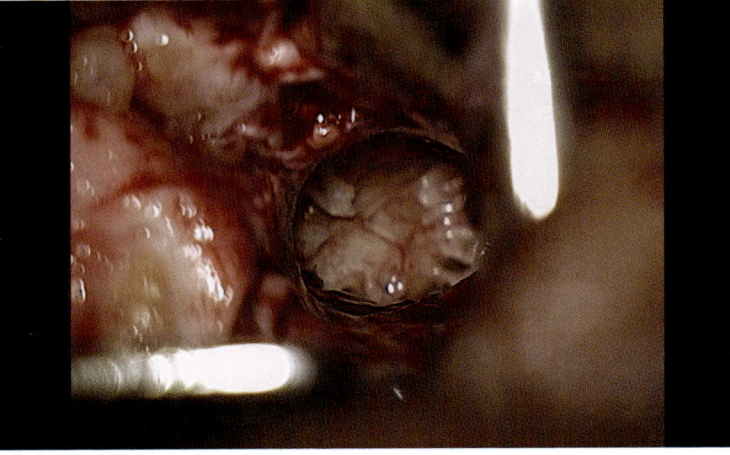

Fig. 20.18 The tympanic cavity with the handle of the malleus (tip destroyed) and the incudostapedial joint is seen.

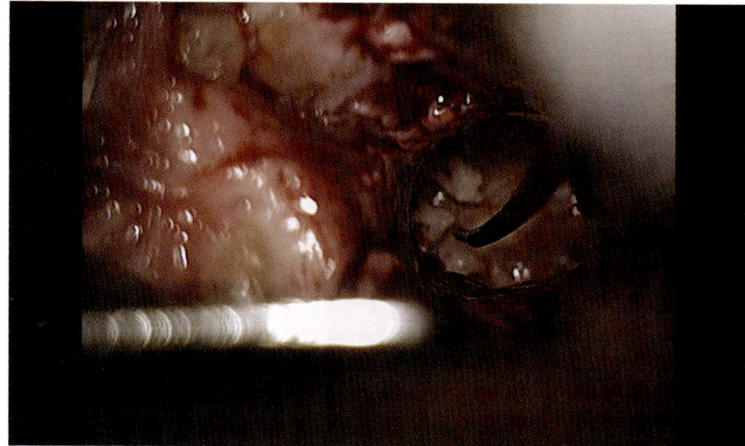

Fig. 20.19 The mobility of the stapes is checked.

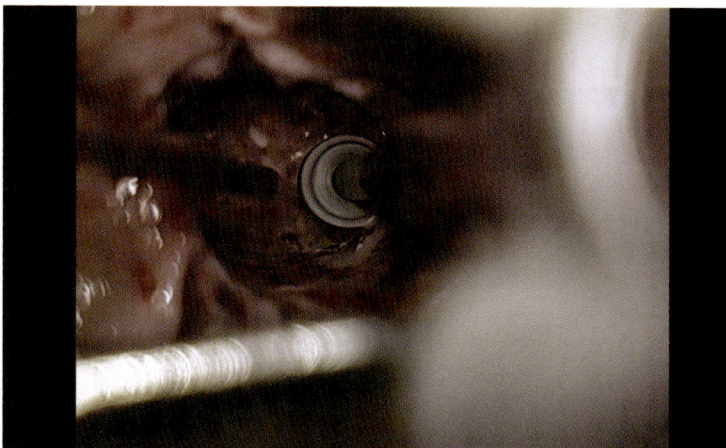

Fig. 20.20 Inferior: canalplasty is done.

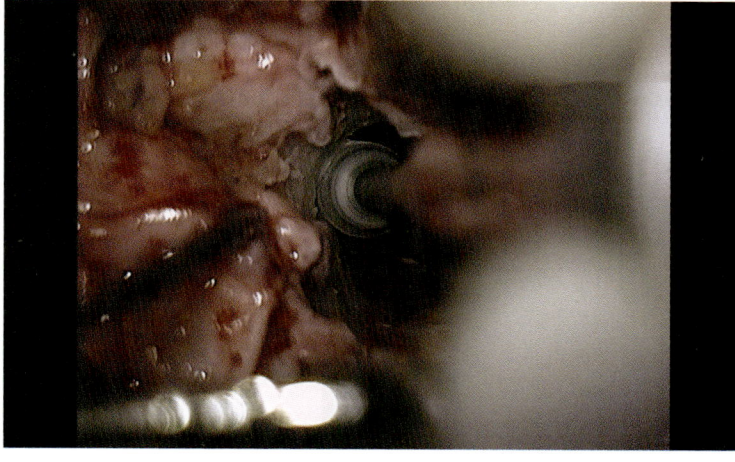

Fig. 20.21 Superior: canalplasty is done.

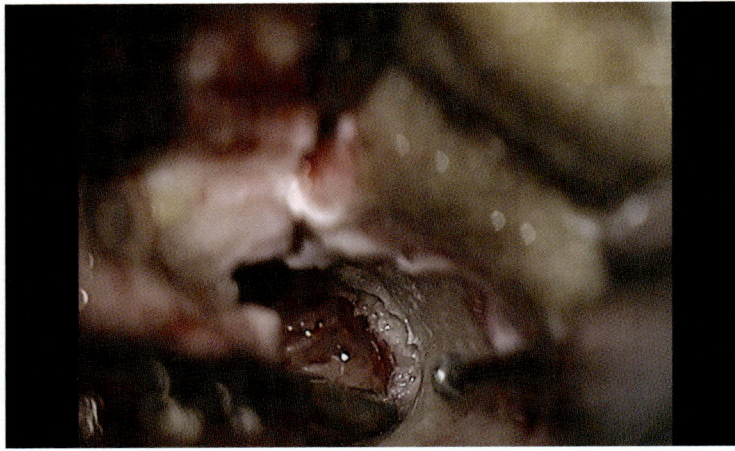

Fig. 20.22 A circumferential groove is made at the level of the inferior sulcus for placement of the cartilage.

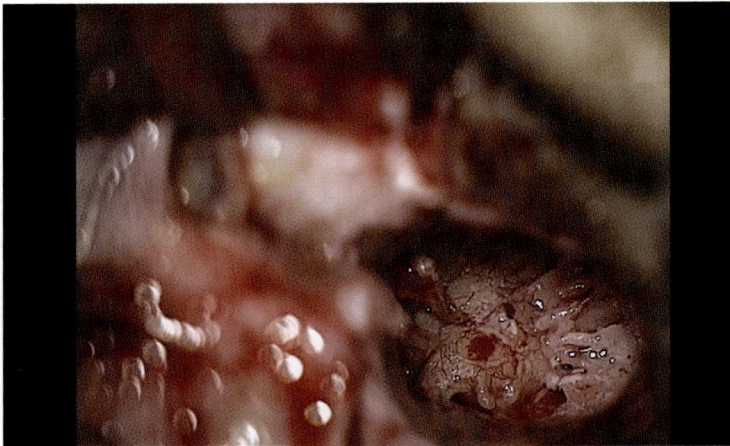

Fig. 20.23 Healthy tympanic cavity is seen nicely after canalplasty.

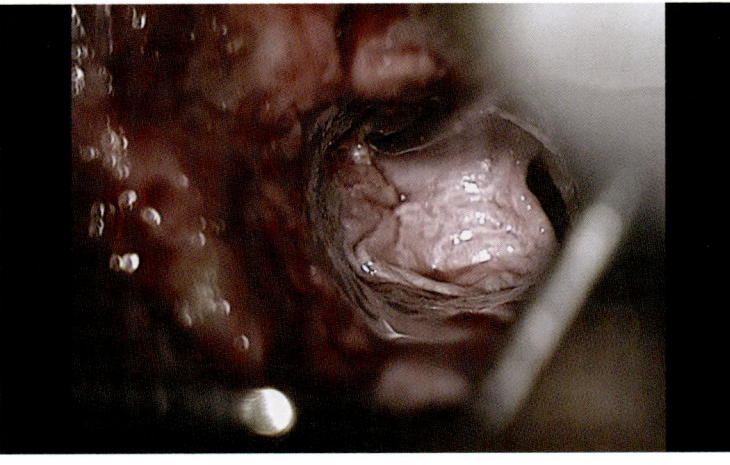

Fig. 20.24 The temporalis fascia underlay graft is placed medial to the handle of the malleus, resting over the bony meatal wall all around.

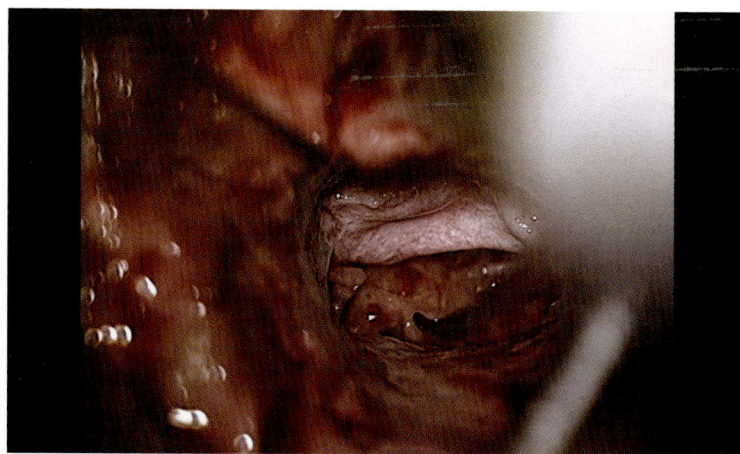

Fig. 20.25 The graft is folded forward and the tympanic cavity is exposed again.

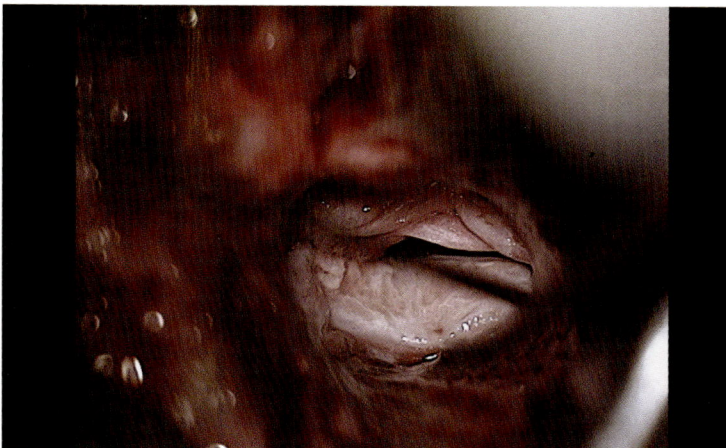

Fig. 20.26 Cartilage with perichondrium is placed horizontally in the middle ear resting inferiorly on the groove made at the level of the inferior sulcus and superiorly resting on the superior canal wall lateral to the incus. Posteriorly its perichondrium is lying on the posterior canal wall.

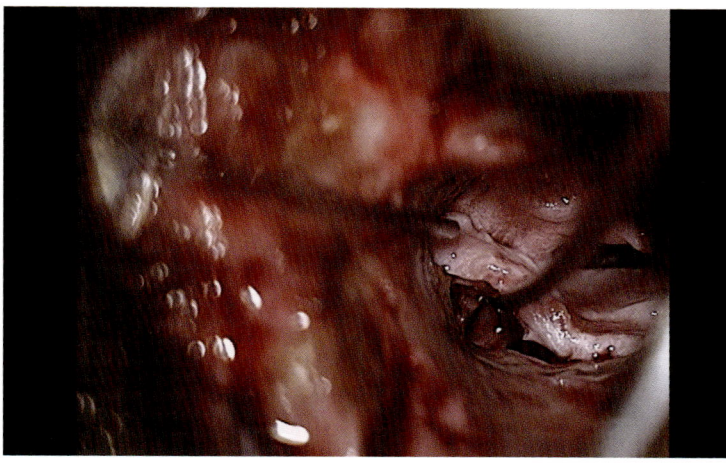

Fig. 20.27 Cartilage is lifted up gently to check the middle ear. It is lying lateral to the incus, maintaining middle ear space, not exerting any pressure over the incus. A small cut is made in the superior part of the cartilage to accommodate the handle of the malleus.

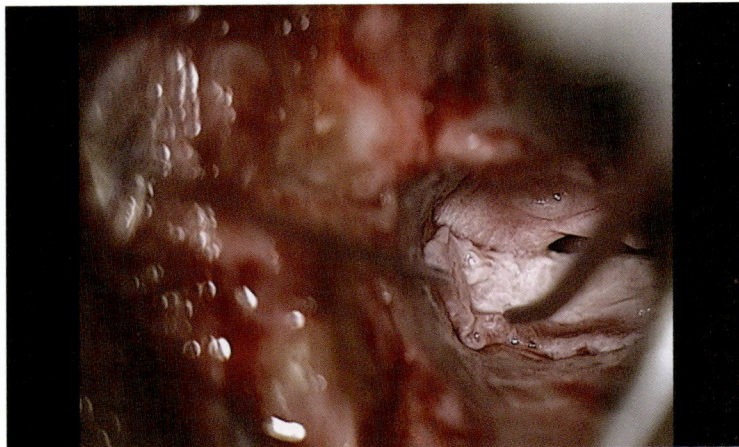

Fig. 20.28 Cartilage is stabilized by the perichondrium on the posterior and superior meatal wall.

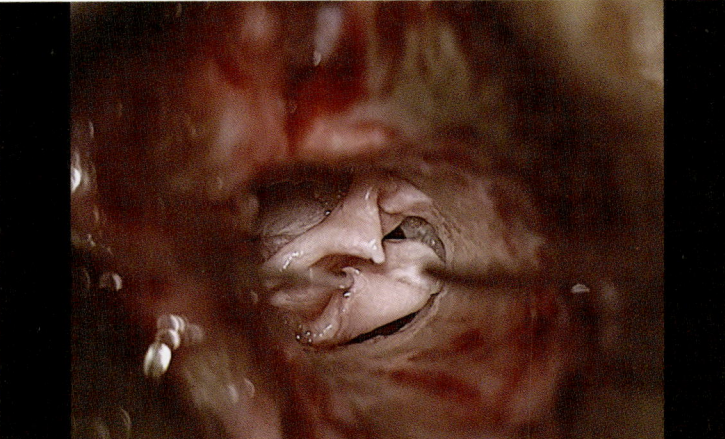

Fig. 20.29 Cartilage with the perichondrium is resting in the groove made at the level of the inferior sulcus.

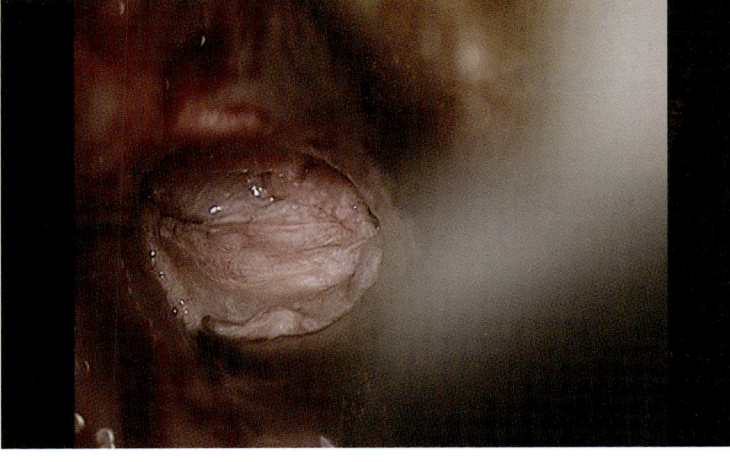

Fig. 20.30 The graft is reposited back. The graft is resting on the bony canal wall on all the sides and on cartilage and remains in contact with the cartilage, which will hold the graft, preventing its lateralization.

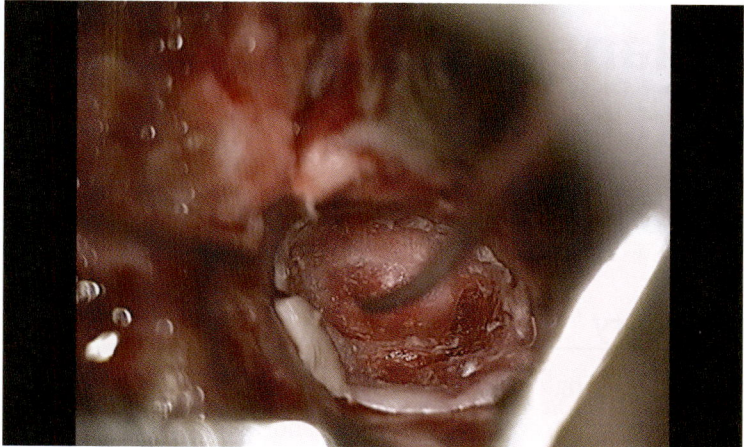

Fig. 20.31   The free tympanomeatal flap, which was taken out earlier, is reposited back lying on the graft and the canal wall.

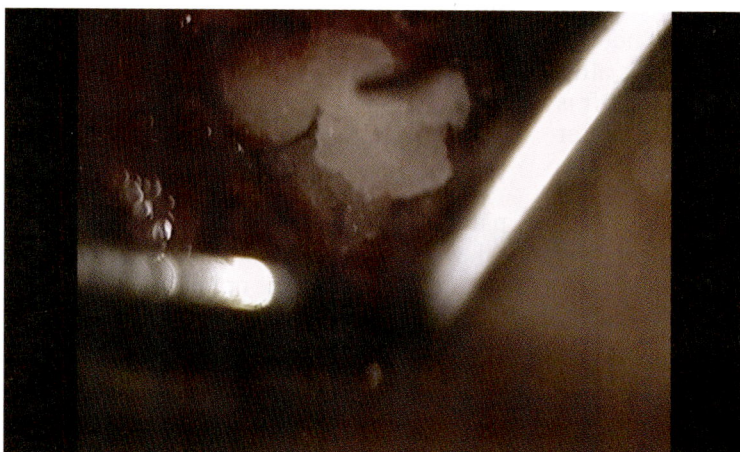

Fig. 20.32   Gelfoam is packed in the exterior auditory canal.

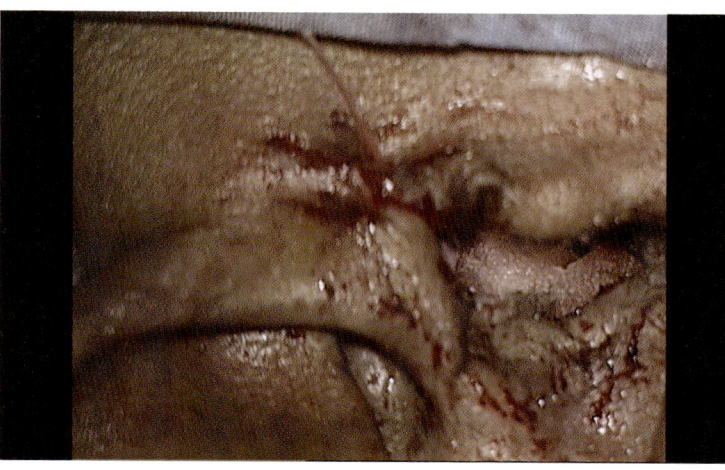

Fig. 20.33   Incision is closed by a single stitch.

21 Miscellaneous Situations Related to Tympanoplasty

Air Travel Following Surgery

Pressure changes, which take place during air travel, may displace the graft, especially when the eustachian tube is blocked and when the patient is suffering from upper respiratory infection (URI).

Hence, these patients should not be allowed air travel for at least 3 weeks after surgery. By these 3 weeks' time, the graft is nicely vascularized and taken up well. After this, the graft will not get displaced with the pressure changes that takes place during air travel. The nose and eustachian tube should be clear and open while traveling. It should be free from any infection.

When Not to Perform Surgery

Patients with otitis media having tinnitus and expecting relief from tinnitus after surgery should not be operated on. Proper counseling is needed for these patients. The exact cause of tinnitus is not known in these patients. Mostly, it is due to associated sensorineural hearing loss (SNHL).

There is a possibility that tinnitus may increase after surgery. Hence, careful consideration should be made before taking the decision to operate on these patients.

Tympanoplasty in the Only Hearing Ear

Ideally, surgery should not be done in the only hearing ear as there is always the possibility of early or late SNHL following surgery.

But these are the patients who require surgery desperately as they have deafness in the only functioning ear. This deafness should be corrected.

While performing surgery in these patients, all possible precautions should be taken, especially while handling the ossicular chain and while opening the mastoid. Your drill should not touch the ossicular chain at any cost.

Another way to help the only hearing ear is to provide bone anchored hearing aid (BAHA) in that ear, especially if there is significant deafness in that ear and these patients are not able to use conventional hearing aid because of recurrent otorrhea. BAHA is very much useful in these patients and unlike surgery there is no risk of SNHL with BAHA.

In bilateral diseases, surgery can be performed in the better hearing ear, if the patient is able to use the hearing aid in the worse hearing ear. Good improvement in hearing is expected in the better hearing ear.

22 Endoscopic Tympanoplasty

The endoscope is used not only for stapes surgery but also for other ear surgeries like tympanoplasty, cholesteatoma surgery, and ossiculoplasty. Zero-degree 4.00-mm endoscopes are commonly used and major work is done with these endoscopes, but to visualize the eustachian tube area and sinus tympani, 70-degree endoscopes are required.

Various advantages of the endoscope over the microscope are as follows:

- Wide angle, sharp visibility with proximity of image, easy visibility of hidden areas like the sinus tympani, facial recess, anterior epitympanic area, and protympanum, which otherwise are difficult to see by microscope.

- As the facial recess, sinus tympani, and footplate area are widely seen by the endoscopes, the need to remove the posterosuperior bony canal wall overhang is less, which otherwise has to be removed while working with the microscope.

Various disadvantages of endoscopic surgery include the following:

- Lack of depth perception is the biggest disadvantage with the endoscope, especially while doing fine work under higher magnification. There is a lack of real three-dimensional pictures with the endoscopes, but with experience the surgeon can overcome this problem.

- An endoscopic surgery is a one-handed surgery. The other hand is occupied in holding the endoscope.

- Risk of thermal injury to the middle and inner ear due to light source. Thermal injury is more with xenon light than with the LED light source.

- Bleeding in the operative field requires repeated suction by one hand. Bleeding can cause fogging and smearing of endoscopes requiring repeated cleaning.

- As these endoscopes are rigid, it is not possible to do endoscopic tympanoplasty in a patient with an extremely curved external auditory canal.

Equipment

Equipment required for an endoscopic tympanoplasty includes a high-definition endoscopic camera with a rigid endoscope 14-cm long and 3 mm in diameter both 0 and 30 degrees, along with standard instruments for ear surgery.

Most of the surgeons use 4-mm 0- and 30-degree nasal endoscopes for ear surgery because these are readily available with them and give better wide-angle view as compared to a 3-mm endoscope (**Fig. 22.1**).

Instruments for endoscopic tympanoplasty are shown in **Fig. 22.1**: (a) suction adapter, (b–e) suction cannula of different sizes, (f) microforceps (crocodile forceps),

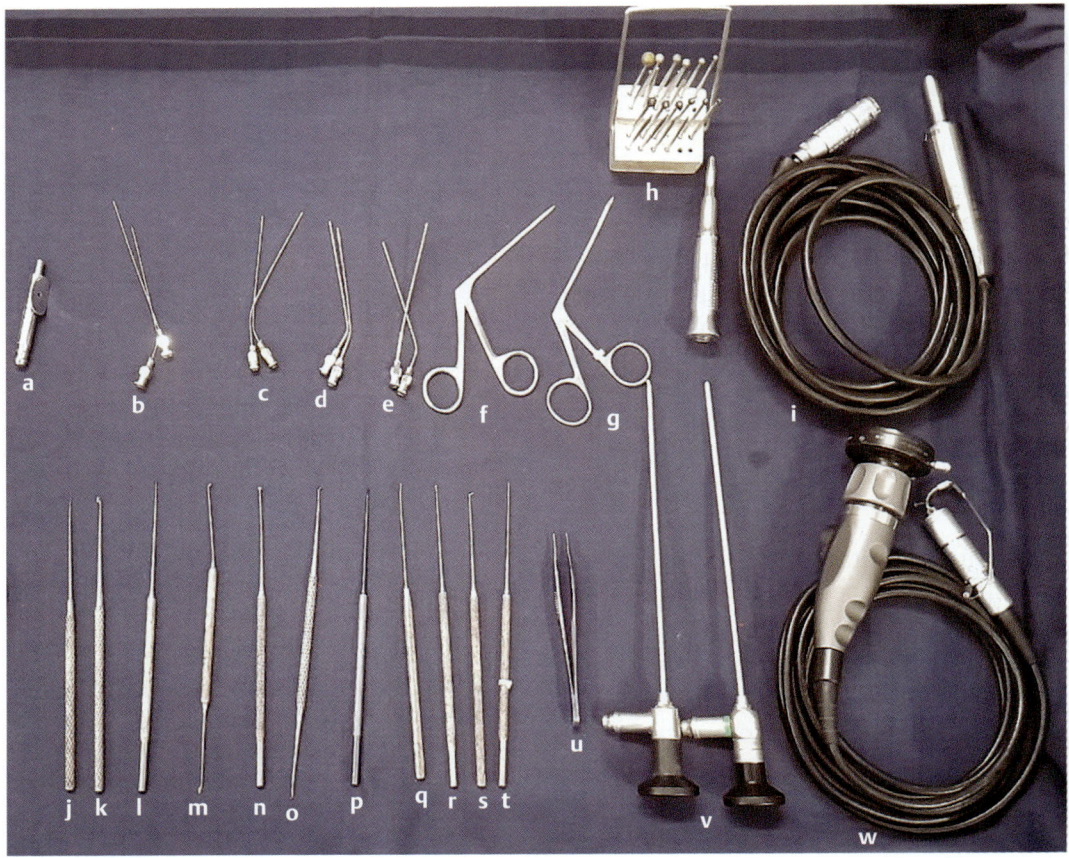

Fig. 22.1 Instrument trolley for endoscopic ear surgery.

(g) microscissors, (h) handpiece with burr, (i) drill machine, (j–t) various picks, side knife, circular knife, and curette; (u) forceps; (v) endoscopes; and (w) camera.

Surgery Technique

Local anesthesia is preferred for tympanoplasty as a bloodless field is required here. Good hemostasis is needed here as the surgeon's one hand is occupied in holding the endoscope and he or she is not able to do repeated suction.

The head end of the operation table should be raised by 15 to 30 degrees to decrease bleeding; simultaneously, the head should be extended at the neck to get better exposure of the middle ear.

Local anesthesia is injected in a similar manner as with microscopic surgery 5 to 6 mL of 2% lignocaine with 1:200,000 adrenaline is enough.

Before starting the surgery, the surgeon should be comfortable with the height of the operation table, with the positioning of the head of the patient, and the height of the monitor.

While using the endoscope, light intensity should be minimum, to prevent thermal damage to the middle ear and inner ear, with intermittent withdrawal of the endoscope for cooling the tissues.

The endoscope provides a wide-angle field, magnified view with the excellent visualization of the entire middle ear, even in the patients with a narrow external auditory canal.

The main problem with an endoscopic ear surgery is the lack of depth perception that makes the work more challenging especially while working under higher magnification.

The surgical steps in endoscopic stapes surgery are the same as microscopic surgery with minor modification.

Visualization of the entire middle ear is achieved without any canal wall removal; however, some canal wall removal is still needed to create more space for easy working especially in anatomically difficult cases.

Thermal injury to the chorda tympani nerve and middle ear is prevented by using an LED light source, using minimum intensity of light with frequent removal of endoscopes for cleaning and defogging. All these reduce the risk of thermal injury by light.

Other steps are the same as a surgery with a microscope.

Results

Results of endoscopic tympanoplasty and microscopic tympanoplasty are compared in a series of patients, and it is found that the success rate is similar in both groups (around 90%).

In patients with a narrow external auditory canal, surgery performed by using a microscope requires endaural incision, which requires an incision. The same patient can be operated by using an endoscope without any incision. That is the advantage of an endoscope over a microscope.

23 Difficult Situations in Tympanoplasty

When ear surgery is planned, all these patients should be examined under a microscope, not only to confirm the findings but also to get an idea about the difficult situations a surgeon may face during surgery. The surgeon will be prepared to handle these situations comfortably if he or she knows them before starting the surgery.

- In general, "exposure" is the biggest problem in all ear surgeries, especially if the ear canal is narrow and there is bulge in the canal wall, making it difficult to visualize the tympanic membrane and perforation fully or completely. These patients require canalplasty, making it easier to see the perforation completely and place the graft. It is said that time spent for canalplasty is time saved while doing tympanoplasty.

- The meatal skin at times is very thin and delicate, having an epithelial lining with very thin periosteal support and no subepithelial connective tissue, making it difficult to elevate this skin, and there is a high possibility of tearing of the tympanomeatal flap. The elevation of the tympanomeatal flap is to be done gently to prevent the flap from getting torn while elevating it. It is equally difficult to reposit this thin tympanomeatal flap properly, especially if it is torn.

- Retracted handle of the malleus is again a problem for placement of the underlay graft especially when the tip of the retracted handle of the malleus is touching the promontory. In few cases, this retracted handle of the malleus is pushed laterally by cutting the tendon of the tensor tympani muscle. At times, slight trimming the tip of the handle of the malleus is done by a malleus head nipper, creating a space to place the underlay graft. Forceful lateralization of the handle of the malleus should not be tried as it may disrupt the incudostapedial joint or may break the lenticular process of the incus.

- Many a time, the posterosuperior part of the tympanic membrane is retracted and adherent to the incus and stapes associated with central perforation of the tympanic membrane. This retracted adherent part of the tympanic membrane is to be dissected from the ossicular chain gently before placing the graft. This posterosuperior part of the tympanic membrane is to be supported by cartilage with the perichondrium to prevent future retraction pocket. Many a time, the posterosuperior retraction of the tympanic membrane is associated with necrosis of the lenticular process of the incus or necrosis of the stapes superstructure, which needs reconstruction.

- The tympanosclerotic plaques are present in the tympanic membrane and around the ossicular chain. The tympanosclerotic plaques in the tympanic membrane should be removed by dissecting it and keeping the epithelium intact. Similarly, if the ossicles are fixed due to tympano-sclerosis, attempt should be made to mobilize the ossicles especially the stapes by removing tympanosclerotic plaques. If stapes mobilization is not successful, then second-stage surgery is required. All these steps are difficult and time-consuming requiring lot of patience.

- Last in the list is ossicular recon-struction, which is difficult especially in patients where the stapes super-structure is missing and the incus is destroyed. Ossiculoplasty results are very good when the stapes superstructure is present and only the lenticular process of the incus is necrosed. Ossiculoplasty results are good when cartilage is used.

24 Postoperative Care after Tympanoplasty

Surgery is done either under local or general anesthesia. Preoperatively before starting surgery, one dose of injectable antibiotic is given intravenously. Third-generation cephalosporin is preferred.

Immediately postoperatively, injectable analgesics can be given to reduce pain if any. Usually, there is not much pain after tympanoplasty and oral analgesic tablet gives good relief.

The patient can have liquids immediately after surgery, when surgery is performed under local anesthesia. If general anesthesia is given, then the patient should be kept nil by mouth for 4 hours after surgery. During that time, intravenous fluids can be given.

Dressing should be changed the next morning and the patient can be discharged. Oral antibiotics are given for 7 days

The patient is given the following instructions:

- Not to wash the head for 10 days.
- Not to blow the nose for at least 1 month. By that time, graft is taken up well and the tympanic membrane heals up.
- While sneezing, the mouth should be kept open.
- As far as possible, avoid catching cold and give them antihistamines with decongestants immediately if the patient catches cold.

Dressing is removed between 7 and 10 days after the surgery and the patient is advised to put antibiotics with steroid ear drops in the operated ear for 6 weeks. Around four to five drops are to be instilled in the ear canal twice a day. These drops will dissolve Gelfoam and clear the ear canal. Steroids locally prevent the formation of any granulations in the ear canal, thus preventing healing with fibrosis and canal stenosis.

Postoperatively, if any granulations are found in the ear canal, it should be cauterized by 50% trichloroacetic acid (TCA).

Full epithelization and complete healing takes place by month 3 and the ear canal with the tympanic membrane heals up completely. Usually, these patients get improvement in the hearing 3 months after surgery and that is the time when an audiogram should be repeated.

25 Complications of Tympanoplasty

Complications can occur following tympanoplasty. These complications can occur during surgery or following surgery. Complications occurring during or immediately after surgery are called immediate complications.

Immediate Complications

- *Facial nerve injury*: This is not common during tympanoplasty. Transient facial nerve palsy can occur secondary to local anesthetic infiltration, which recovers within a few hours.

  Accidental injury to the tympanic part of the facial nerve is the only possibility in tympanoplasty especially when the fallopian canal is dehiscent.

  The most common situation where the facial nerve palsy can occur during tympanoplasty is while performing simple mastoidectomy, which is performed as a part of tympanoplasty. The most common site is the second genu of the facial nerve while working inside the mastoid. The chances of getting this injury are higher when there are associated facial nerve anomalies.

  All these injuries are preventable by acquiring better knowledge of the anatomy of the temporal bone by doing more and more temporal bone dissections.

  If the facial nerve has been damaged during surgery, if the surgeon is quite sure about partial damage of the nerve, and if the continuity of the nerve is maintained, these cases recover within a few months.

  If the surgeon is not sure about the integrity and continuity of the nerve, it should be explored. The nerve should be decompressed. Direct anastomosis or nerve grafting may be required.

- *Chorda tympani nerve injury*: The chorda tympani nerve should be preserved as far as possible. If the nerve is stretched, then transecting the nerve will be the better choice as the patients are more symptomatic with the stretched nerve than with the transected nerve.

- *Bleeding during surgery*: Usually bleeding problem is not there in tympanoplasty due to local anesthetic infiltration with adrenaline. Under general anesthesia, hypotensive anesthesia gives a very good bloodless field.

  The dehiscent high jugular bulb, if accidentally damaged, can cause profuse bleeding, which can be controlled by packing with Gelfoam and waiting for some time. All the bleeding should be perfectly controlled before placing the graft.

When surgery is performed under local anesthesia, local anesthetic with adrenaline infiltration should be repeated at regular intervals (usually every 45 minutes) to avoid rebound congestion with bleeding.

- *Infection*: Infection is not a problem if proper aseptic precautions are taken during and after surgery.

The following factors are responsible for infection:

- ○ Poor aseptic technique is always associated with infection.
- ○ Prior contamination of the middle ear tissues and graft by hair or thread particles invites foreign body reaction and infection.

Immediate postoperative infection occurs if aseptic precautions are not taken. With good asepsis, and good antibiotic coverage, postoperatively infections are rare. If it occurs, broad-spectrum intravenous antibiotics covering especially *Pseudomonas* infection should be given to prevent failure of tympanoplasty. Perichondritis can also occur due to lack of aseptic precautions. This can be very well prevented.

- *Sensorineural hearing loss (SNHL) and vertigo after surgery*: These complications are usually not there with tympanoplasty and ossiculoplasty. High-speed drill touching the intact ossicular chain or excessive manipulation of the ossicles can lead to SNHL. Accidental dislocation of the stapes usually does not occur with experienced surgeons.

Late Complications

- Persistent or increased conductive hearing loss after surgery can occur. This could be due to the following:
  - ○ Unrecognized eroded incudostapedial joint; hence, ossicular discontinuity remains after surgery.
  - ○ Unrecognized stapes fixation and malleus and incus fixation especially in the attic. If missed, severe conductive hearing loss remains.
  - ○ Blunting of the anterior sulcus is the problem with the overlay technique.
  - ○ Lateralization of the graft from the handle of the malleus can occur during healing with fibrosis. The graft falls away from the handle of the malleus if not placed medial to it.
- *External auditory canal stenosis*: This is not very common. Stenosis of the external auditory canal following tympanoplasty is due to inflammatory reaction with formation of granulations in the external auditory canal followed by healing with fibrosis causing narrowing of the external auditory canal.

In the beginning, this narrowing can be prevented by gently widening the external auditory canal under local anesthesia and lining the canal by a thick silastic sheet. Local steroid ear drops are given to these patients to be instilled for few months. These drops decrease the inflammatory reaction in the external auditory canal and prevent the formation of granulations. If stenosis has already taken place, it requires surgical excision.

26 Ossiculoplasty

Surgery for otosclerosis has become standard now, but surgery for chronic otitis media, especially ossiculoplasty, is still quite variable and techniques for ossiculoplasty depends upon the following:

- Individual experience of the surgeon.
- The disease process especially the presence of residual ossicles.
- The status of the middle ear mucosa and eustachian tube patency.

The ossicular chain acts as a middle ear transformer mechanism.

In ossiculoplasty, the ossicular chain that has been destroyed by the disease is reconstructed to connect the tympanic membrane to the cochlea so that sound from the outer ear is transmitted to the inner ear.

The reconstruction of the ossicular chain is more difficult than any other otology procedures. If the ossiculoplasty is not successful, around 40 to 45dB hearing loss (40–45 dB air–bone gap) remains, and these patients will not be happy, even though tympanic membrane reconstruction is successful.

Ossiculoplasty in cases of otitis media is performed either as a first-stage operation along with tympanic membrane reconstruction or as a second-stage operation after the tympanic membrane has been reconstructed in the first operation. The second-stage procedure is performed few months after the myringoplasty (first

procedure), and by that time, the middle ear has completely healed up.

Remember that in ossiculoplasty, it is the long-term results that are important than the immediate results.

26a: History

Ossiculoplasty was started in year 1957. Earlier it was the autografts that were most commonly used for ossiculoplasty. In addition to autografts, homografts were also used for ossicular reconstruction. These homografts were discontinued later due to fear of human immunodeficiency virus (HIV) infection, but autografts are still being used and are very popular as an ossiculoplasty material.

Later on, various prosthesis made up of metals like stainless steel and platinum were used for ossicular reconstruction but discontinued because of high extrusion rate.

Partial plastipore ossicular replacement prosthesis (PORP) and total plastipore ossicular replacement prostheses (TORP) were very popular ossiculoplasty material because of their high biocompatibility and nonreactivity. Their extrusion is very less if they are covered by a piece of cartilage. They are not very costly.

Later on, ceramics were used for ossiculoplasty but discontinued due to high extrusion rate. Another very popular ossiculoplasty material being used since 1970 is hydroxylapatite, which is very much biocompatible, lightweight with good osteointegration, and easy to handle with no extrusion if covered by cartilage. Hydroxylapatite is very brittle, but it can be shaped according to the situation by using a diamond burr.

Since 1993, titanium is being used for ossicular reconstruction. It is very a popular ossiculoplasty material. It is biocompatible, has good osteointegration, lightweight, strong, and is an ideal ossiculoplasty material but costly. It is widely used, and there is no extrusion if it is covered by cartilage.

Nowadays titanium and hydroxylapatite are the most popular ossiculoplasty material and are widely used. Another ossiculoplasty material commonly used is the cartilage with perichondrium taken out from the tragus or from the concha. This cartilage has got many advantages, which are discussed later in the chapter.

26b: Intraoperative Assessments

Ossicles are either destroyed by disease or removed because they are eroded by disease.

Before reconstruction of the ossicular chain, the status of each ossicle should be assessed by gentle palpation after elevating the tympanomeatal flap. Gently palpate the handle of the malleus, incus lenticular process, and stapes, especially its footplate for the mobility. Look for the integrity of the incudostapedial joint. At times, the stapes crura are not healthy. They are intact but weak to stand ossicular reconstruction.

Round window reflex should be checked to confirm the mobility of the stapes footplate.

The head of the malleus and the body of the incus may be fixed in the attic due to adhesions, calcification, or ossification.

Calcification may also be seen in the tendon of the tensor tympani and the stapedius muscle.

The stapes footplate may be fixed due to fibrosis, tympanosclerosis, or otosclerosis. There may be congenital fixation of the stapes footplate.

All these pathologies may coexist. These situations should be managed nicely to get successful results and good hearing.

All the cases of otitis media with central or subtotal perforation should be assessed for the possibility of ossicular defect, either ossicular discontinuity or ossicular fixation, especially stapes fixation.

Routine patch test by closing the perforation by filter paper and Gelfoam patch test by keeping a piece of Gelfoam in the middle ear will be the most reliable test for assessment of the integrity of the ossicular chain, especially stapes.

26c: Various Situations for Ossiculoplasty

There are three situations that a surgeon usually come across when the middle ear is entered.

- *Situation one*: Intact malleus and intact mobile stapes, with the incus either partially or completely destroyed by disease.

- *Situation two*: Intact malleus and mobile stapes footplate (no stapes superstructure), with the incus either partially or completely destroyed.

- *Situation three:* Only mobile stapes or footplate; no malleus and no incus.

- Ossiculoplasty in situation one is comparatively easier and results are better than situations two and three. In situations two and three, ossiculoplasty is difficult and results are not very encouraging.

26d: Ossiculoplasty Materials

Various ossiculoplasty materials used for the ossiculoplasty are autografts, homografts, and alloplasts.

Autografts

Autografts are graft materials from the patient's own body. Various autograft materials used are either the patient's own residual ossicle if healthy or cartilage with perichondrium from the tragus or the concha. Autografts are well accepted by the body and are biocompatible with no cost.

Homografts

Various homograft materials used for ossiculoplasty are again ossicles and cartilage.

Homografts are not used for ossiculoplasty nowadays because of the risk of infection especially viral infection transmission from the donor to the recipient.

Alloplasts

Various alloplasts used for ossiculoplasty are either metallic or nonmetallic.

Metallic

Various metallic prostheses used for ossiculoplasty are either gold or titanium.

Among these, titanium is the most ideal ossiculoplasty material because it is lightweight, biocompatible, and has a very good osteointegration property with very low extrusion rate, which can be further minimized by keeping cartilage between the prosthesis and the tympanic membrane.

Nonmetallic

Various nonmetallic prostheses used for ossiculoplasty are ceramics or hydroxylapatite.

Of these, hydroxylapatite is the best alloplastic material. It is made up of bonelike material having calcium base with low extrusion rate. Even though it is very brittle, it can be shaped according to the situation by using a diamond burr. After titanium, hydroxylapatite is the second most popular ossiculoplasty material.

The material used should satisfy certain physical and structural qualities:

- The material used for ossiculoplasty should have certain qualities through which sound can be transmitted efficiently from the tympanic membrane to the oval window.

- The ossicle used should be rigid enough to transmit high-frequency sound from the tympanic membrane to the oval window, but it should not be too hard to cause subluxation of the footplate into the vestibule whenever there is an inward pressure. The autograft ossicles and cartilage are ideal for this purpose.

- The ossicle should be at right angle to the stapes footplate or stapes.

- The wide surface area of the ossicle should be in contact with the eardrum.

- The ossicle should be stable and should not have a tendency to get displaced from its contact with the stapes.

- The ossicle should have excellent damping properties to prevent transmission of unwanted vibrations to the footplate.

26e: Situation 1 for Ossiculoplasty

This is the most common situation, and it is also easier to handle. In this situation, the malleus is normal, and the stapes is normal and mobile. The incus is either partially eroded or there is no incus (totally destroyed)

Ideal ossiculoplasty is by the following:

1. Incus transposition (autograft incus).

2. Cartilage ossiculoplasty (cartilage columella).

3. Titanium or hydroxylapatite prosthesis can be used if the incus is not available.

Incus Transposition (Autograft Incus)

Many a time, the continuity of the ossicular chain is broken either due to necrosis of the lenticular process of the incus or due to destruction of the long process of the incus. The remaining incus can be used for transposition (**Fig. 26e1–26e18**). The incus remnant is taken out, refashioned, and transposed between the malleus handle and the stapes head. The main requirement for this arrangement is that sufficient healthy incus remnant should be available for refashioning.

If the incus is not available, the malleus head can be used in place of the incus but the main problem here is that the malleus handle becomes very unstable after removal of its head and it is difficult to give a stable assembly when the handle of the malleus is unstable.

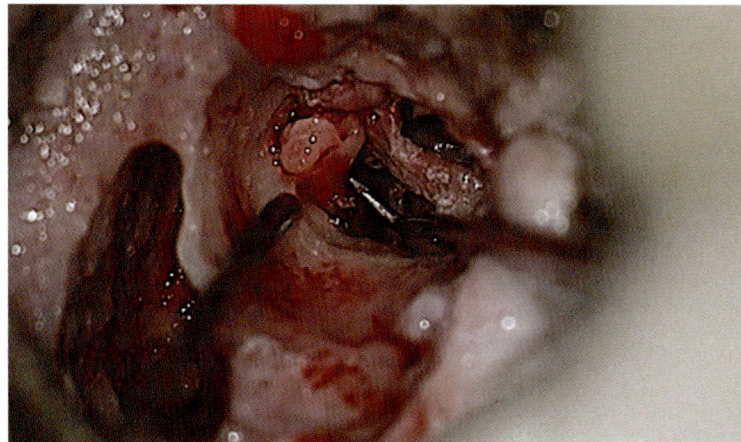

Fig. 26e1   Incus remnant is separated from malleus by right angle hook and taken out.

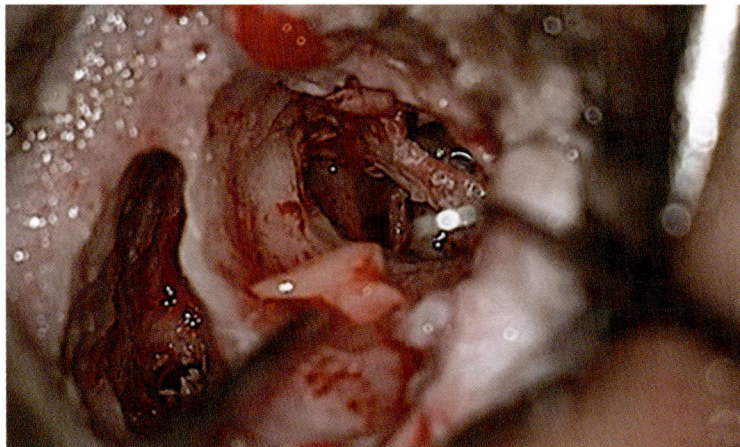

Fig. 26e2   Incus remnant is taken out. The lenticular process with long process of incus is necrosed.

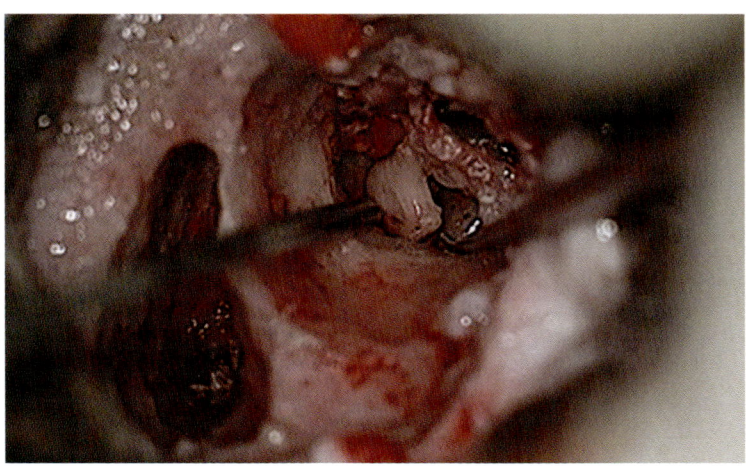

Fig. 26e3   The removed incus is placed between handle of malleus and head of stapes, just to get an idea about distance between head of stapes and malleus.

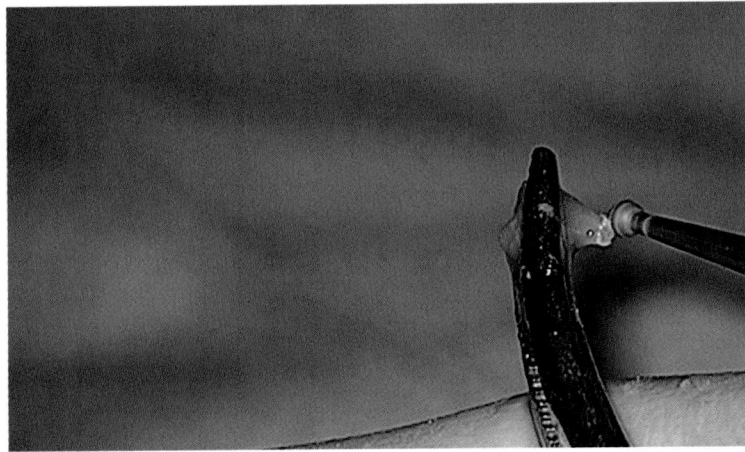

Fig. 26e4 The short process of the incus is reduced and a circular facet is made over the short process of incus.

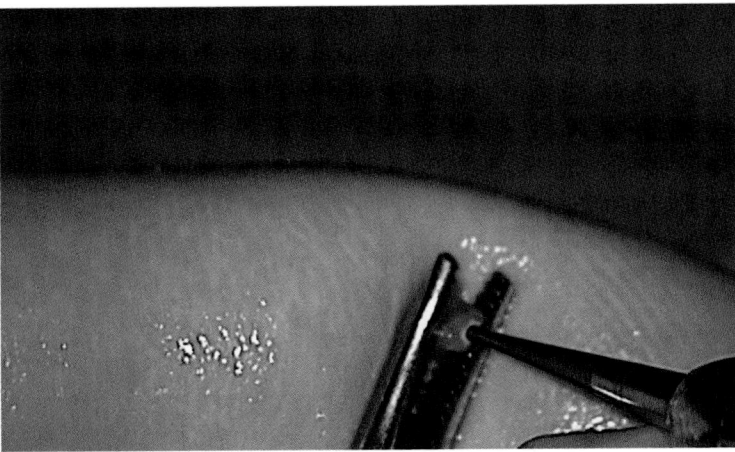

Fig. 26e5 A small rounded socket is made in the smooth facet of short process of the incus for head of the stapes by using 0.8-mm cutting burr.

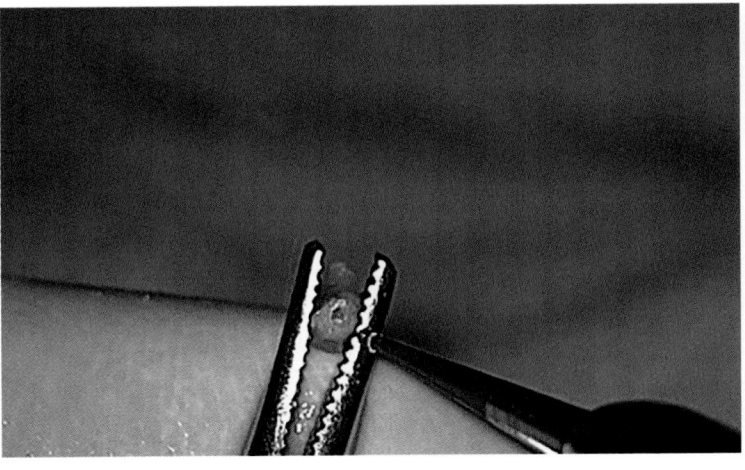

Fig. 26e6 A small symmetrical socket has been made in the short process of incus for the head of the stapes.

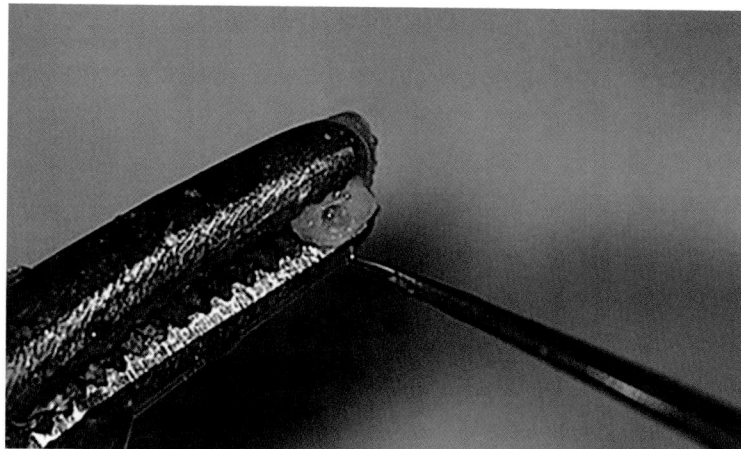

Fig. 26e7 Socket for stapes head under higher magnification.

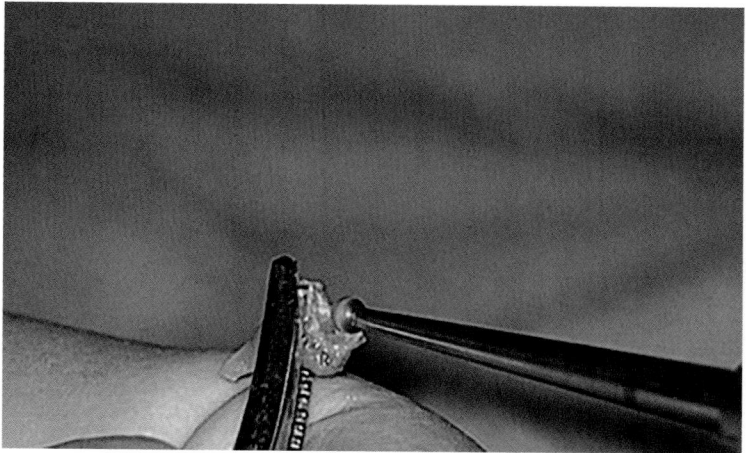

Fig. 26e8 The mallear surface of incus is smoothened.

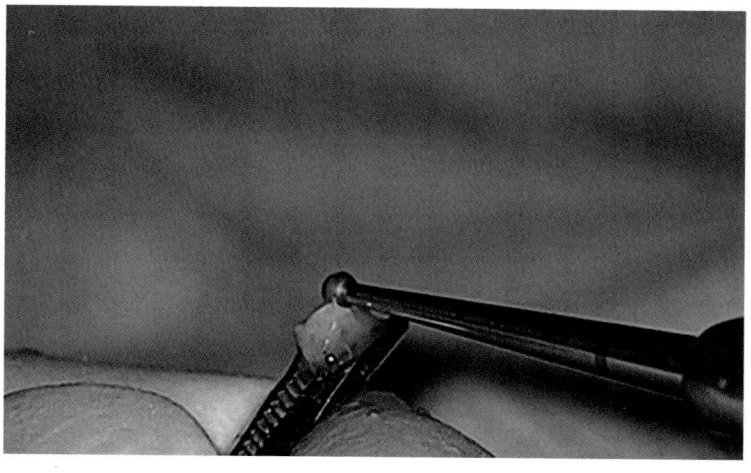

Fig. 26e9 The bulk of body of incus is reduced.

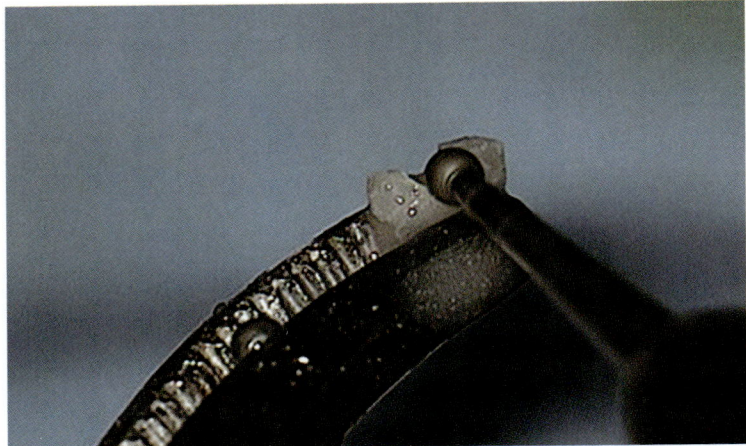

Fig. 26e10 The mallear surface of incus is smoothened and a small groove is made in the body of the incus for handle of malleus.

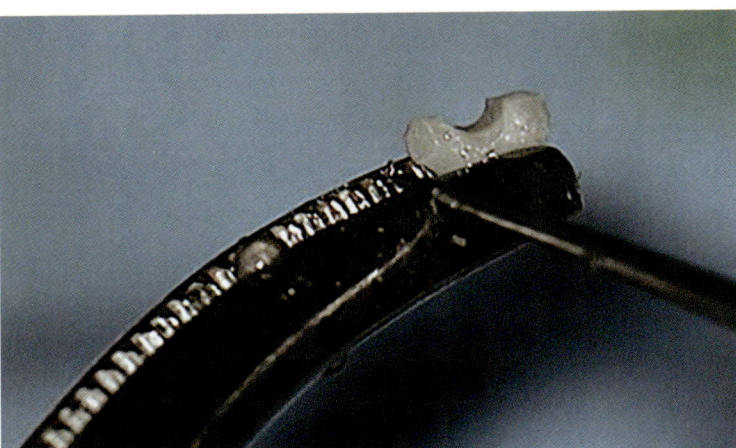

Fig. 26e11 The incus is ready to be transposed between handle of malleus and head of stapes.

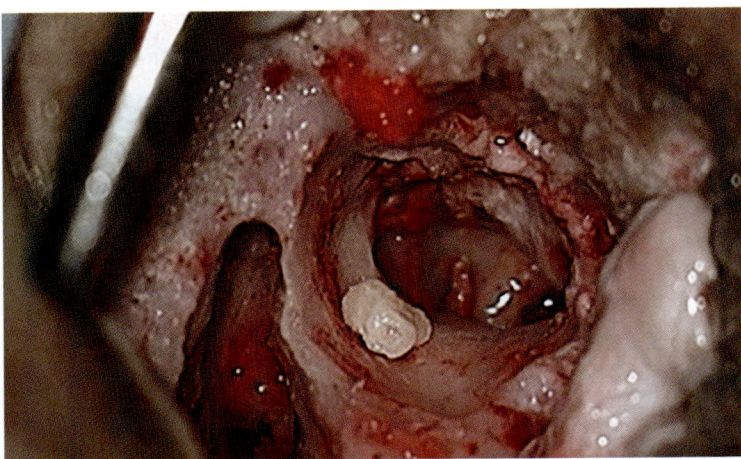

Fig. 26e12 The refashioned incus is placed in the ear canal. Before transposition of incus, mobility of stapes and malleus is confirmed and underlay graft is placed.

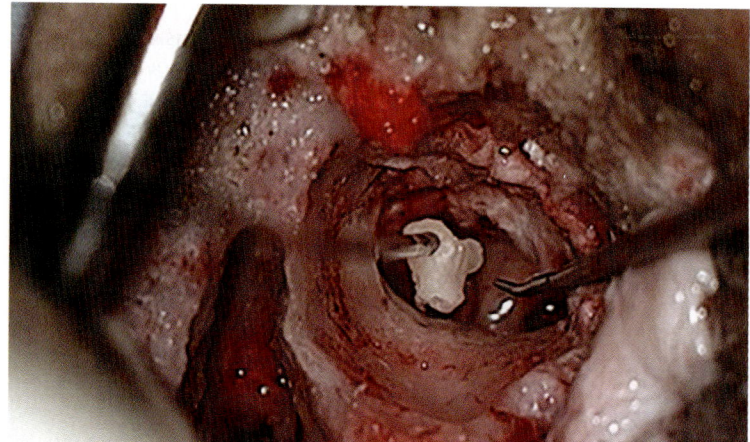

Fig. 26e13 The refashioned incus is introduced in the middle ear with groove for malleus is facing handle of malleus.

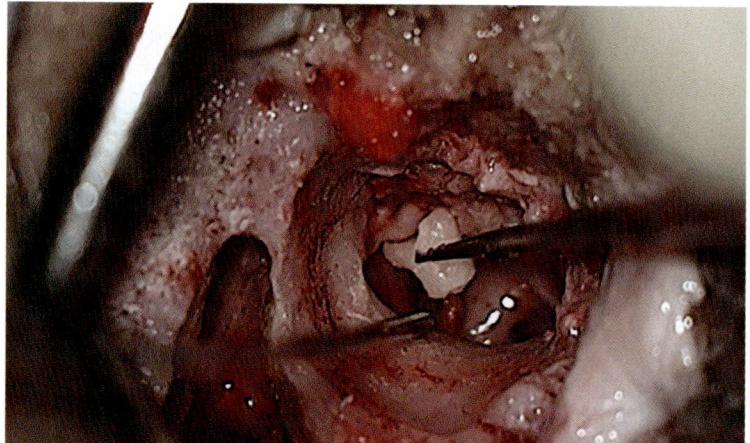

Fig. 26e14 The groove for malleus is engaged under handle of malleus near its neck.

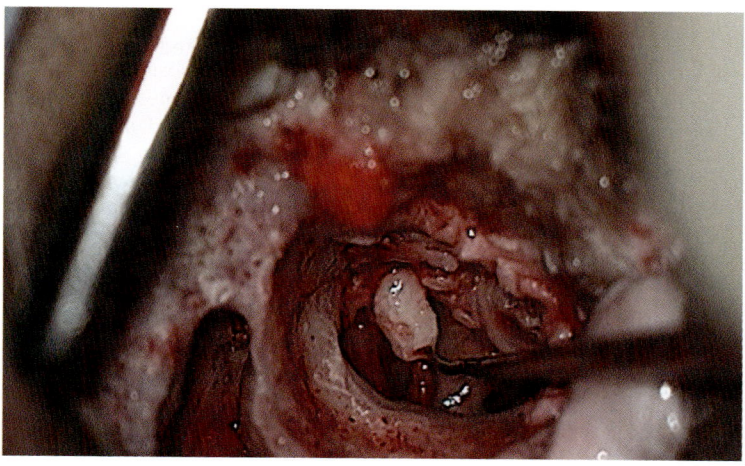

Fig. 26e15 The transposed incus after engaging under handle of malleus is gently placed/slided over the head of the stapes by right angle hook.

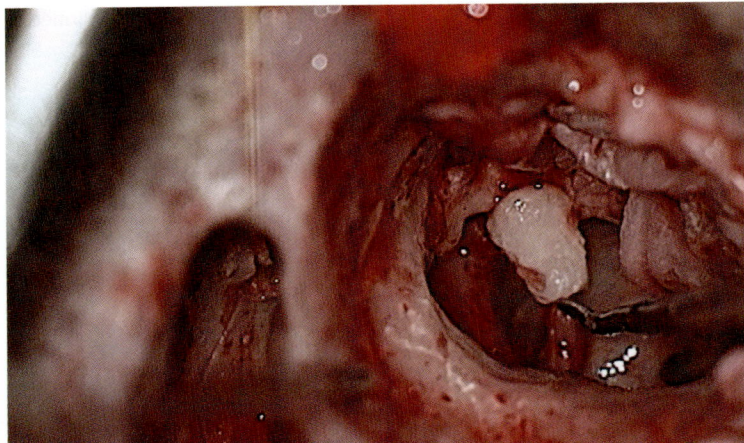

Fig. 26e16 The transposed incus after engaging under handle of malleus is gently placed/slided over the head of the stapes by right angle hook (under higher magnification).

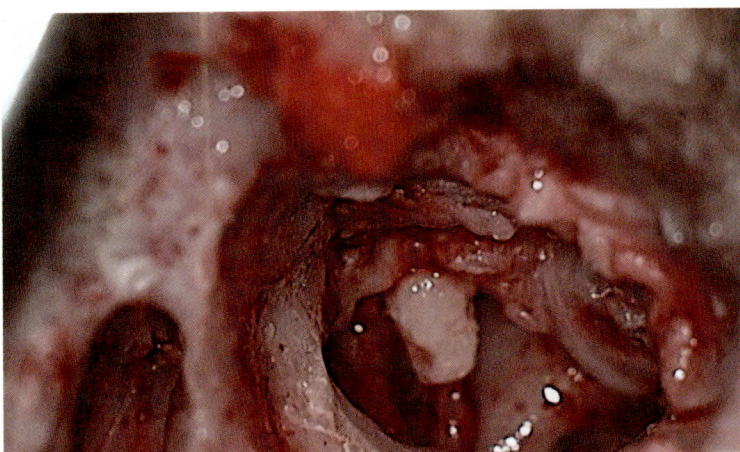

Fig. 26e17 Incus is well transposed between handle of malleus and head of the stapes, not touching fallopian canal and promontory.

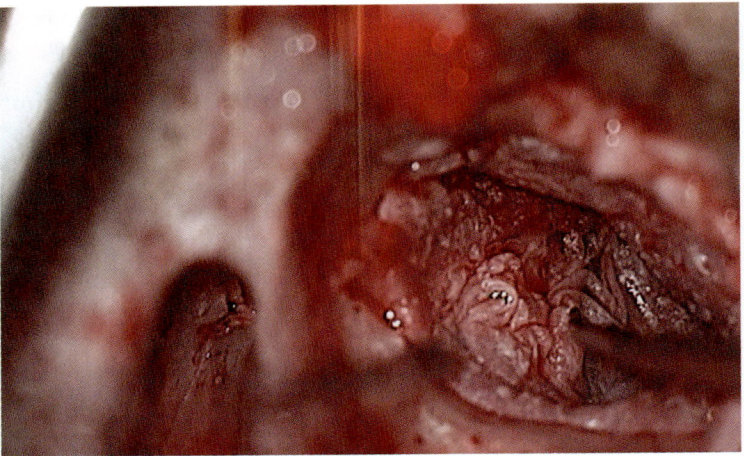

Fig. 26e18 Tympanomeatal flap is reposited back.

Certain Rules to Follow

- Check for the mobility of malleus. If it is fixed in the attic, it should be mobilized by performing posterior atticotomy and the tympanosclerotic plaque or the bone that is fixing the malleus head should be removed. The malleus head should be preserved. The purpose is to keep the malleus stable so that it will be easier to transpose the incus between the malleus handle and the stapes.

- Tensor tympani tendon should be preserved, but if it is calcified and restricting the movement of the handle of the malleus, it should be cut with scissors.

- The distance between the stapes head and the malleus handle is variable and should be measured. The incus should be of perfect length to be fitted between the stapes head and the malleus handle.

- The malleus and stapes are not in the same plane. The malleus is anterior to the stapes. If the malleus is too anterior to the stapes, it is difficult to place the incus and a significant tilting of the incus takes place, causing a decrease in hearing improvement. Here cartilage will be the most stable.

- Before the incus is handled, always look for the dehiscent facial nerve. If it is dehiscent, due care should be taken while working in that area.

- If incus removal is planned, to start with, first dislocate the incudomalleolar joint, thus separating the incus from the malleus. Then, by right angle hook lateralize the incus; now hold the long process of the incus by crocodile forceps and pull it down inferiorly toward the hypotympanum, and then remove the incus for refashioning. Lateralization of the long process of the incus is important, so that it can be held nicely by forceps and will not slip into the attic or aditus or will not be lost.

- The integrity of the stapes is important. If the stapes superstructure is intact and healthy with a mobile footplate, incus transposition between the stapes head and the malleus will be successful. If the stapes superstructure is destroyed or if it is very weak and delicate, the incus is transposed between the malleus and the stapes footplate. The problem here is that the distance between the malleus and the stapes footplate is longer as compared to the distance between the malleus and the stapes head. Hence, the ossicle required will be longer and thinner for it to stay on the footplate. This longer and thinner ossicle will be very unstable and the success rate is less as compare with the intact stapes superstructure.

If the stapes is fixed, check for calcification in the stapedius muscle. If the stapedius muscle is calcified, the mobility of the stapes can be achieved by cutting the stapedius muscle. If the footplate of the stapes is fixed due to tympanosclerosis around the stapes, attempt is made to mobilize the stapes by removing these tympanosclerotic plaques around the stapes superstructure and footplate. This type of dissection is dangerous and should be carried out very gently along the long axis of the stapes. If the stapes gets mobilized by removing the tympanosclerosis around it, incus transposition can be done and if stapes mobilization is not successful, second-stage surgery, in which stapedectomy can be planned, should be done if the incus is healthy.

The main problem with incus transposition is that this assembly looks very stable while operating but after reposition of the tympanomeatal flap and after packing the external auditory canal by Gelfoam, there is pressure over the malleus handle, pushing it more medially. Hence, the assembly tends to become more horizontal, causing dislocation of the transposed incus from the head of the stapes. Hence, checking and rechecking the transposed incus by lifting the tympanomeatal flap is very important while packing the external auditory canal by Gelfoam.

In addition, when middle ear healing takes place, this healing with fibrosis may change the position of the transposed incus and the incus may lose contact with the stapes. The transposed incus develops adhesions with the surrounding bone of the fallopian canal and the cochleariform process, causing conductive deafness. Finally, this transposed incus undergoes atrophy in due course leading to conductive hearing loss.

Cartilage Transposition

When the incus is completely eroded, destroyed, and not useful, a **Y**-shaped tragal cartilage piece can be transposed between the malleus neck and the stapes footplate.

Malleus Relocation Technique

When the malleus is very much anterior in relation to the stapes, it can be brought back by the malleus relocation technique described by Dr. Robert Vincent.

In this technique, the malleus handle is completely separated from the tympanic membrane, the tensor tympani muscle is divided at its insertion, and the neck of the malleus is pulled back by a right angle hook. This allows stretching of the anterior mallear ligament and placing the handle of the malleus more posteriorly in the plane of the stapes head so that prosthesis can be placed easily between the malleus and the stapes, which are in the same plane after relocation.

Cartilage Columella

This type of arrangement is done when the stapes is intact and mobile, and the malleus is normal but the incus lenticular process or the tip of long process of incus is necrosed.

A columella effect is created by keeping a cartilage piece over the head of the stapes, which is stabilized by the pressure of the necrosed long process of the incus. The tympanic membrane rests over this cartilage, thus creating a columella.

A triangular piece of cartilage with perichondrium is harvested from the tragus The lower end of this triangular piece of cartilage is placed over the groove made at the inferior sulcus. This triangular piece of the cartilage lies horizontally over the middle ear with its upper end under the long process of the incus, touching the stapes head and supporting the tympanic membrane (columella effect).

This type of arrangement is only possible when there is minimal destruction of the long process of the incus and the gap between the long process of the incus and the stapes head is very less. This type of arrangement is not possible when there is major destruction of the incus long process and there is a big gap between the stapes head and the incus long process. Here the cartilage will be unstable and hearing improvement is unpredictable.

Some surgeons use bone cement or bone pate to close this defect, but results are not long lasting.

Clinical Case

Case 1: Cartilage Columella

Clinical case 1 is depicted in **Fig. 26e19–26e28**.

Case 2: Cartilage Columella

Clinical case 2 is depicted in **Fig. 26e29–26e34**.

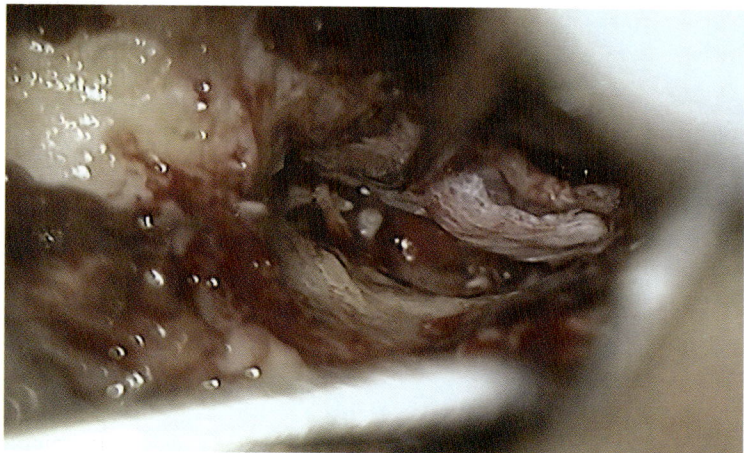

Fig. 26e19 Lenticular process of the incus is necrosed, the stapes is intact and mobile, and the malleus is normal. An underlay graft has been placed.

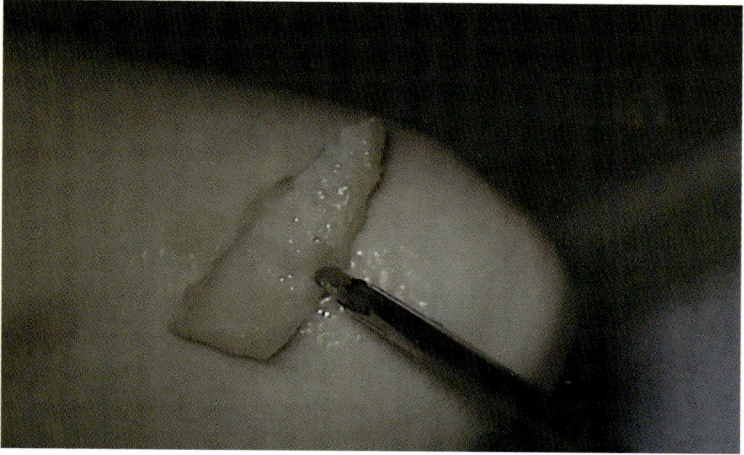

Fig. 26e20 A triangular piece of cartilage with perichondrium is taken out from the tragus.

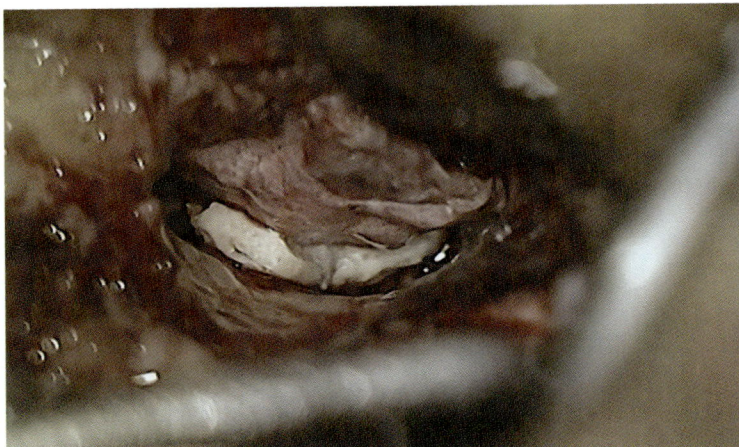

Fig. 26e21 Cartilage is introduced in the middle ear after placing an underlay graft.

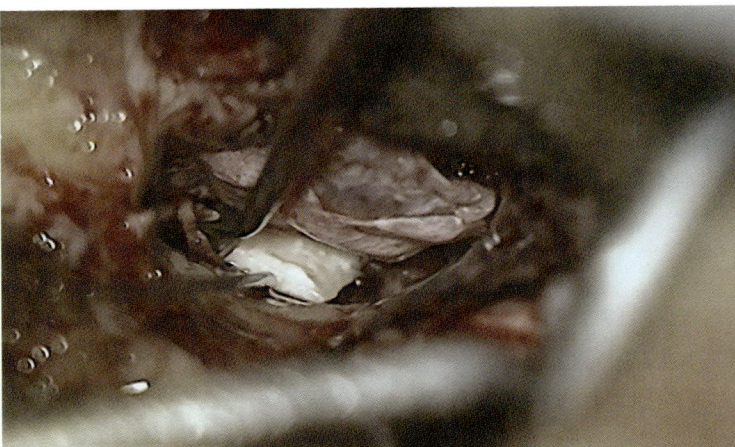

Fig. 26e22 Cartilage is placed horizontally in the middle ear after placing an underlay graft.

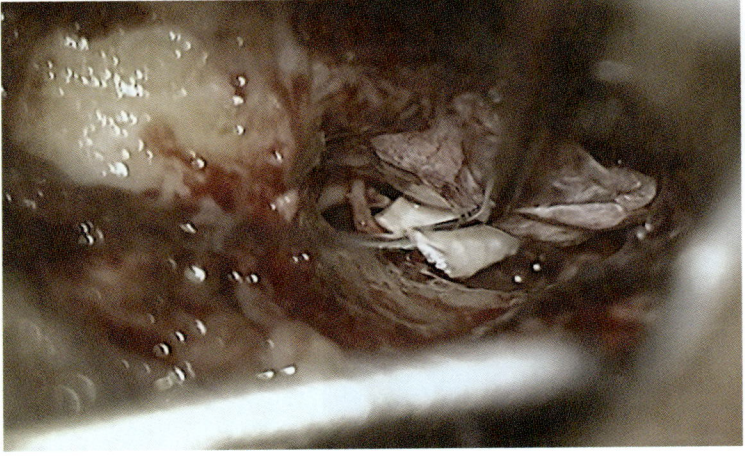

Fig. 26e23 Cartilage is placed in the middle ear horizontally, Attempt is made to slide this triangular piece of cartilage under the long process of the incus and over the stapes head.

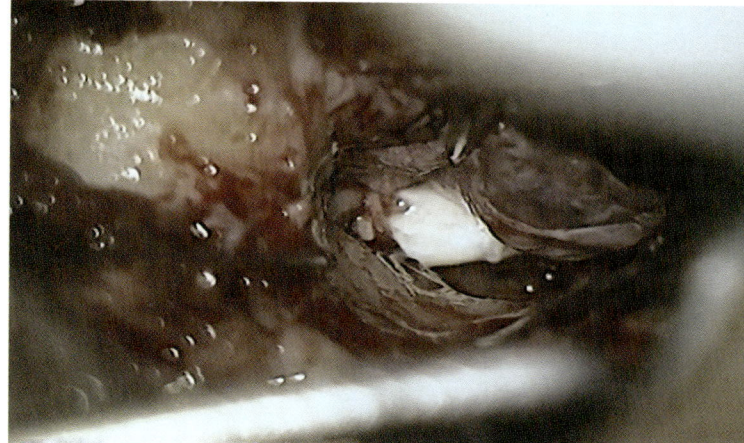

Fig. 26e24 Cartilage is slided under the long process of the incus touching the stapes head.

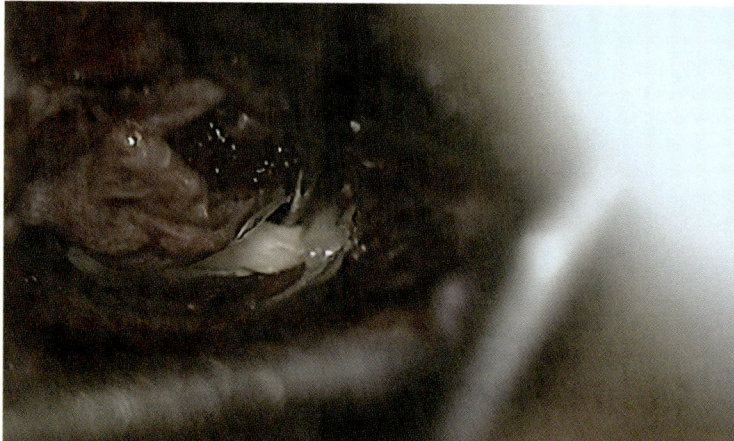

Fig. 26e25 The lower end of the cartilage is to be placed into the groove made at the inferior sulcus.

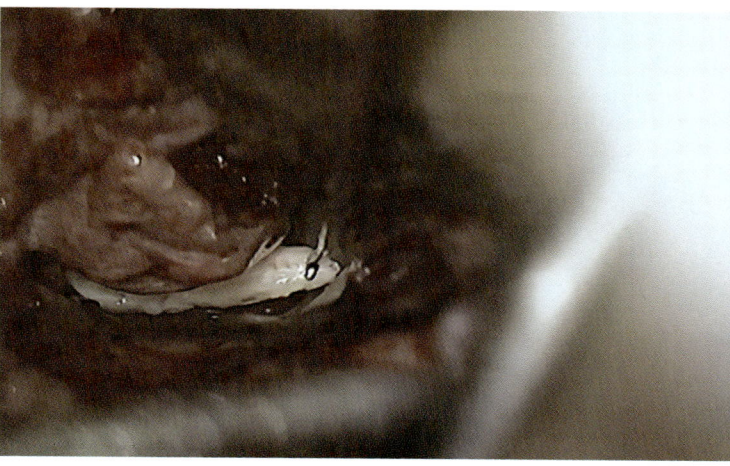

Fig. 26e26 The lower end of the cartilage is placed into the groove made at the inferior sulcus.

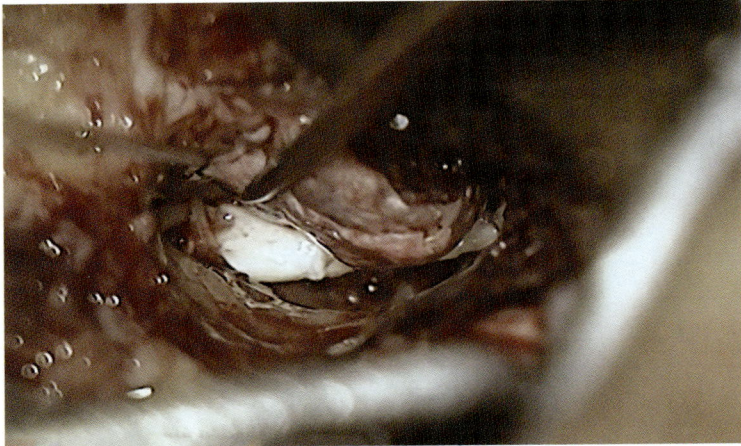

Fig. 26e27 Final position of the cartilage, lying horizontally in the middle ear lying over the stapes head, stabilized by the pressure of the long process of the incus and supporting graft (columella effect).

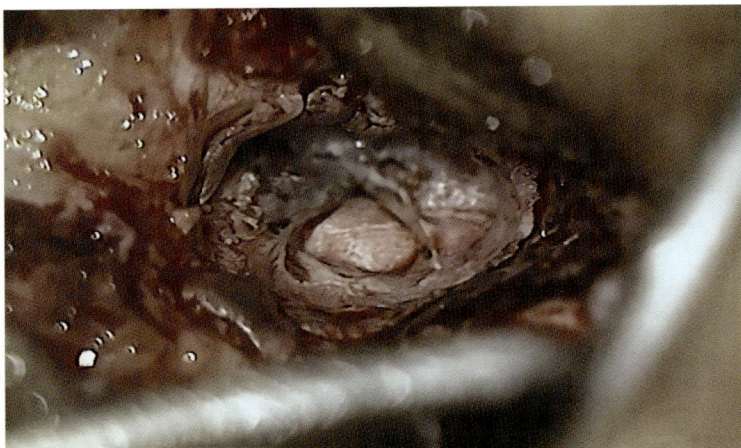

Fig. 26e28 The tympanomeatal flap is reposited back.

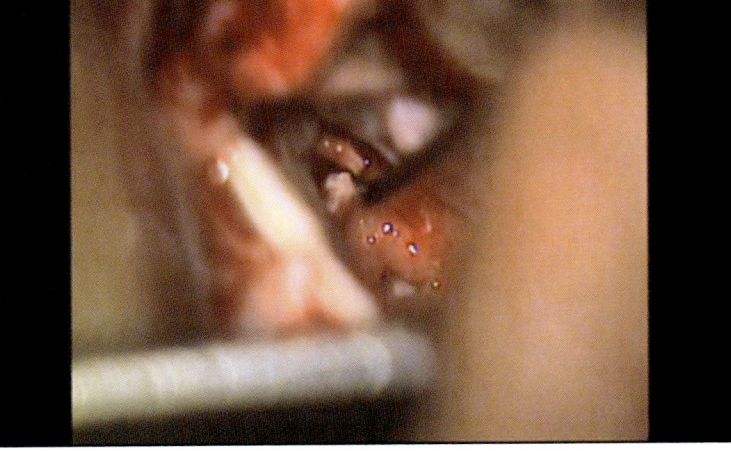

Fig. 26e29 Lenticular process of the incus is necrosed, the stapes is intact and mobile, and the malleus is normal.

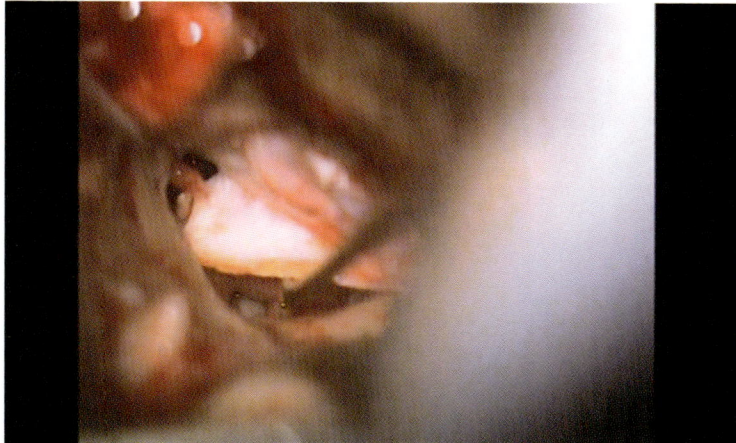

Fig. 26e30 A triangular piece of cartilage is introduced horizontally in the middle ear after placing an underlay graft.

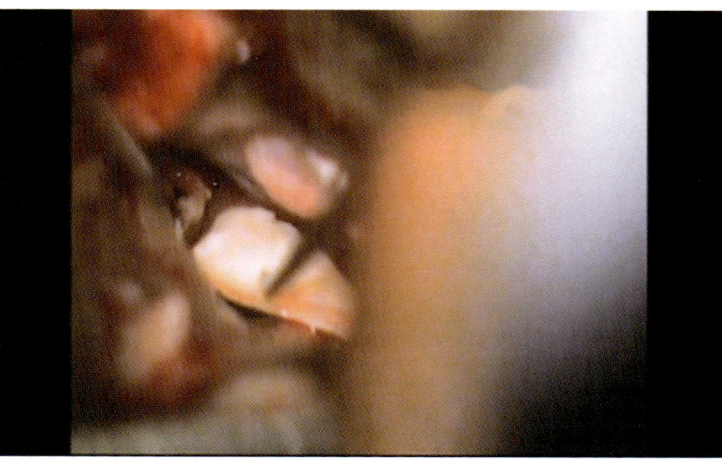

Fig. 26e31 An attempt is made to slide the cartilage under the long process of the incus touching the stapes head.

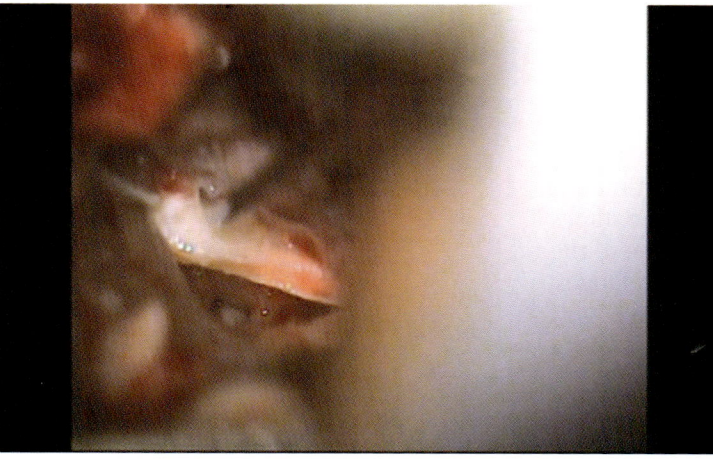

Fig. 26e32 Cartilage is slided under the long process of the incus touching the stapes head, and its lower end is resting over the groove made at the inferior sulcus.

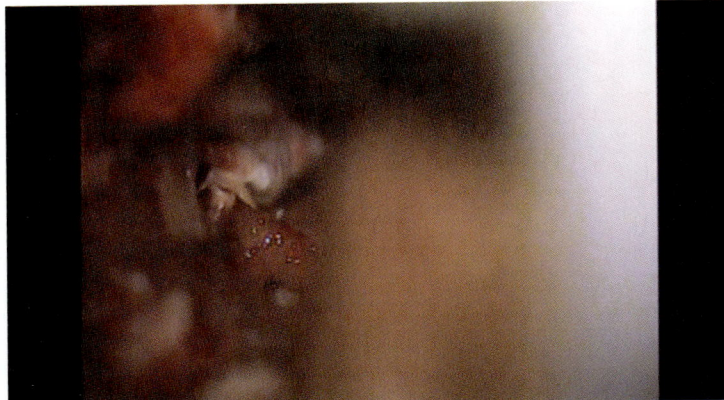

Fig. 26e33 Cartilage is seen touching the stapes head and good pressure contact is maintained by the long process of the incus keeping the cartilage in place.

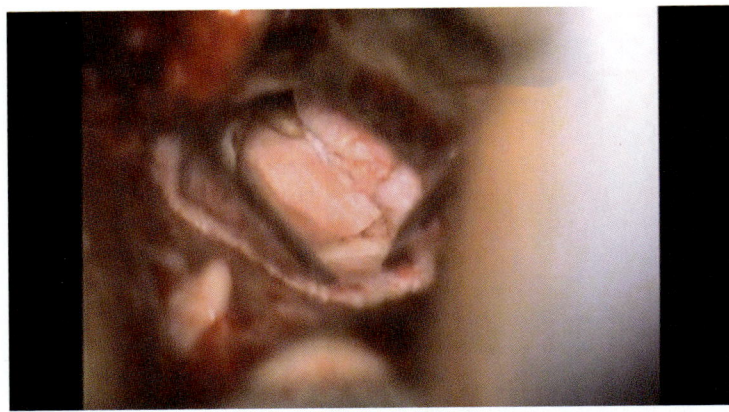

Fig. 26e34 Tympanomeatal flap is reposited back.

26f: Situation 2 for Ossiculoplasty

In this situation, there is intact malleus and mobile stapes footplate (no stapes superstructure), and the incus has been destroyed or missing.

Ossiculoplasty in this situation is unstable due to lack of stability at the stapes footplate, and the distance between the stapes footplate and the malleus is longer, making it more prone to displacement especially when the eustachian tube is not functioning well.

Ossiculoplasty in this situation is:

1. Auto-incus or partial Plastipore ossicular replacement prosthesis (PORP) can be used.

2. Titanium prosthesis is also useful here.

3. Cartilage (two-cartilage technique) is the best (demonstrated later).

The incus is transposed between the handle of the malleus and the stapes footplate, which is covered by the perichondrium (**Fig. 26f1–26f13**).

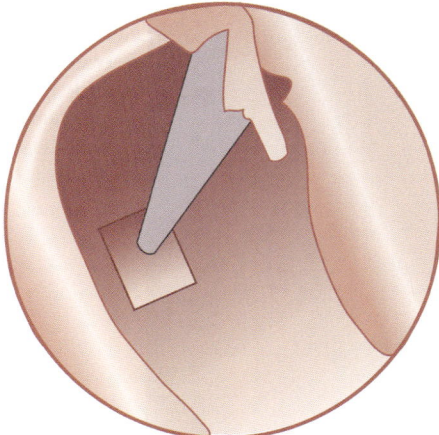

Fig. 26f1   Auto-incus is refashioned and transposed between the handle of the malleus and the footplate of the stapes covered by the perichondrium. The incus is placed under the handle of malleus very close to the lateral process of the malleus, where the lateral movement of the malleus handle is minimum, thus protecting the stapes footplate from the pressure of unwanted movement of the handle of the malleus, which takes place while cleaning the ear.

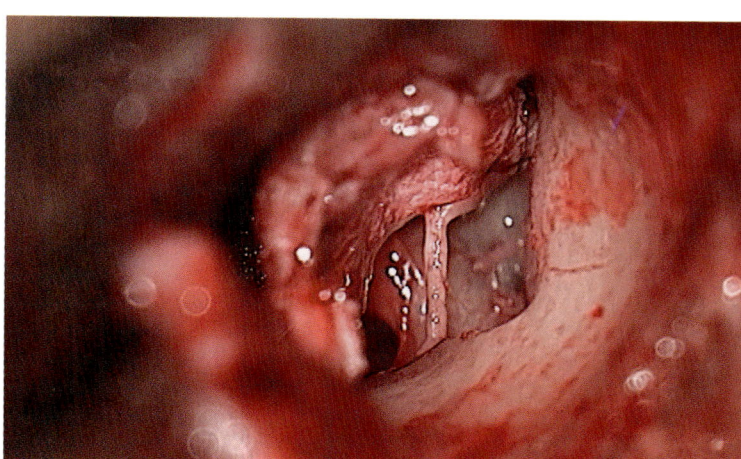

Fig. 26f2   Middle ear is exposed. There is no stapes superstructure, the footplate of the stapes is intact and mobile, the long process of the incus is necrosed, and the malleus is normal.

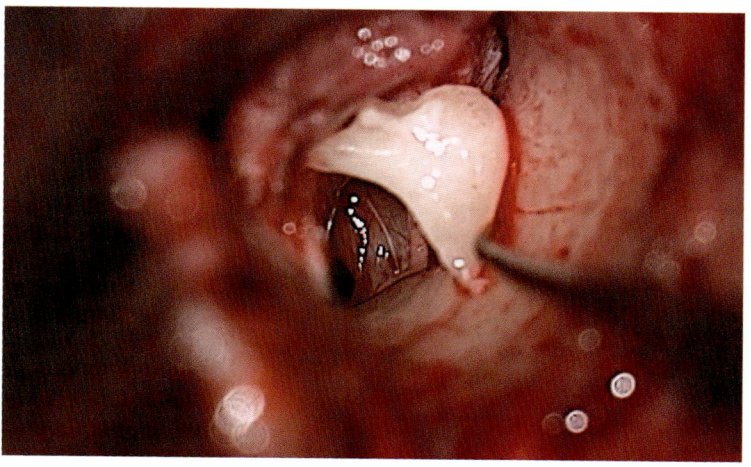

Fig. 26f3   Necrosed incus is taken out.

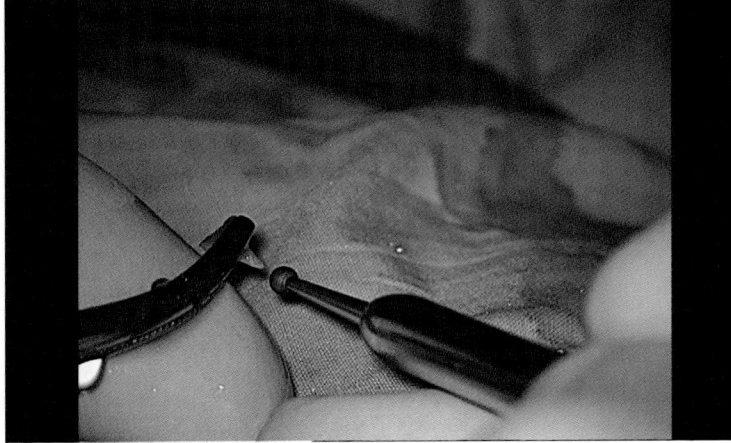

Fig. 26f4   Necrosed incus is taken out to be transposed between the malleus handle and the footplate of the stapes. The distance between the malleus handle and the stapes footplate is measured.

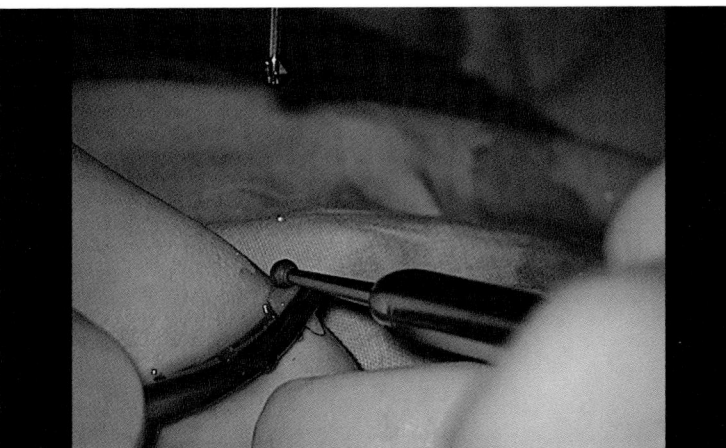

Fig. 26f5   The mallear surface of the incus has been smoothened.

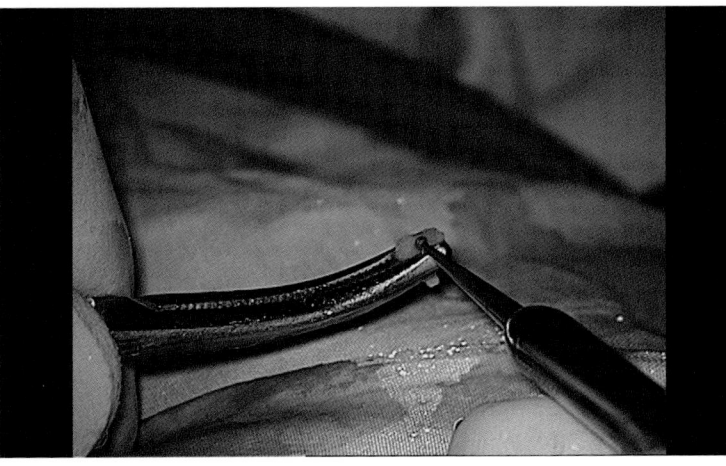

Fig. 26f6   A 1-mm diamond burr is used for making the groove in the body of incus for the malleus handle.

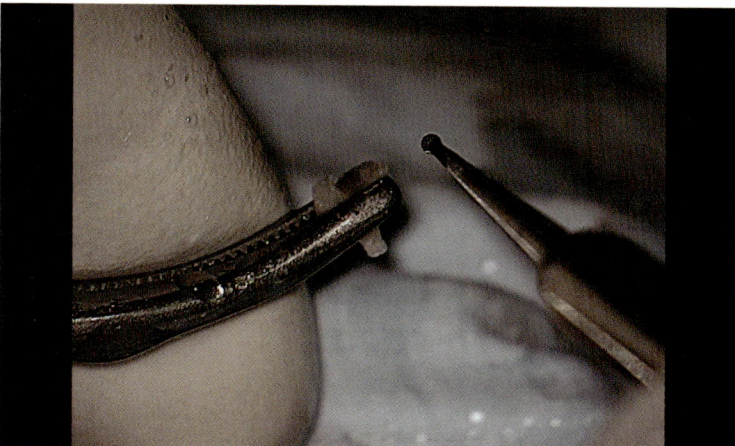

Fig. 26f7 Groove is made on the mallear surface of the incus for the handle of the malleus.

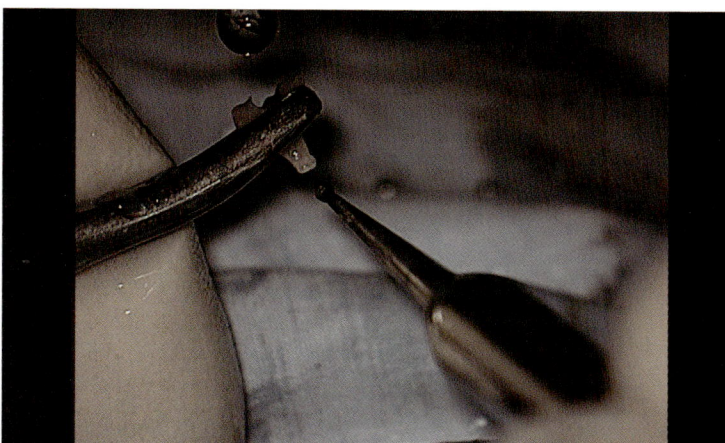

Fig. 26f8 The short process of the incus is smoothened and flattened to be placed over the stapes footplate.

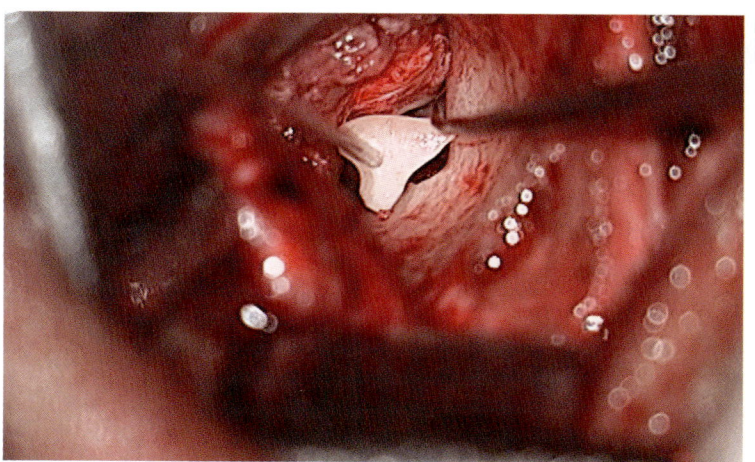

Fig. 26f9 Refashioned incus is placed in the middle ear.

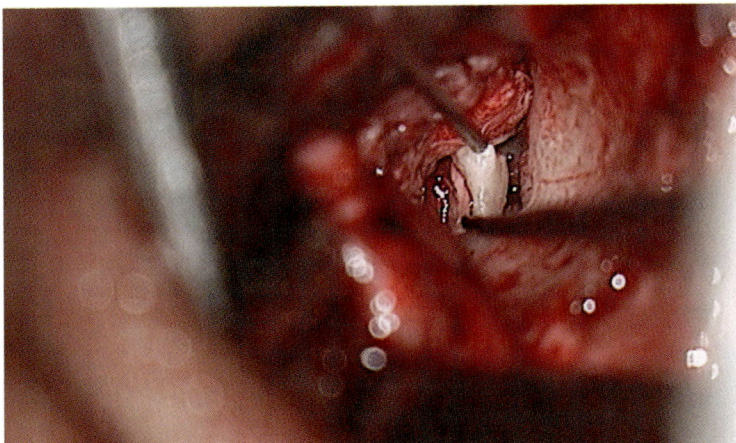

Fig. 26f10 The groove for the malleus is engaged under the handle of the malleus.

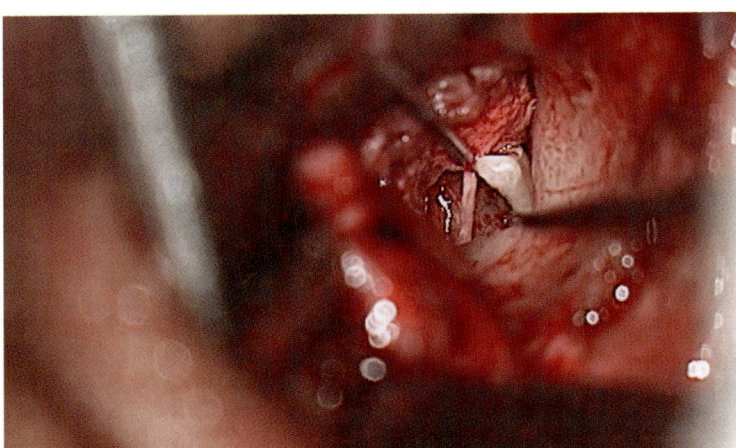

Fig. 26f11 The short process of the incus is placed over the footplate of the stapes.

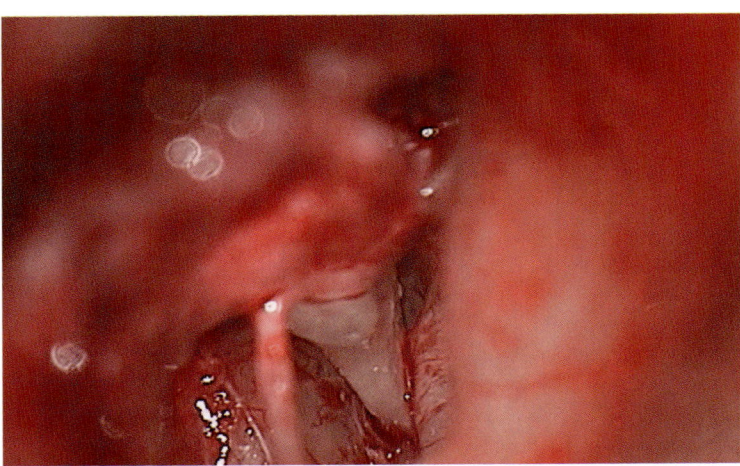

Fig. 26f12 Transposed incus between the handle of the malleus and the footplate of the stapes under higher magnification.

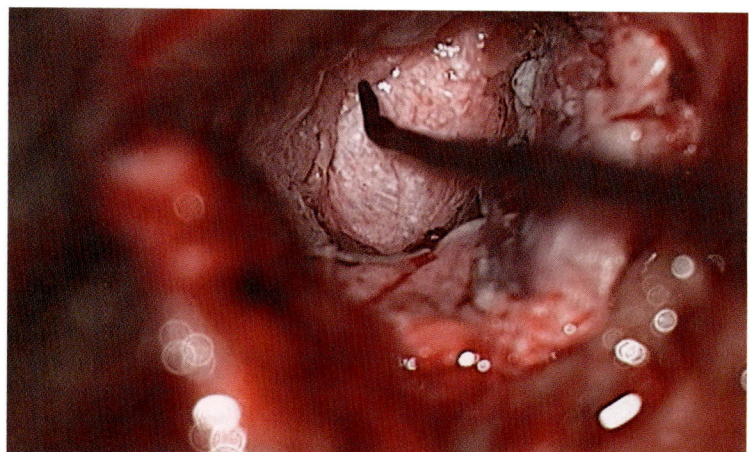

26g: Situation 3 for Ossiculoplasty

In this, there is mobile stapes or footplate. There is no malleus and no incus.

Whenever there is absent malleus or malleus handle, ossiculoplasty results are not good, due to lack of lateral support to the transposed ossicle.

There are various alternatives:

- *Neomalleus*: Here the neomalleus is made by using either the cortical bone or cartilage. This neomalleus gives good lateral support to the ossicle or prosthesis for good hearing improvement.

- *Malleus replacement prosthesis*: This is developed by Dr. Robert Vincent to get good hearing improvement as compared to the reconstruction without the malleus.

Various arrangements commonly practiced are the following:

- TORP is the suitable material (**Fig. 26g1**).

- Titanium prosthesis is equally good (**Fig. 26g2**).

- Autograft ossicle can be used (**Fig. 26g3**).

- The two-cartilage technique is the best here (**Figs. 26g4–26g24**).

The two-cartilage technique, pioneered by Dr. A.B.R. Desai, has the highest success rate as compared to other techniques. There is no chance of any complication with this technique. There is no possibility of any displacement, as the cartilage assembly is very stable. It is very safe as no pressure is exerted over the footplate of the stapes as cartilage is soft and elastic.

Case 1: The two-cartilage technique. Only mobile stapes and no malleus or incus (**Fig. 26g4–26g14**).

Case 2: The two-cartilage technique. Only mobile stapes footplate. There are no stapes superstructure, malleus, or incus (**Fig. 26g15–26g24**).

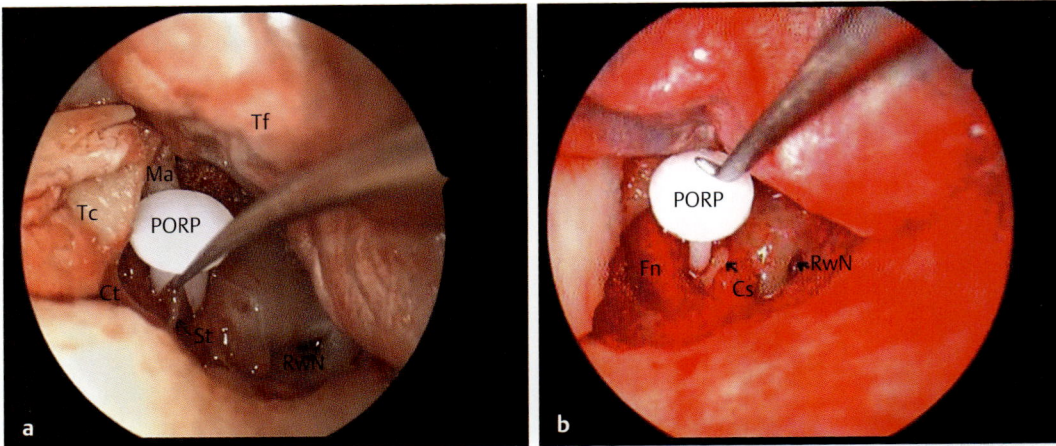

Fig. 26g1 Plastipore **(a)** PORP and **(b)** TORP are comparatively cheaper and popular.

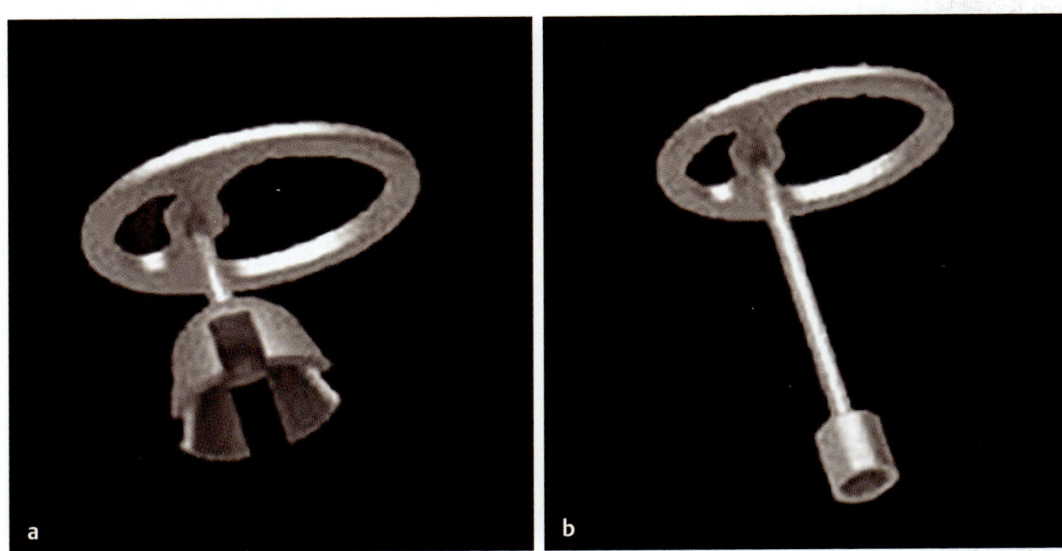

Fig. 26g2 Titanium prosthesis. **(a)** PORP. **(b)** TORP.

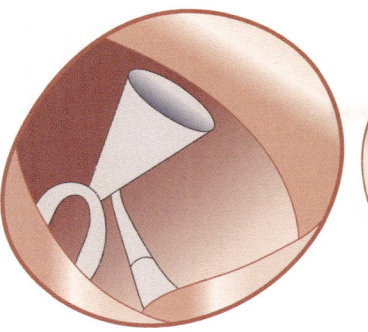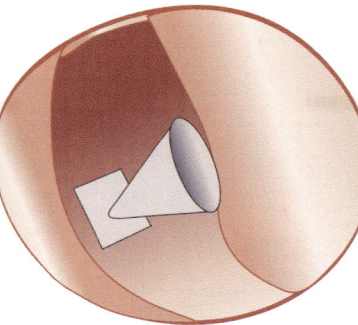

Fig. 26g3 Autograft ossicle is used between the stapes head or the footplate and the tympanic membrane. The footplate is covered by perichondrium.

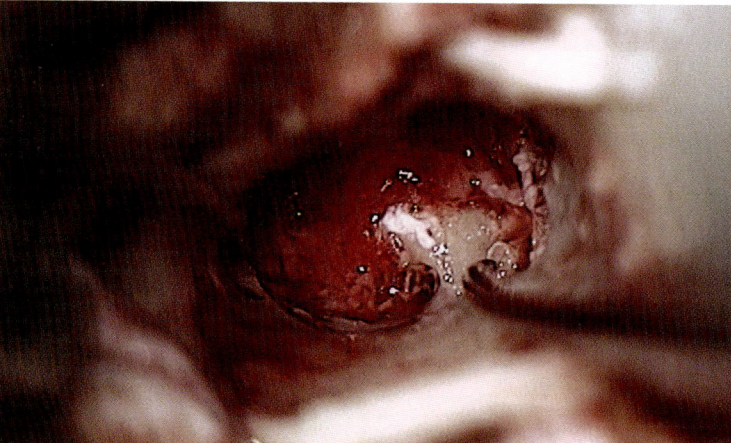

Fig. 26g4 Circumferential (360-degree) tympanomeatal flap has been elevated and taken out as free graft. No malleus or incus; only intact and mobile stapes.

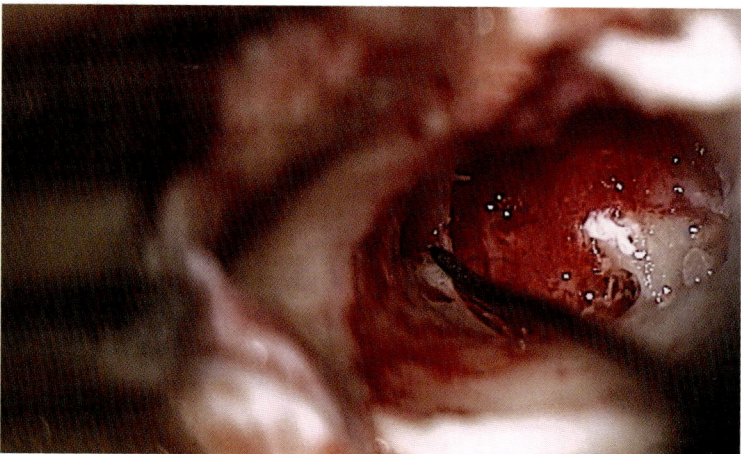

Fig. 26g5 Groove (depression) is made at the level of inferior sulcus for placing the cartilage.

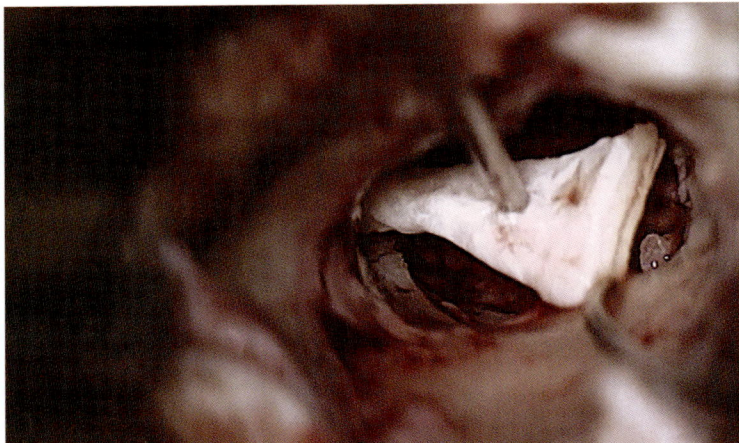

Fig. 26g6 A triangular piece of cartilage is placed lying horizontally in the middle ear touching the stapes head and resting over the groove made at the inferior sulcus.

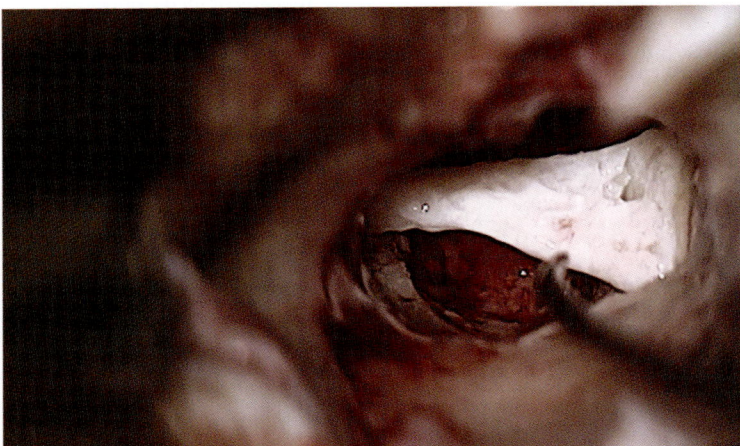

Fig. 26g7 A triangular piece of cartilage is placed horizontally in the middle ear (first cartilage). A small hole is made in this cartilage, in its upper end for placing the second cartilage.

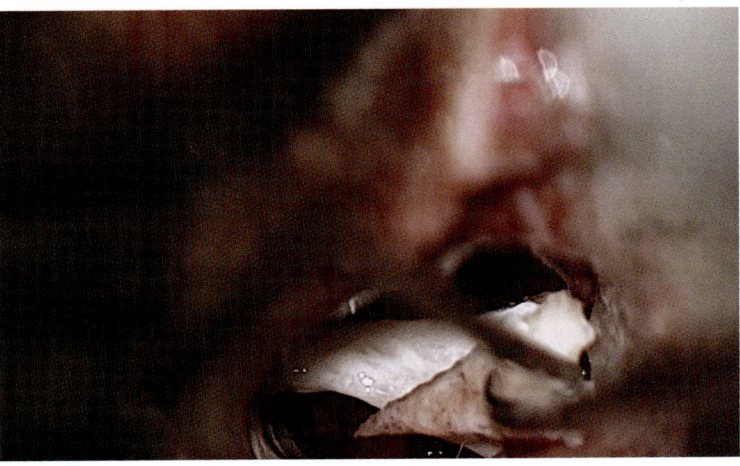

Fig. 26g8 A Y-shaped second cartilage is placed in the middle ear.

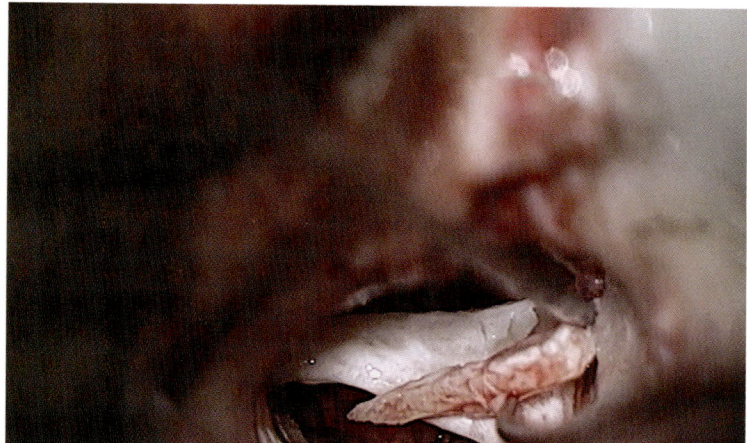

Fig. 26g9 A Y-shaped second cartilage is hooked at the lateral attic wall with its lower end to be engaged into the hole made in the first cartilage.

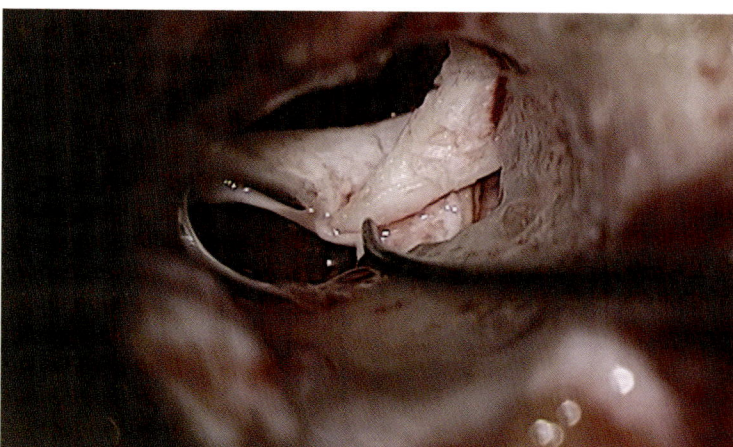

Fig. 26g10 A Y-shaped second cartilage is hooked at the lateral attic wall with its lower end, to be placed into the hole made in the first cartilage.

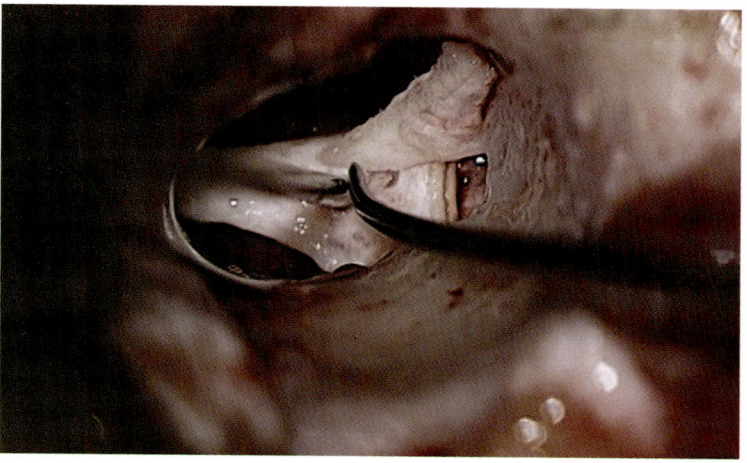

Fig. 26g11 A Y-shaped second cartilage is hooked at the lateral attic wall with its lower end gently slided by a curved pick into the hole made in the first cartilage.

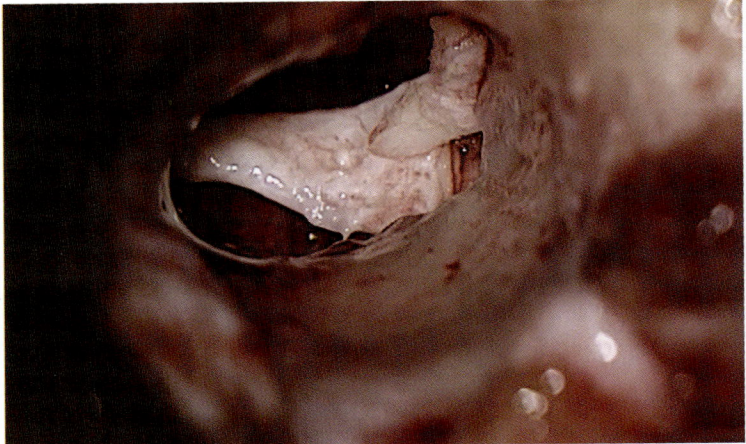

Fig. 26g12 A Y-shaped cartilage is hooked at the lateral attic wall exerting pressure over the first cartilage, hence making good pressure contact between the first cartilage and the stapes head. For this, the Y-shaped cartilage should be of perfect length.

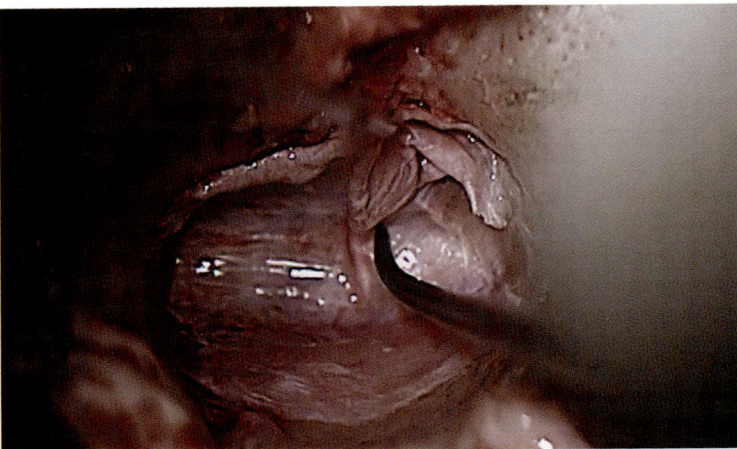

Fig. 26g13 Temporalis fascia graft is placed, lying over the middle ear, touching the cartilage, resting over the meatal wall all around.

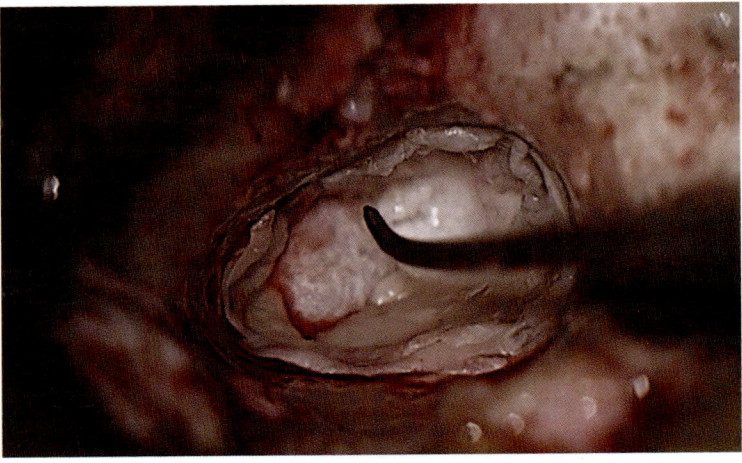

Fig. 26g14 Free tympanomeatal skin flap, which was elevated earlier, is reposited back into its original position. Gelfoam packed. Incision closed.

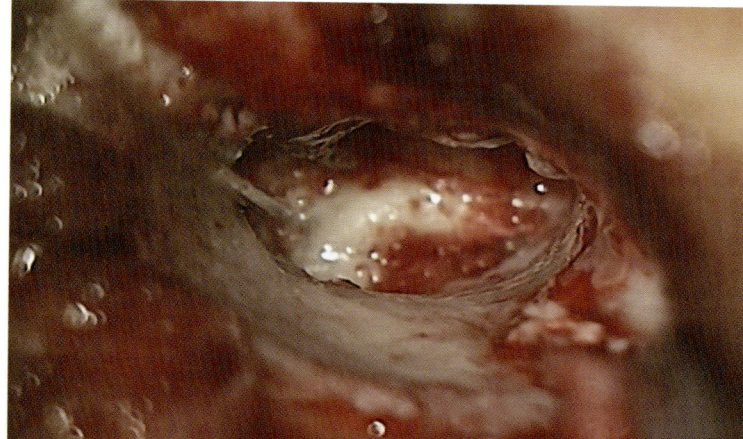

Fig. 26g15   Only stapes footplate; no superstructure, malleus, or incus (tympanomeatal flap has been elevated and taken out as free graft).

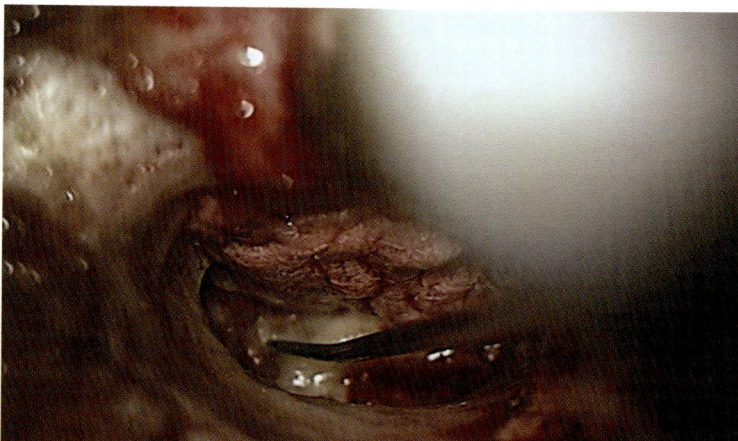

Fig. 26g16   Mobile stapes footplate; no superstructure. Underlay graft has been placed and folded forward with tympanomeatal flap exposing the middle ear.

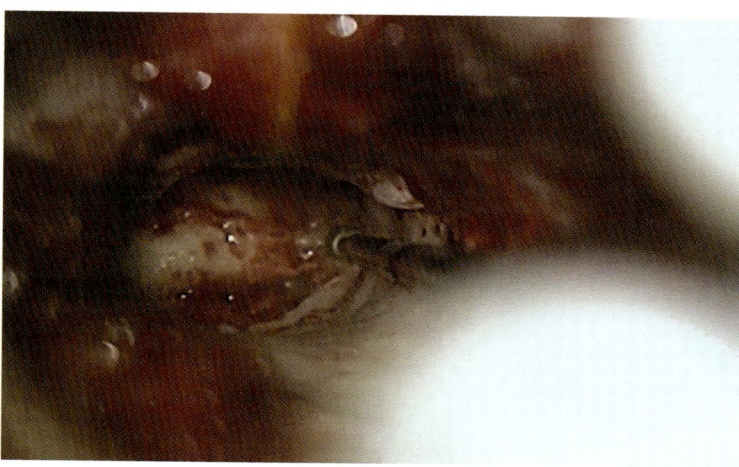

Fig. 26g17   A small groove is made at the hypotympanum by a 1-mm cutting burr.

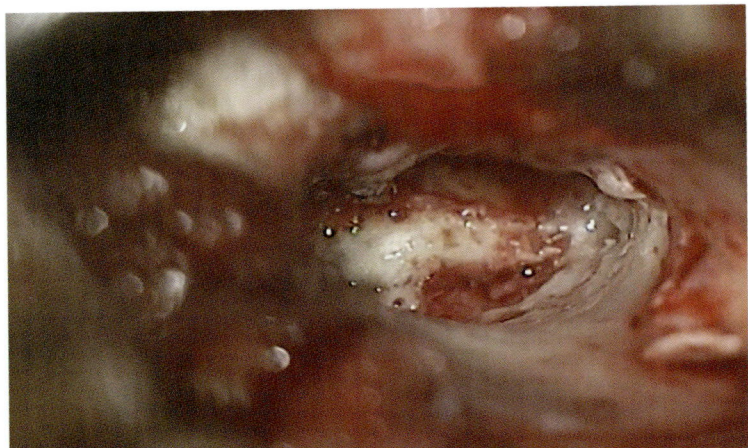

Fig. 26g18 A small groove is been made in the hypotympanum for placement of the cartilage.

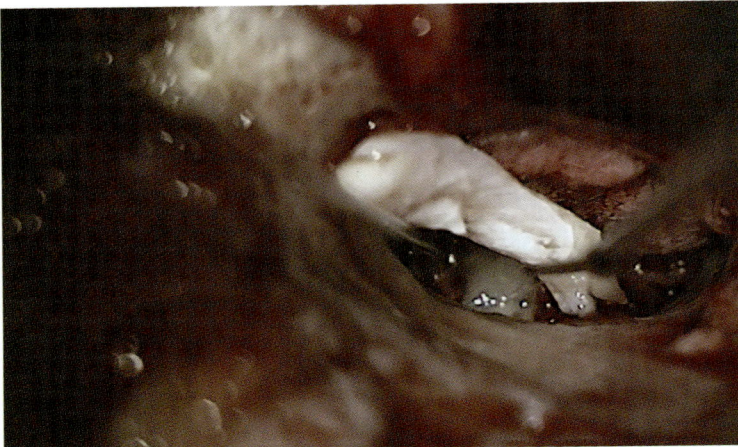

Fig. 26g19 A spindle-shaped cartilage is placed in the middle ear with its lower end into the groove in the hypotympanum.

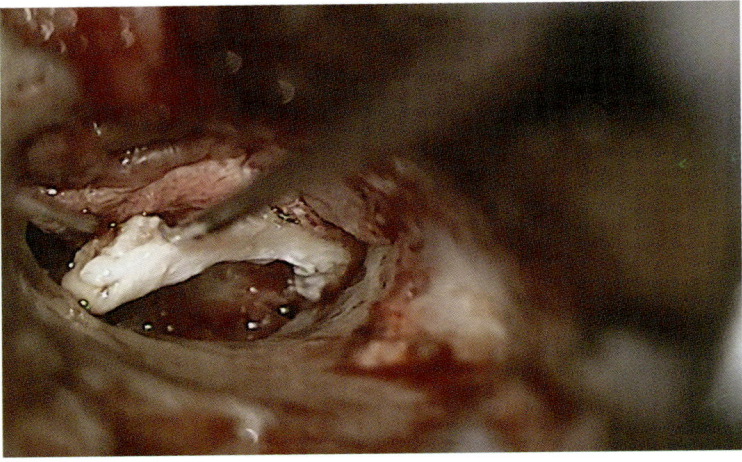

Fig. 26g20 A spindle-shaped cartilage is placed in the middle ear, with its lower end into the groove in the hypotympanum, arching over the promontory with its upper end to be placed over the stapes footplate.

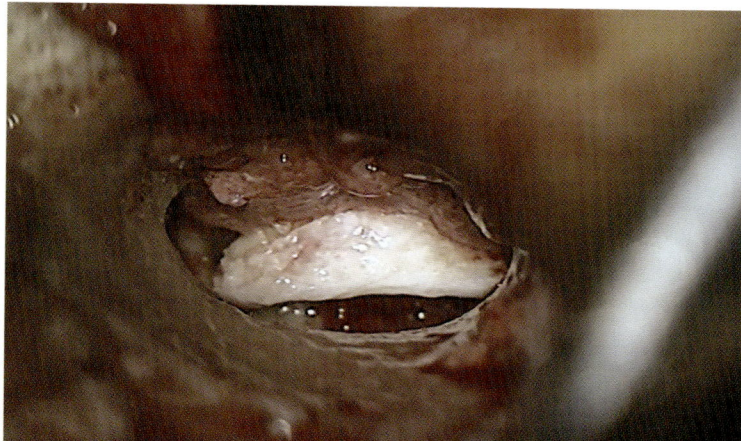

Fig. 26g21 Cartilage is arching over the tympanic cavity, with its lower end into the hypotympanum and upper end placed over the stapes footplate. Cartilage has a hole near its upper end.

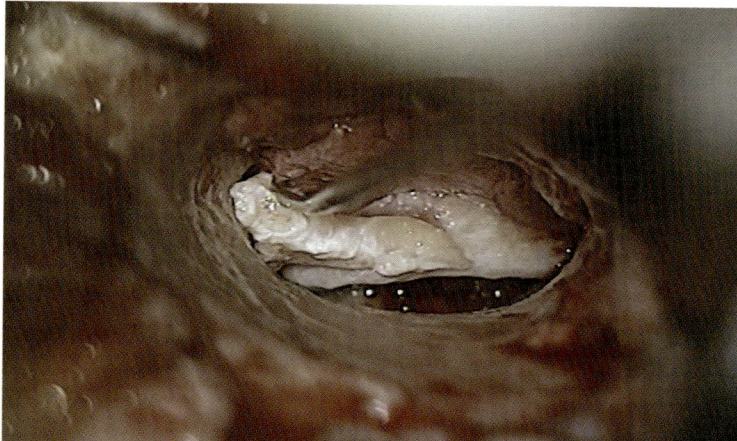

Fig. 26g22 The Y-shaped cartilage is placed in the middle ear. Its upper end is hooked at the lateral attic wall with its lower end to be placed into the hole made in the first cartilage.

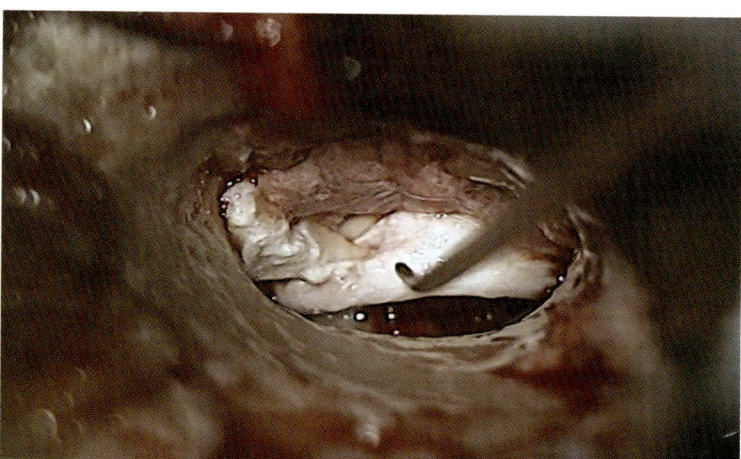

Fig. 26g23 A Y-shaped cartilage is hooked at the lateral attic wall with its lower end tip placed into the hole made in the first cartilage. The Y-shaped cartilage should be of perfect length to exert gentle pressure over the first cartilage to maintain good pressure contact between the first cartilage and the stapes footplate.

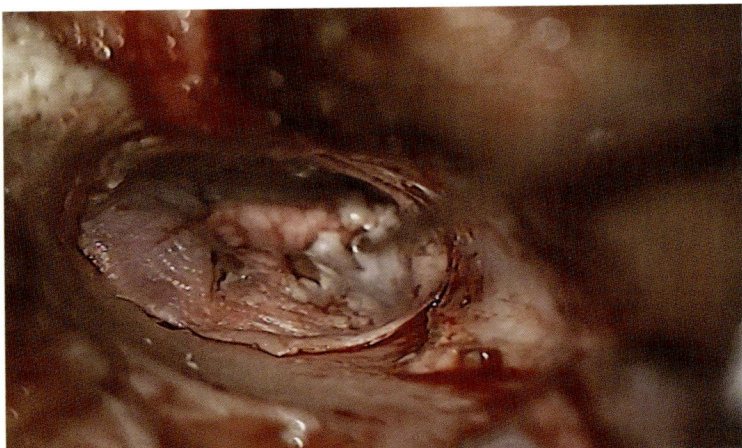

Fig. 26g24   Underlay graft with tympanomeatal flap is reposited back. Gelfoam is packed and the incision is closed.

26h: Ossiculoplasty in Canal Wall Down Surgery

Cholesteatoma is removed from the middle ear either by intact canal wall technique or by canal wall down technique. In the intact canal wall technique, the ossicular reconstruction is easier and effective as the normal anatomy of the middle and external ear is preserved or restored. In the canal wall down technique, the ossicular reconstruction is difficult as the posterosuperior bony canal wall has been removed and normal anatomy of the external and middle ear is lost.

In the canal wall down technique, in addition to dry ear, good hearing improvement can be achieved by creating a neotympanum in which the small tympanic cavity is reconstructed by cartilage. This neotympanum is covered by cartilage and fascia. This neotympanum is ventilated by the eustachian tube anteriorly leaving the mastoid cavity draining into the external auditory canal by meatoplasty (**Fig. 26h1–26h12**).

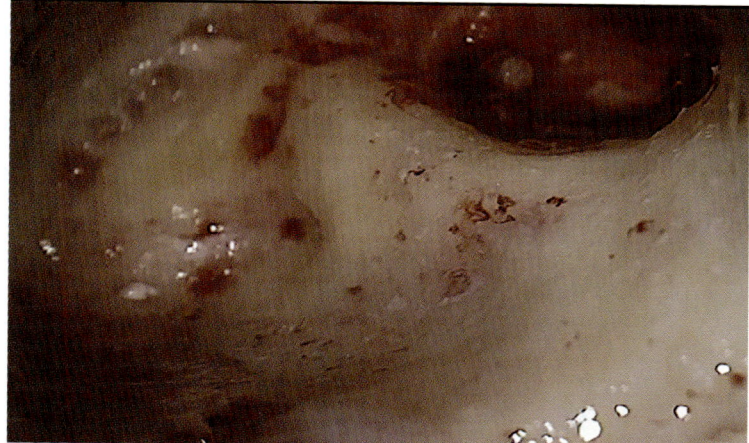

Fig. 26h1   Canal wall down mastoidectomy has been performed for cholesteatoma. The malleus and incus invaded by the cholesteatoma are removed. The stapes is intact and mobile.

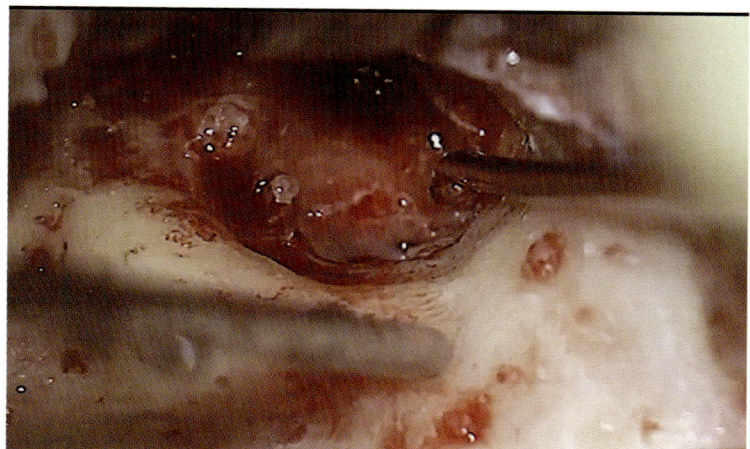

Fig. 26h2   Tympanic cavity is healthy with patent eustachian tube with mobile stapes.

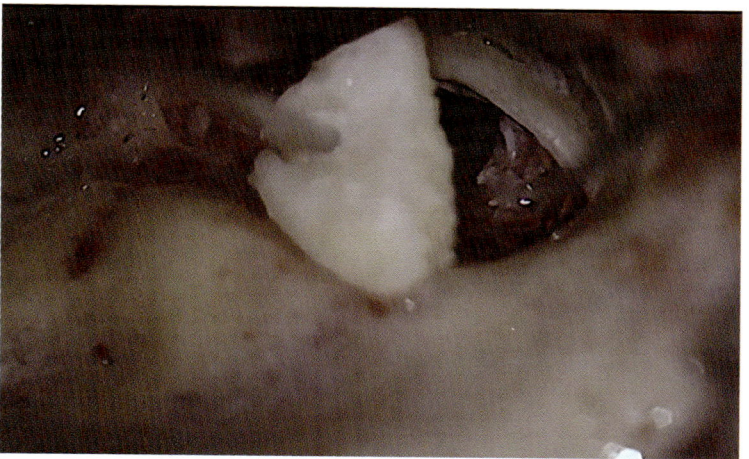

Fig. 26h3   Cartilage pieces from the concha are used to create neotympanum.

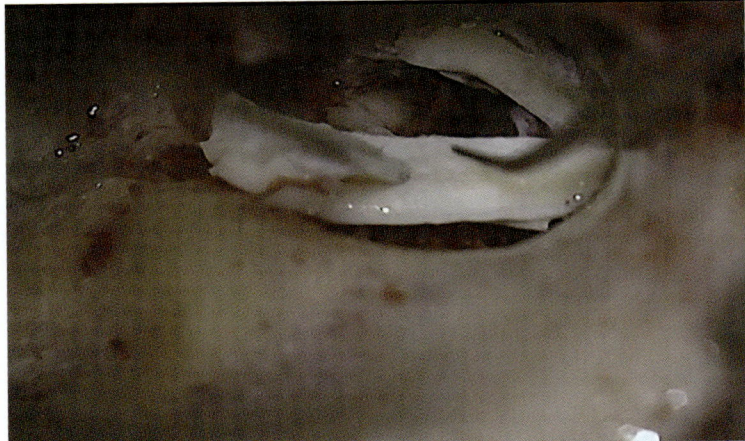

Fig. 26h4 Cartilage piece lying horizontally over the tympanic cavity, resting over the groove made at the level of the inferior sulcus touching the stapes head (columella effect).

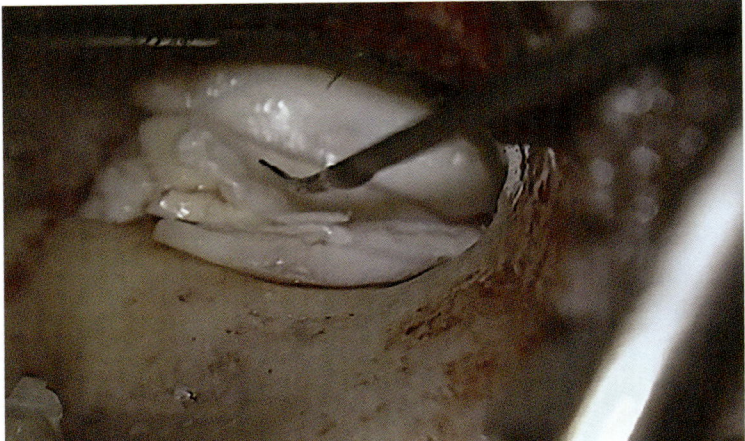

Fig. 26h5 Multiple cartilage pieces are kept horizontally, covering the tympanic cavity, resting inferiorly over the groove made at the level of the inferior sulcus with neotympanum medially with an air space communicating with the eustachian tube. This horizontal cartilage is touching the stapes head giving good improvement in hearing (columella effect).

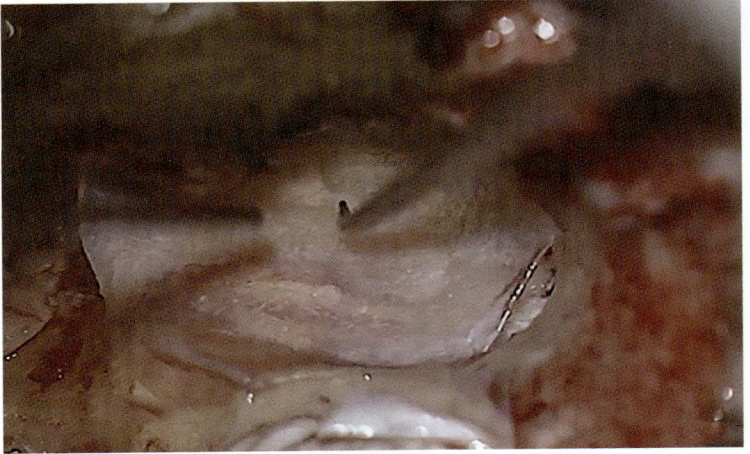

Fig. 26h6 Cartilage is covered by the fascia.

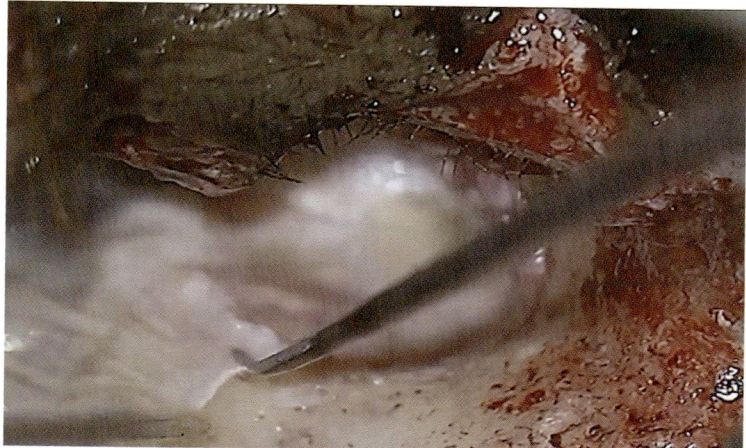

Fig. 26h7   Big fascia is used to cover the tympanic cavity and mastoid cavity.

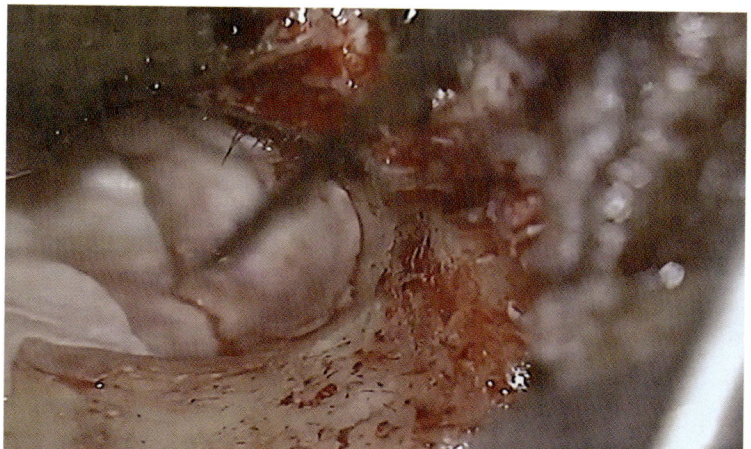

Fig. 26h8   Skin is reposited back over the fascia and the meatal wall.

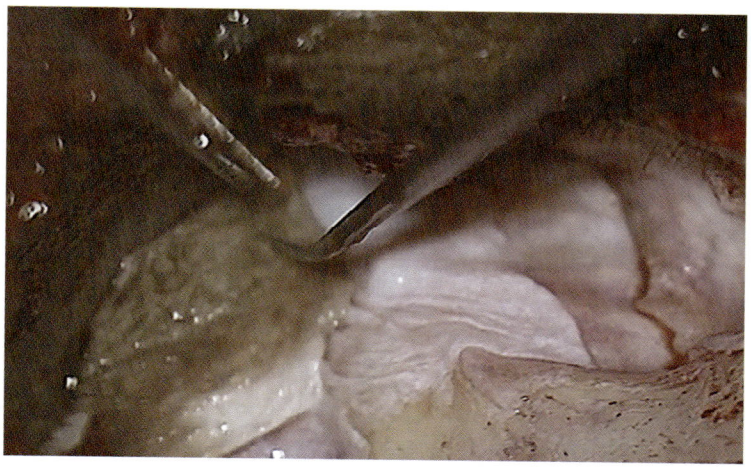

Fig. 26h9   Skin is used to cover the mastoid cavity for fast epithelialization.

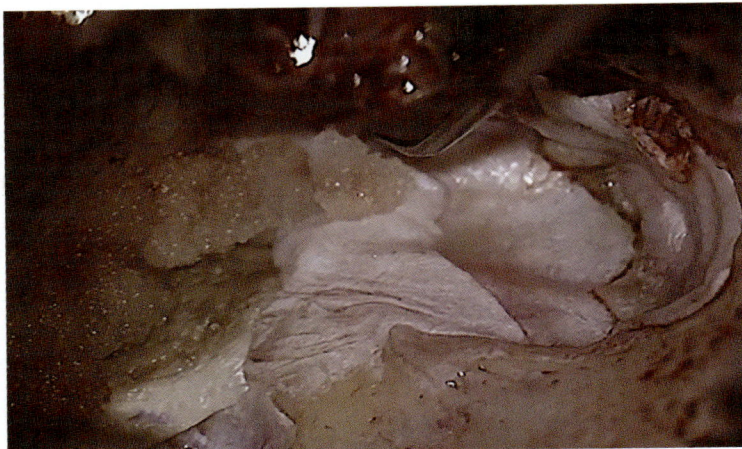

Fig. 26h10 Mastoid cavity is packed by Gelfoam.

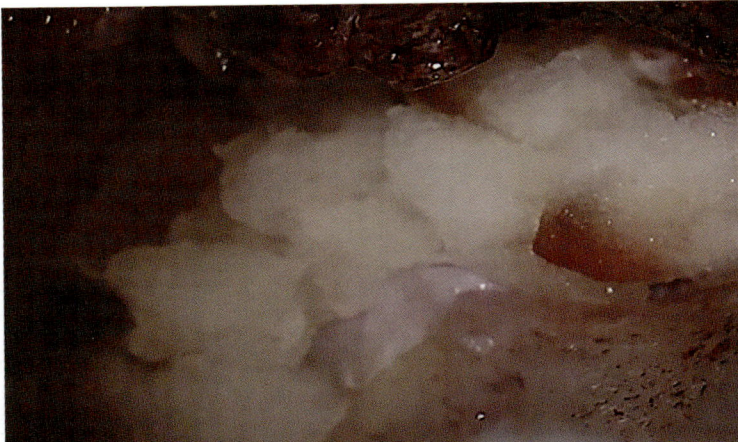

Fig. 26h11 Mastoid cavity is packed by Gelfoam and the incision is closed.

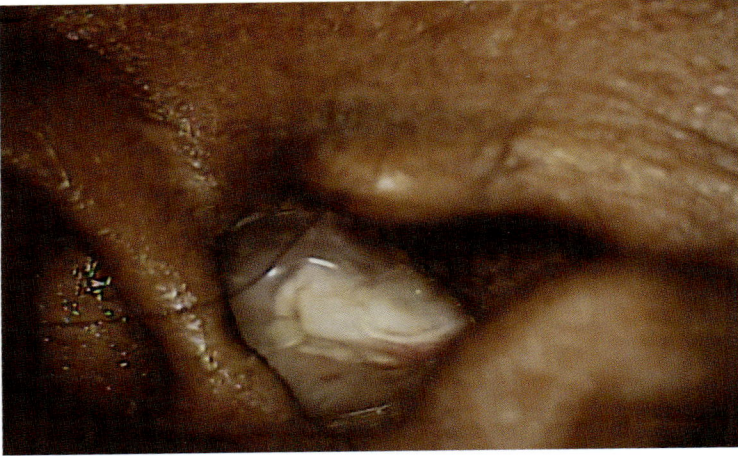

Fig. 26h12 After 6 months. Nicely healed and dry mastoid cavity with the neotympanum made by the cartilage with an adequate meatoplasty. Good improvement in the hearing as the cartilage is touching the stapes head and giving good columella effect.

26i: Tympanoplasty with Canal Wall Reconstruction in Patients with Cholesteatoma

Cholesteatoma removal by the canal wall down technique is the most popular technique, but it is followed by open cavity problems with not much successful ossiculoplasty. Hence, removal of cholesteatoma by the canal wall down technique followed by reconstruction of the canal wall and ossicular chain by cartilage is the most useful technique. It gives a dry, disease-free ear with near normal hearing with no cavity problems. The only care to be taken is to preserve as much as bony canal wall as possible while removing the cholesteatoma, which helps in reconstruction (**Fig. 26i1–26i29**).

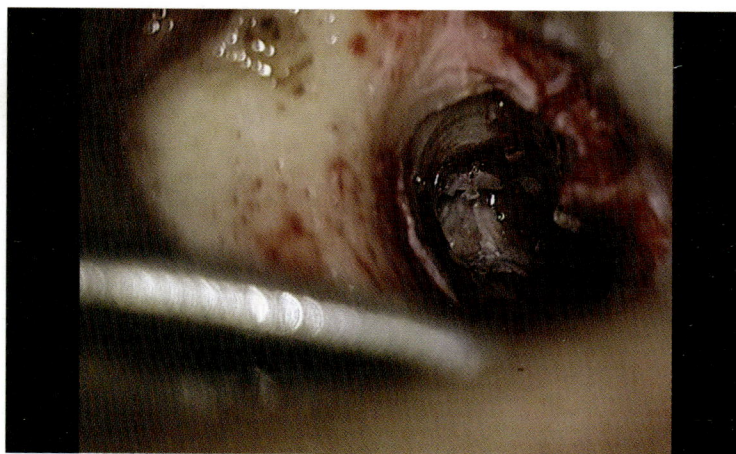

Fig. 26i1 Cholesteatoma, endaural incision, and posterior and superior meatal wall skin is excised, taken out as free graft.

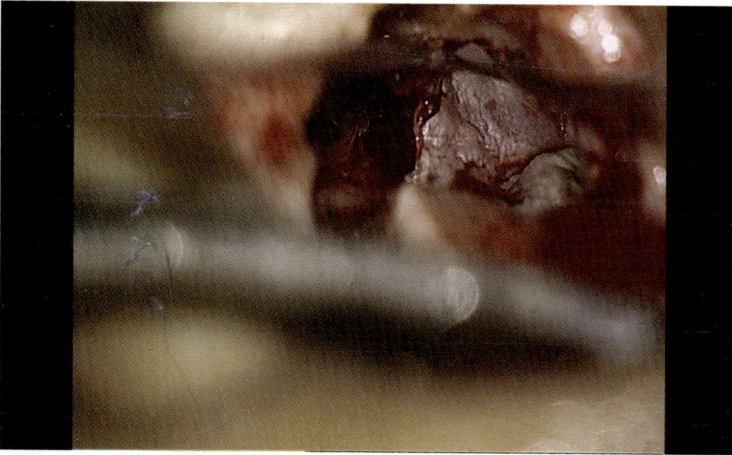

Fig. 26i2 Cholesteatoma has been removed after removing the posterosuperior bony canal wall (atticoantral mastoidectomy is done). Attempt is made to preserve the posterior canal wall as much as possible, which helps during reconstruction. Healthy tympanic membrane is seen.

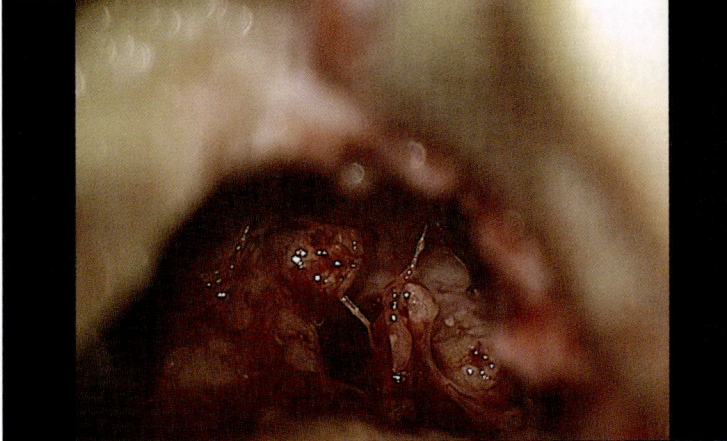

Fig. 26i3 Cholesteatoma has been removed, and the malleus and incus are removed as they are eroded by the cholesteatoma. Tympanomeatal flap has been reflected forward exposing the healthy tympanic cavity with intact and mobile stapes.

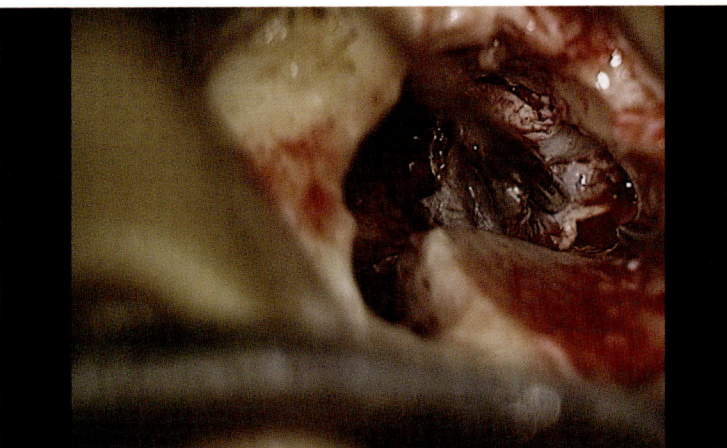

Fig. 26i4 Tympanomeatal flap has been elevated inferiorly.

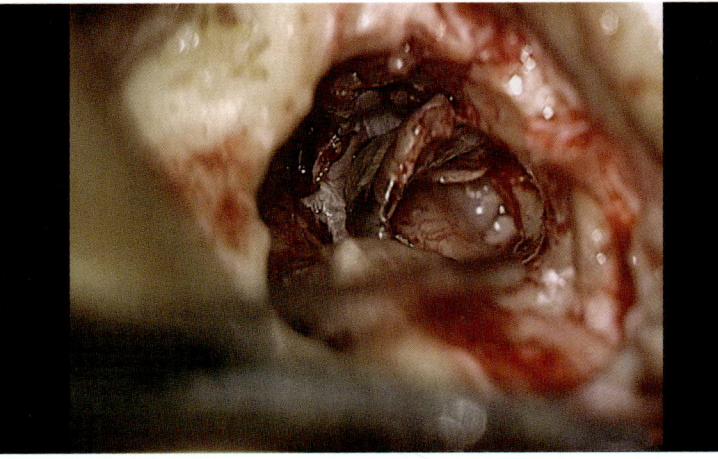

Fig. 26i5 Posterior and inferior tympanomeatal flap has been elevated for placement of the underlay graft. Inferior bony meatal wall and inferior part of the tympanic cavity are exposed.

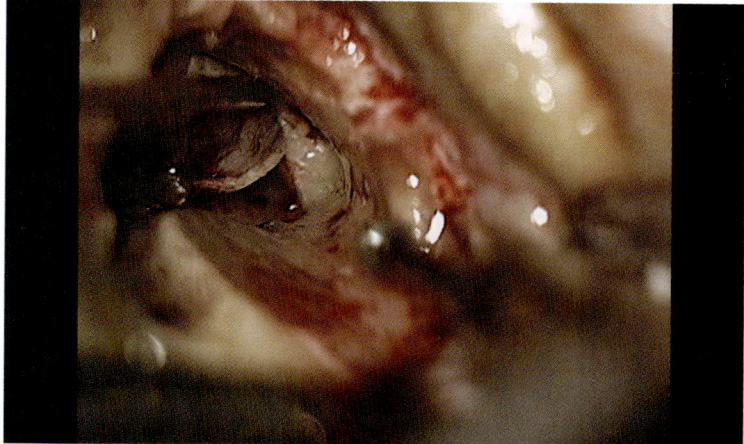

Fig. 26i6   A depression is made at the inferior sulcus for placement of the cartilage.

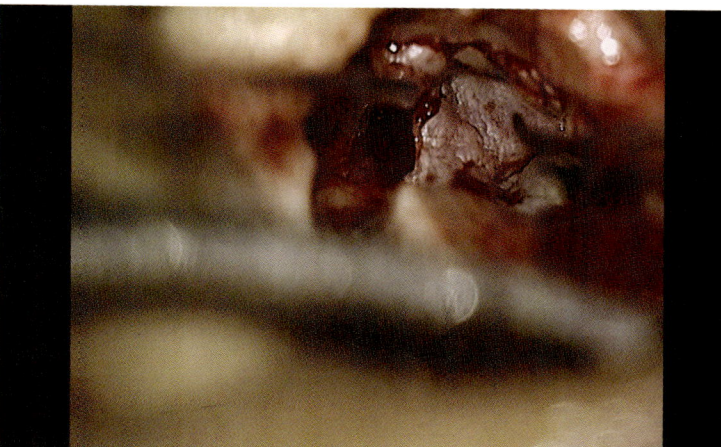

Fig. 26i7   Inferior tympanomeatal flap is reposited back.

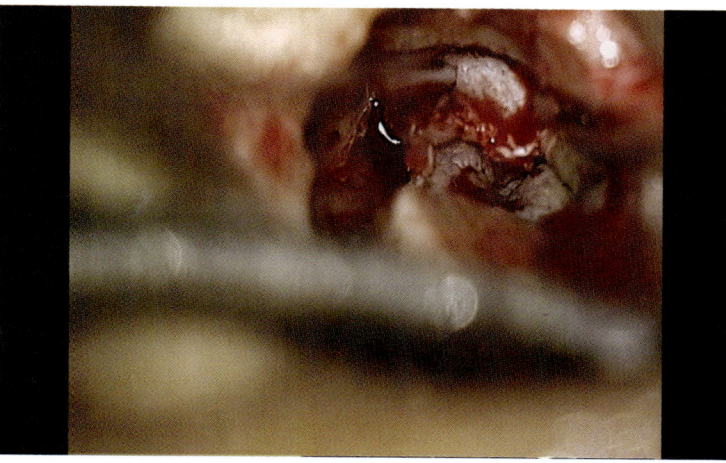

Fig. 26i8   Anterior meatal wall skin is elevated.

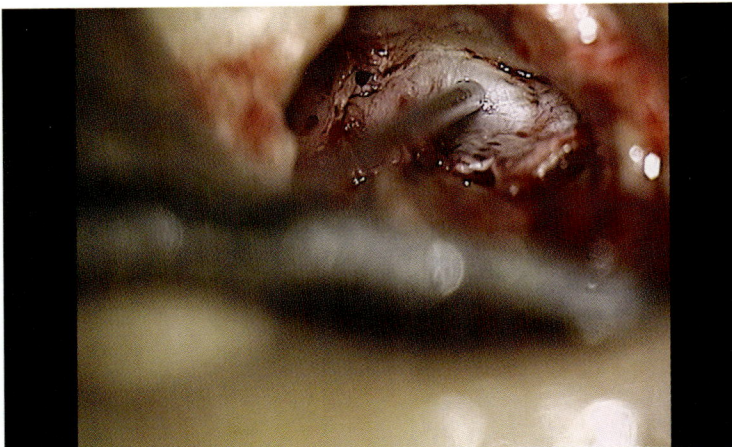

Fig. 26i9   Anterior meatal wall skin is elevated up to the annulus.

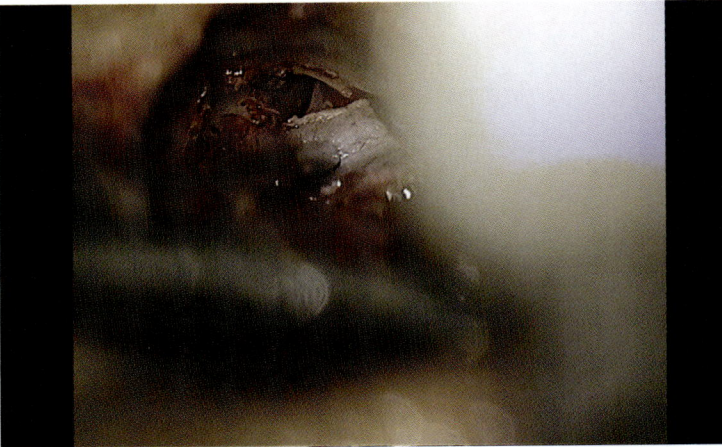

Fig. 26i10   Anterior tympanomeatal flap is elevated for anterior placement of the underlay graft. The annulus is elevated from the sulcus, thus exposing the eustachian tube opening, which is healthy.

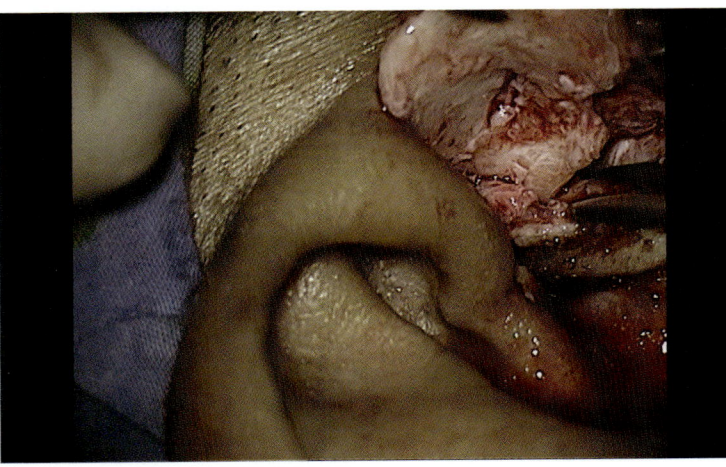

Fig. 26i11   A big piece of cartilage is removed from the tragus from the same endaural incision, for reconstruction of the canal wall and ossicle.

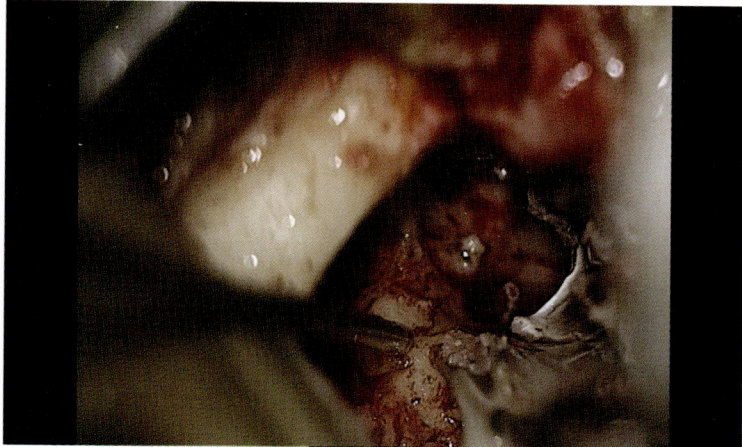

Fig. 26i12 A groove is made in the posterior bony meatal wall for placement of the cartilage for meatal wall reconstruction.

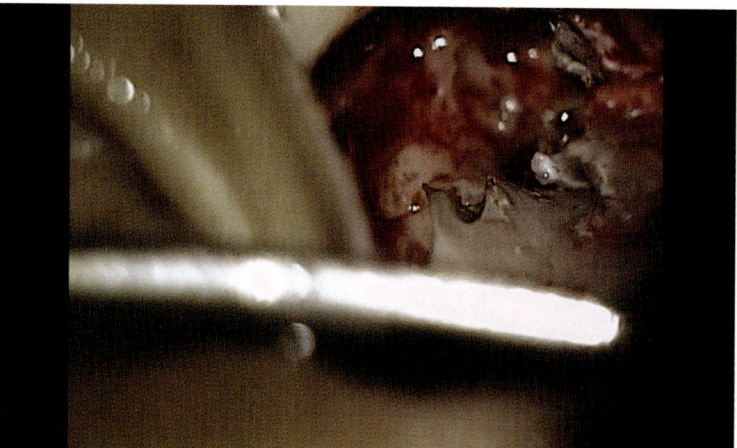

Fig. 26i13 The depth of the groove in the posterior bony meatal wall is increased.

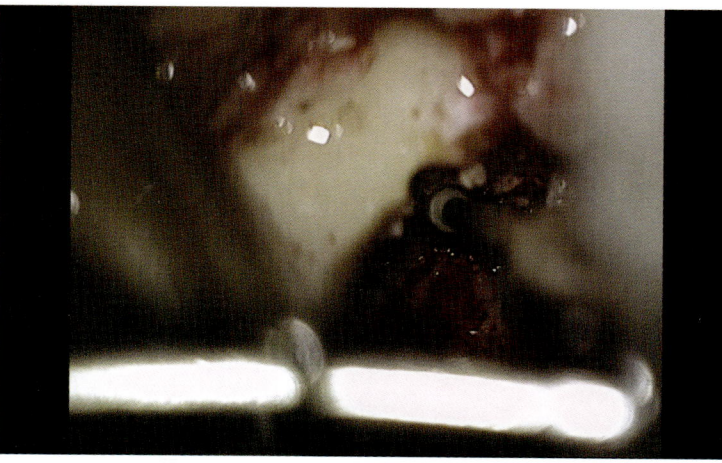

Fig. 26i14 Parallel groove is made on the anterior bony meatal wall for placement of the cartilage for meatal wall reconstruction.

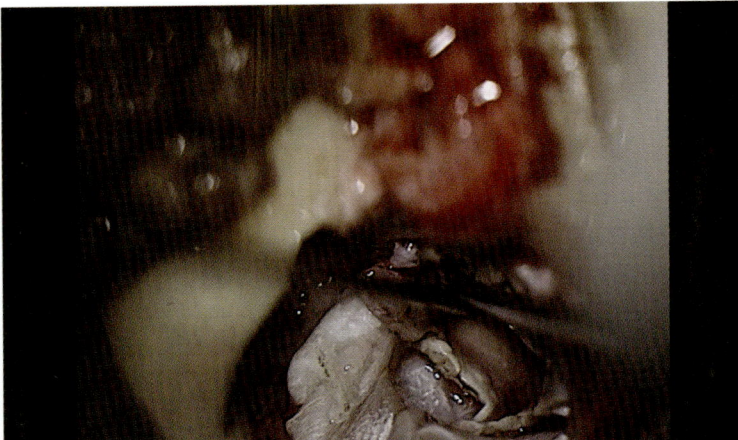

Fig. 26i15 Underlay graft has been placed under the tympanic membrane, supported by anterior and posterior bony meatal wall.

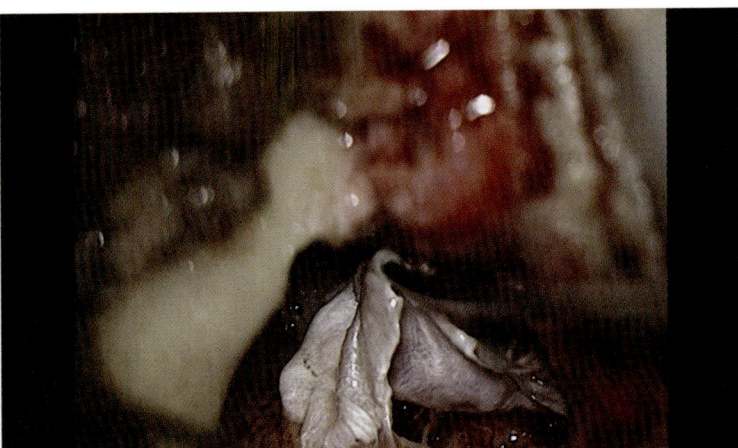

Fig. 26i16 Underlay graft with posterior tympanomeatal flap is lifted up for placement of the cartilage columella in the middle ear.

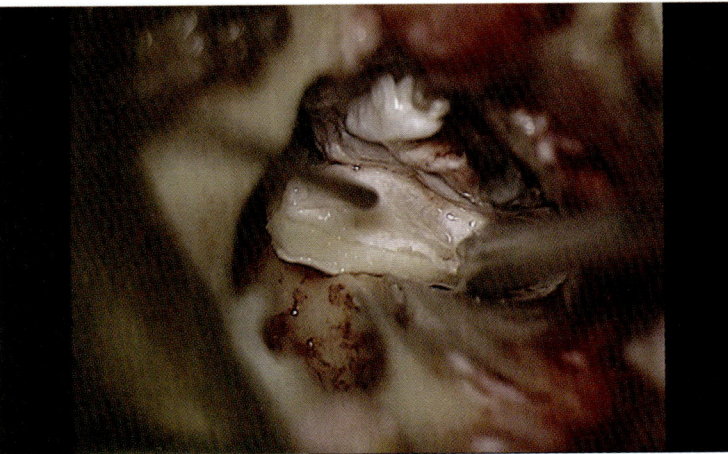

Fig. 26i17 A triangular piece of cartilage is placed in the middle ear horizontally with its lower end resting over the groove made at the inferior sulcus and the upper end touching the stapes head, resting over it and maintaining the middle ear space medial to it. This cartilage acts as a columella with tympanic membrane resting over it (ossiculoplasty).

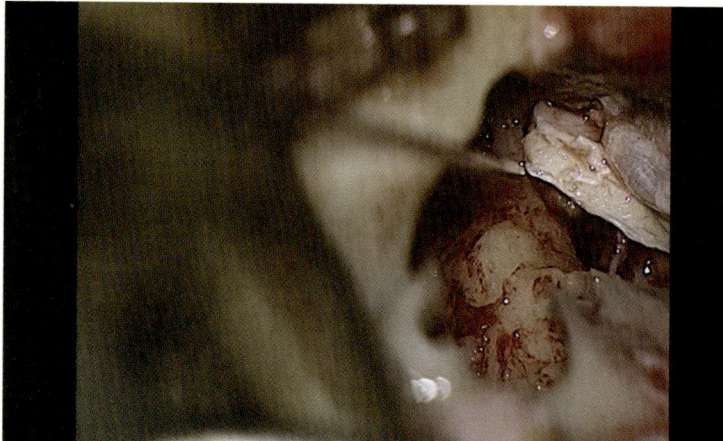

Fig. 26i18 The cartilage acts as a columella touching the stapes head with tympanic membrane resting over it (ossiculoplasty). The middle ear space is maintained medial to the cartilage.

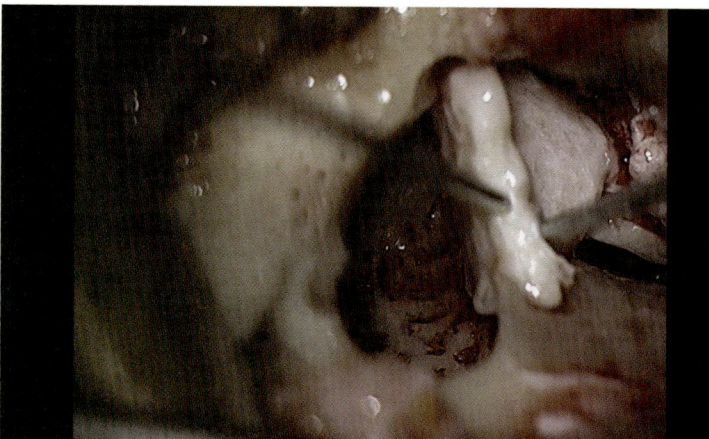

Fig. 26i19 The distance between the grooves on the anterior and posterior bony meatal wall is measured and a proper size cartilage piece is fixed between these two grooves, with its medial end touching and resting over the first cartilage and exerting very gentle pressure over the first cartilage to maintain good pressure contact between the stapes head and the first cartilage, creating a very effective columella.

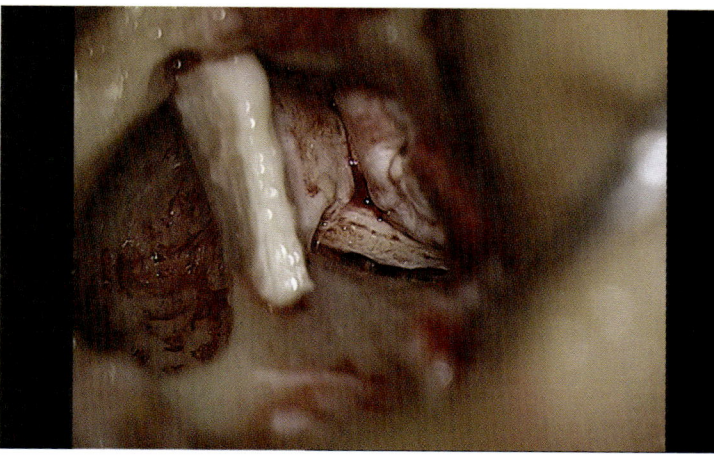

Fig. 26i20 The medial end of the second cartilage is touching and resting over the first cartilage. It is exerting very gentle pressure over the first cartilage to maintain good pressure contact between the stapes head and the first cartilage, creating a very effective columella. This second cartilage is reconstructing the canal wall, hence separating the tympanic cavity from the mastoid cavity. Normal anatomy of the middle ear cleft is achieved.

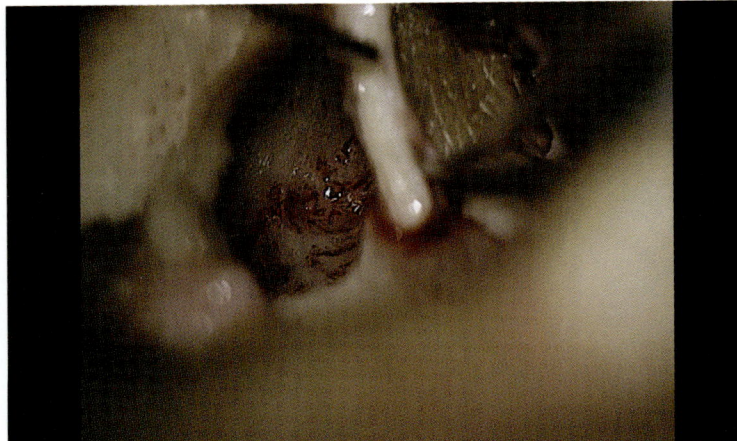

Fig. 26i21   Graft is reposited back. The external auditory canal is lined by the free full-thickness skin graft taken from the postaural region for fast epithelialization of the canal.

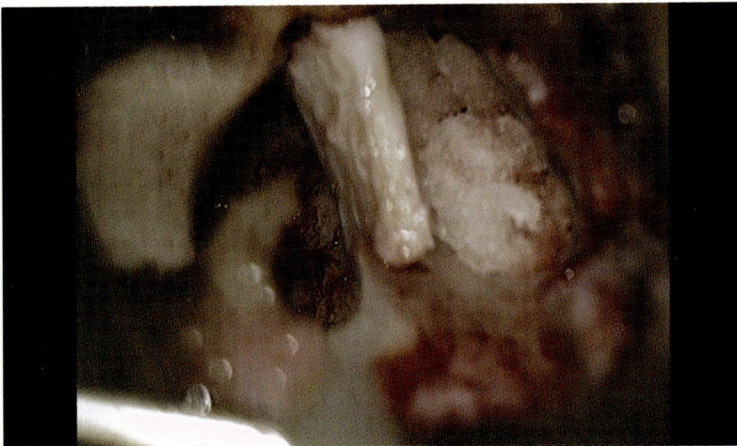

Fig. 26i22   The external auditory canal is packed by Gelfoam.

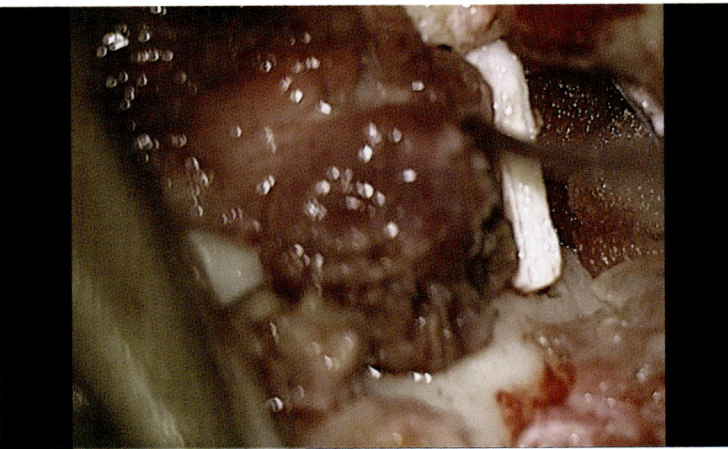

Fig. 26i23   The mastoid is covered by the periosteal and pedicled temporalis muscle flap.

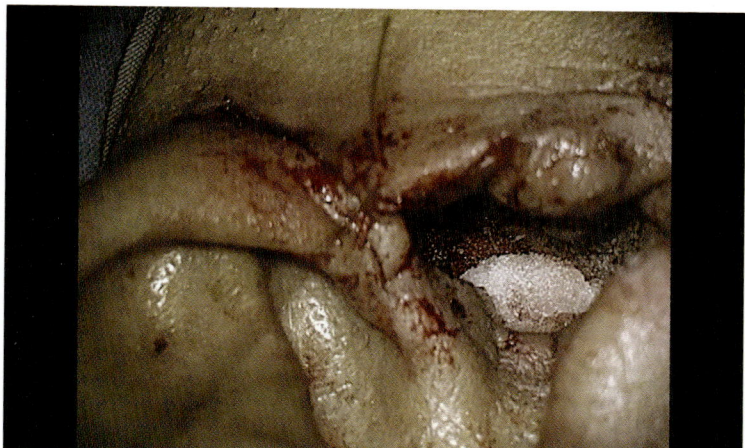

Fig. 26i24 Endaural incision is closed.

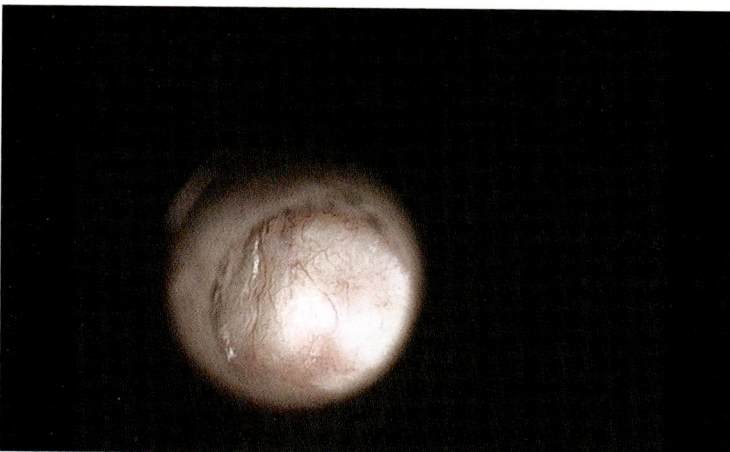

Fig. 26i25 Six months after surgery. Nicely healed external auditory canal and tympanic membrane.

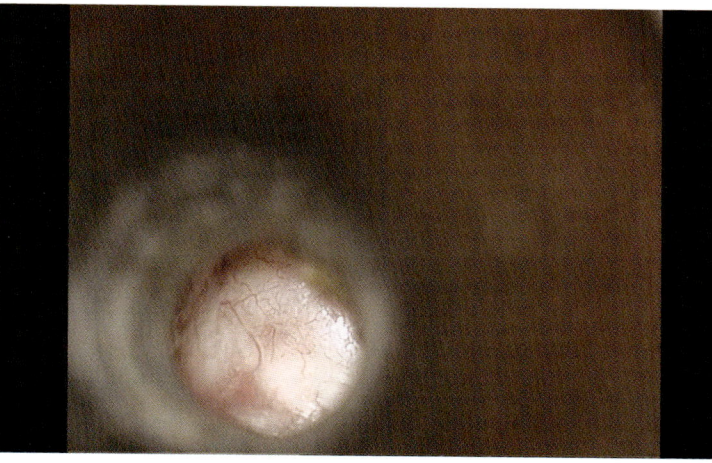

Fig. 26i26 Tympanic membrane is touching the cartilage, which is lying horizontally in the middle ear touching the stapes head (columella effect) with good improvement in hearing. The middle ear space is well maintained.

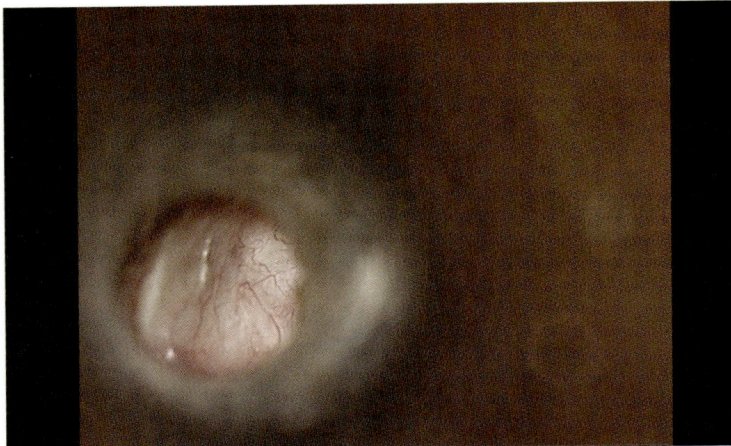

Fig. 26i27 Tragal cartilage is seen, which is used for the canal wall reconstruction after removal of cholesteatoma.

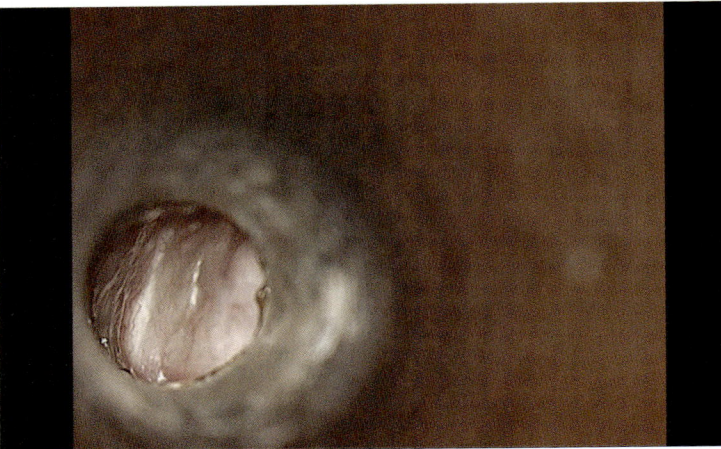

Fig. 26i28 The canal wall defect is closed and the external auditory canal is nicely healed and well epithelialized.

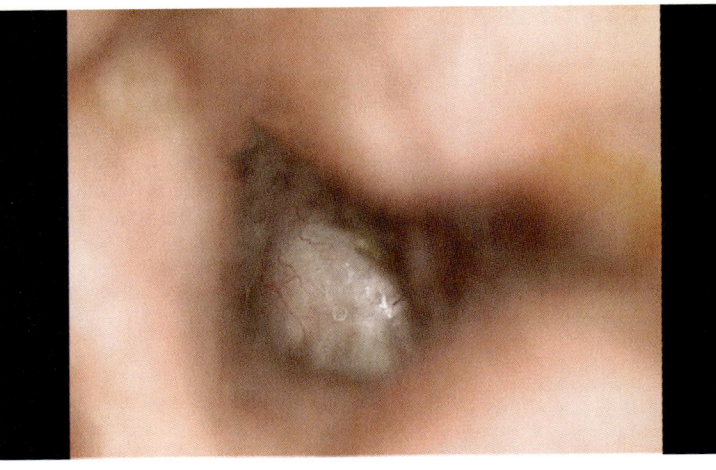

Fig. 26i29 Well-reconstructed external auditory canal.

26j: Tympanoplasty in Atelectatic Middle Ear

Middle ear atelectasis occurs due to reduction in the volume of the middle ear because of eustachian tube block followed by absorption of air from the middle ear causing retraction of the tympanic membrane medially. The tympanic membrane becomes very thin and atrophic with loss of the middle fibrous layer of the pars tensa.

Various causes of eustachian tube dysfunction are the following:

- Infection: nose and sinus infection.
- Allergy: Nasal allergy causing edematous nasal mucosa, hypertrophied inferior turbinate, nasal polypi, all blocking the eustachian tube opening.
- Mechanical: Adenoids are the most common cause of mechanical eustachian tube obstruction. Any mass in the nasopharynx can cause eustachian tube block.
- Congenital.
- Iatrogenic.

Classification

Depending upon the site of retraction, it is classified into the following:

- Retraction of the pars tensa.
- Retraction of the pars flaccida.

Retraction of the pars flaccida is more common than that of the pars tensa as the former has got less collagenous support and hence is more prone to retraction.
Sade's classification:

- Grade 1: The eardrum is retracted but not touching the middle ear structure.

- Grade 2: The eardrum is retracted and touches the incus or stapes.
- Grade 3: The eardrum retraction progresses further and touches the promontory. It may just touch the promontory or it may get adherent to the promontory.
- Grade 4: The eardrum is retracted around the edge of the scutum and all aspects of the drum is not seen.

Treatment

Medical or surgical treatment depends upon the following:

- Atelectatic grade of the tympanic membrane.
- Whether the pathology is progressive or stable.

Better results are obtained in patients diagnosed early than those with more advanced disease. In general, it is found that patients with grade 3 and 4 atelectasis are associated with ossicular chain erosion with conductive hearing loss. These bigger atelectatic pockets are associated with secondary infection with recurrent otorrhea. This conductive deafness and otorrhea require surgery and there is no conservative treatment for this.

The surgery is to exteriorize the atelectatic tympanic membrane first by canalplasty and then elevate the atelectatic tympanic membrane by dissecting and separating it from the promontory and ossicular chain. Then cartilage tympanoplasty with ossicular chain reconstruction is performed to prevent recurrence.

This ossicular chain reconstruction can be done either as first-stage surgery or as a second-stage surgery depending upon the status of the middle ear mucosa. The cartilage tympanoplasty is very effective to prevent future retraction pockets and there is no possibility of adhesion between the tympanic membrane and the promontory so that the middle ear space is well maintained.

Treatment in Grade 1 and 2 Patients

- Keep them under observation.

- Decongestants, both oral and nasal, should be tried for a short time. Patients should be taught to perform the Valsalva maneuver, which they should continue.

- Treat the nasal allergy by nasal steroids or by desensitization. This is difficult.

- Treatment of any mechanical obstruction in the nose and nasopharynx.

Treatment in Grade 3 Patients

- Treatment is similar to that for grade 1 and 2 patients.

- If drum fails to improve, grommet insertion is done to equalize the pressure, but here it hardly works.

- If the above treatment is not successful, cartilage tympanoplasty is the final treatment.

Treatment in Grade 4 Patients

- These patients do not respond to medical treatment.

- Surgical treatment is by doing cartilage tympanoplasty and if needed combined with simple mastoidectomy.

- Treatment of any associated mechanical obstruction in the nose and nasopharynx is to be done before performing ear surgery.

Summary

- Various treatment options are available.

- Early stages can be controlled by medical treatment.

- In advanced disease, especially where recurrent infections have weakened the tympanic membrane, surgical correction is the treatment.

Tympanoplasty in the atelectatic drum (grade 3 according to Sade's classification) is depicted in **Fig. 26j1–26j22**.

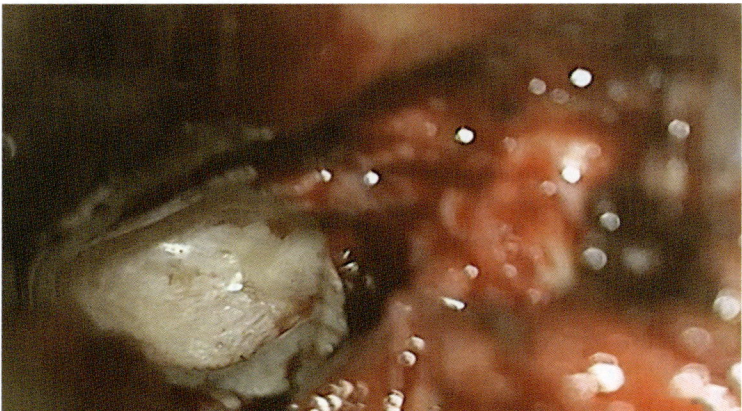

Fig. 26j1 Retracted and atelectatic tympanic membrane (grade 3). Tympanic membrane is retracted, adherent to the promontory and ossicular chain. Surgery is by endaural incision.

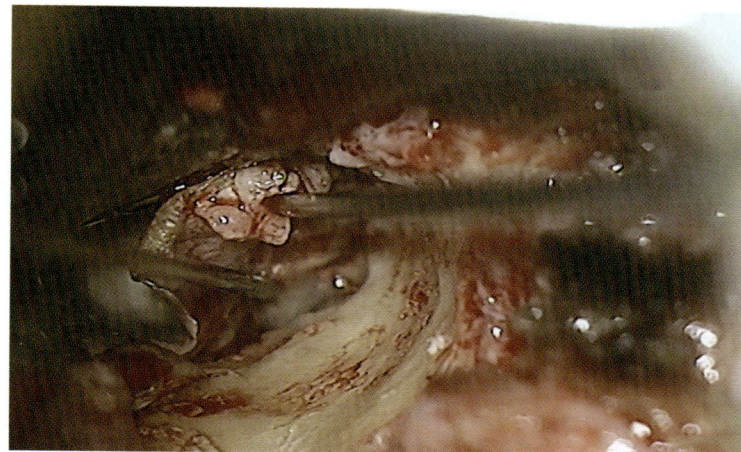

Fig. 26j2 Posterior tympanomeatal flap is elevated. Posterosuperior overhang is removed to find the middle ear space.

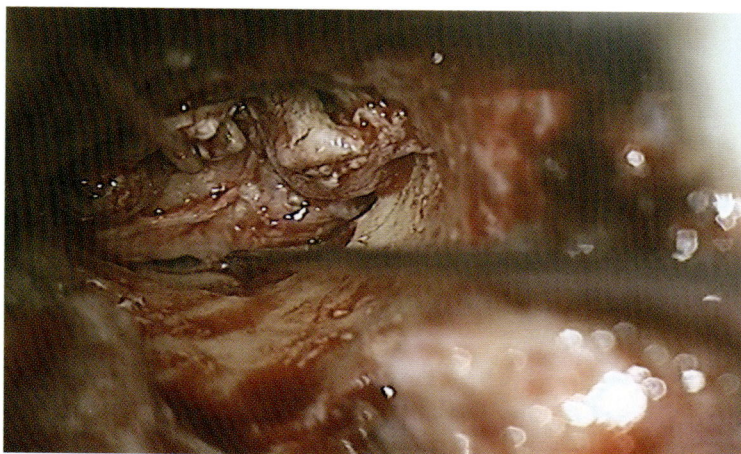

Fig. 26j3 Middle ear is entered in the inferior part (inferior to the retraction pocket).

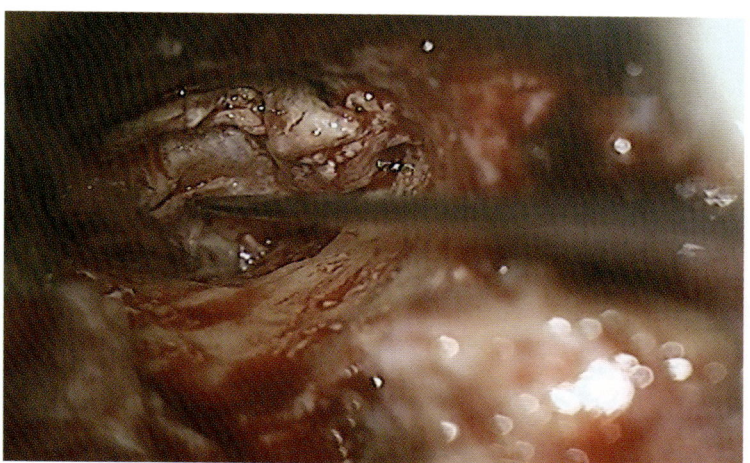

Fig. 26j4 Adherent drum is elevated from the promontory by a side knife.

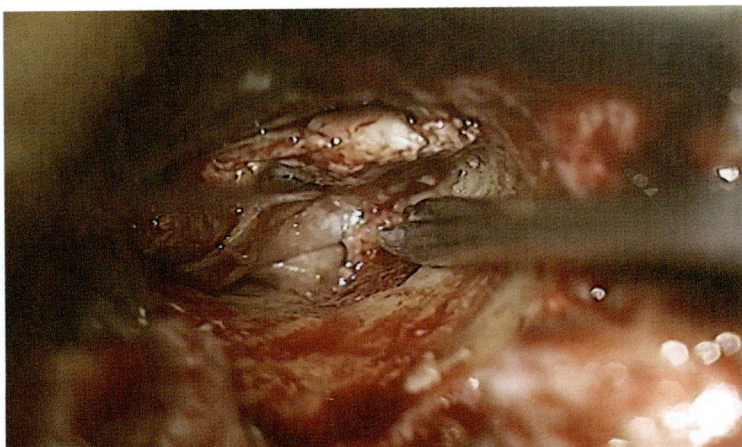

Fig. 26j5 Adhesions around the stapes and incus are dissected by scissors.

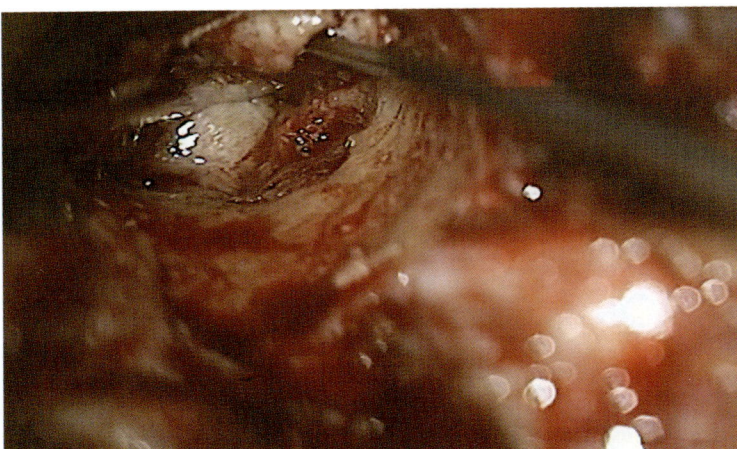

Fig. 26j6 Tympanic membrane is separated from the incus and promontory. The incus and stapes are covered by the edematous mucosa.

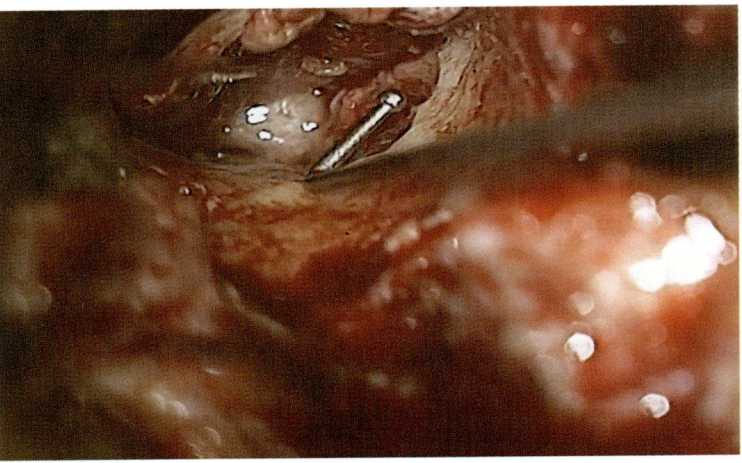

Fig. 26j7 A ball probe is going to be inserted under the anterior part of the tympanic membrane to see for any adhesions.

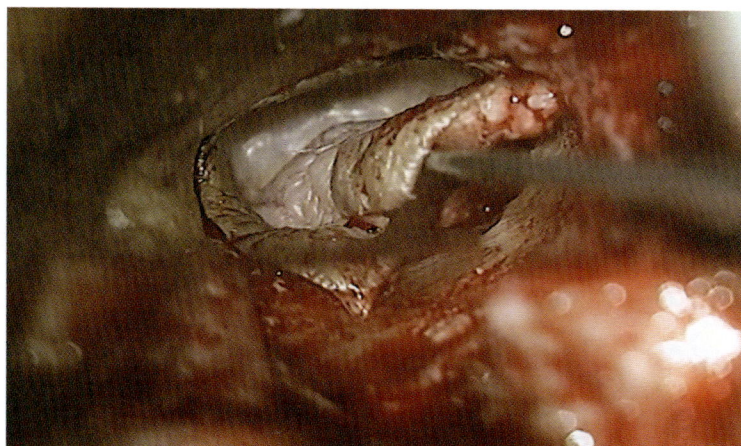

Fig. 26j8 A ball probe is inserted under the anterior part of the tympanic membrane to see for any adhesions.

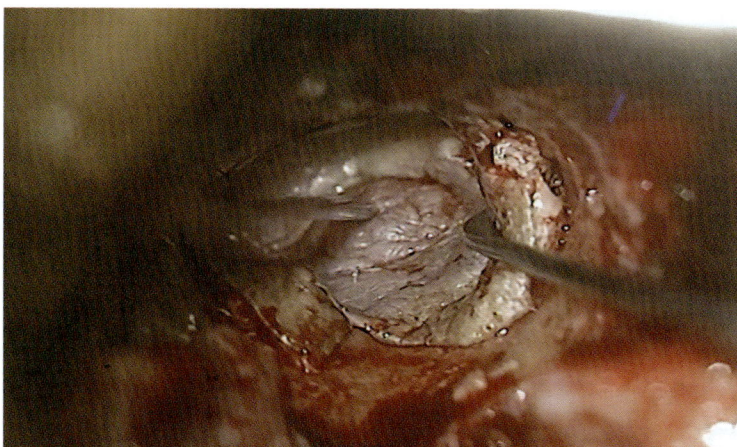

Fig. 26j9 Complete atelectatic and adherent tympanic membrane is elevated without any tear in the tympanomeatal flap.

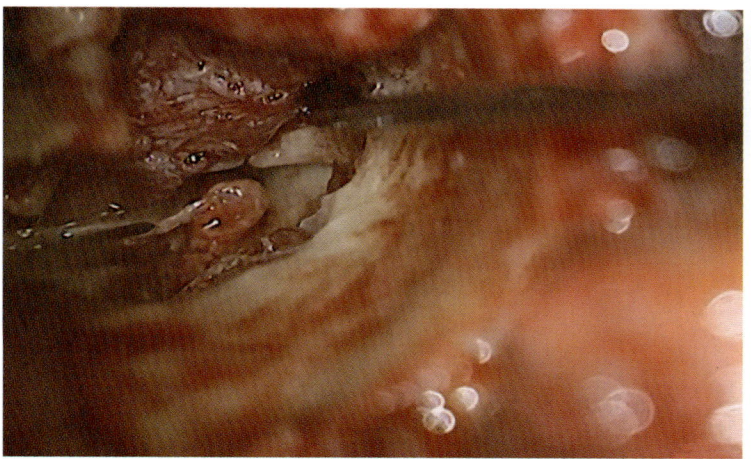

Fig. 26j10 The stapes is found to be intact and mobile. The incus lenticular process is necrosed.

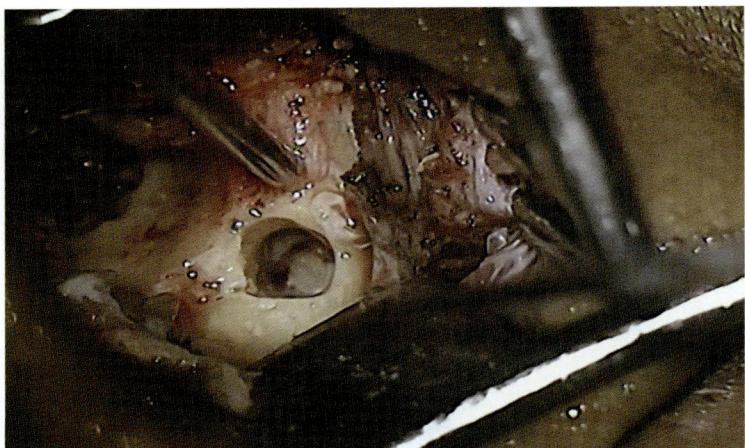

Fig. 26j11 The mastoid is opened and the antrum is found to be healthy.

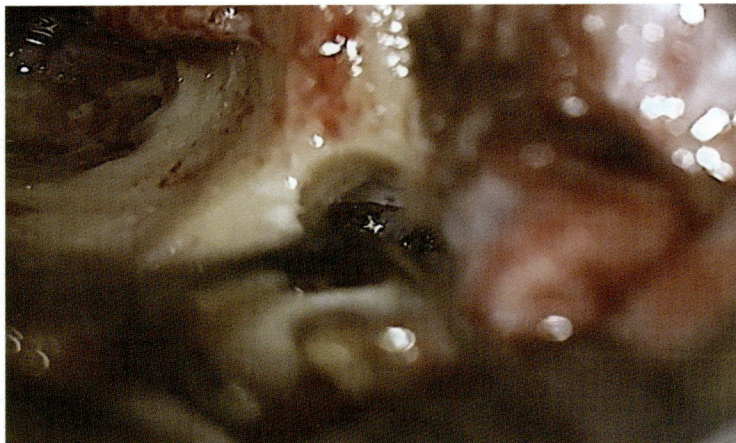

Fig. 26j12 The mastoid is opened. Water test is positive.

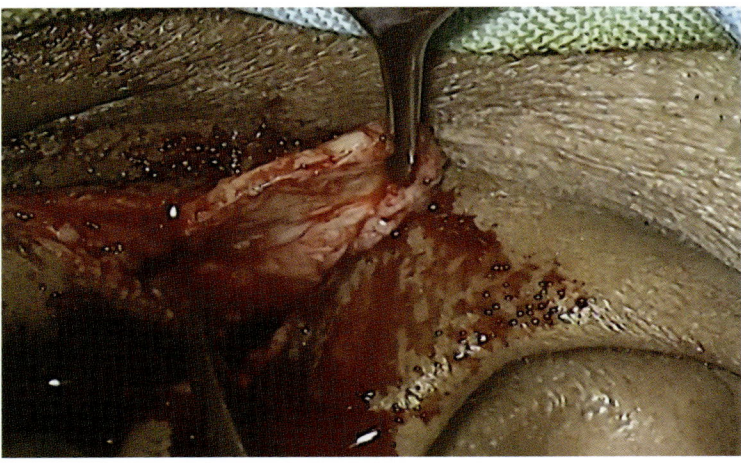

Fig. 26j13 Tragal cartilage is removed from the same endaural incision.

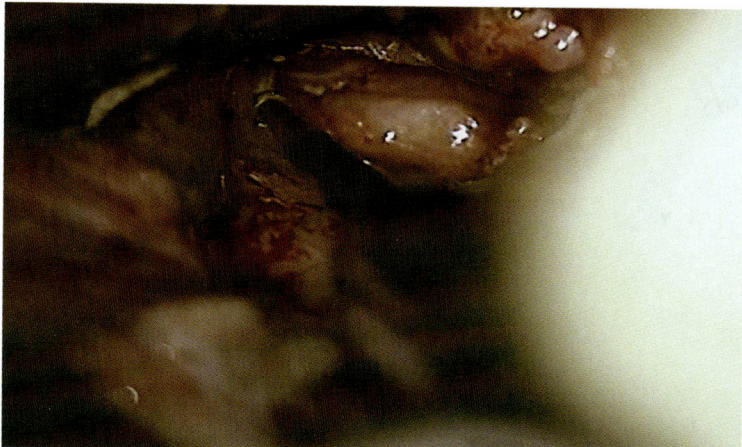

Fig. 26j14   A groove is made in the inferior part of the external auditory canal near the sulcus.

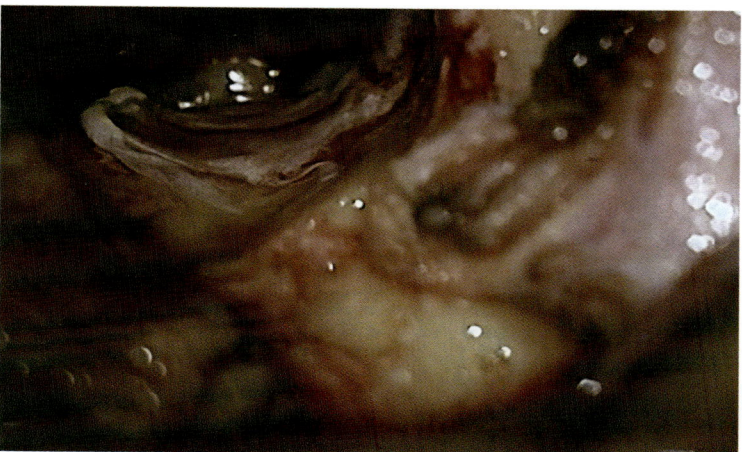

Fig. 26j15   An underlay graft is placed. The mastoid opening is closed by a periosteal flap.

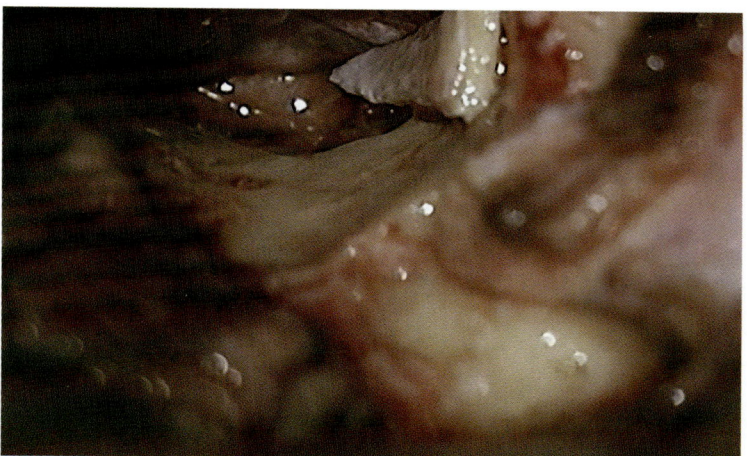

Fig. 26j16   Tympanomeatal flap with graft is elevated to expose the middle ear. A triangular piece of cartilage is to be placed in the middle ear.

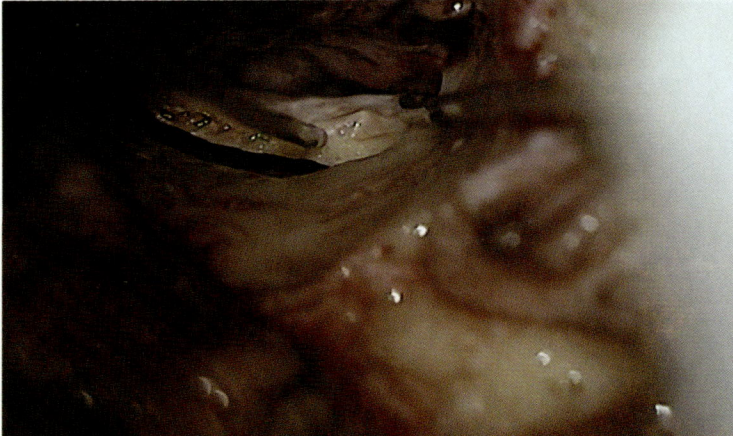

Fig. 26j17 Cartilage is placed horizontally in the middle ear with its lower end resting over the groove at the inferior sulcus and the upper end is placed under the necrosed long process of the incus touching the stapes head (columella effect).

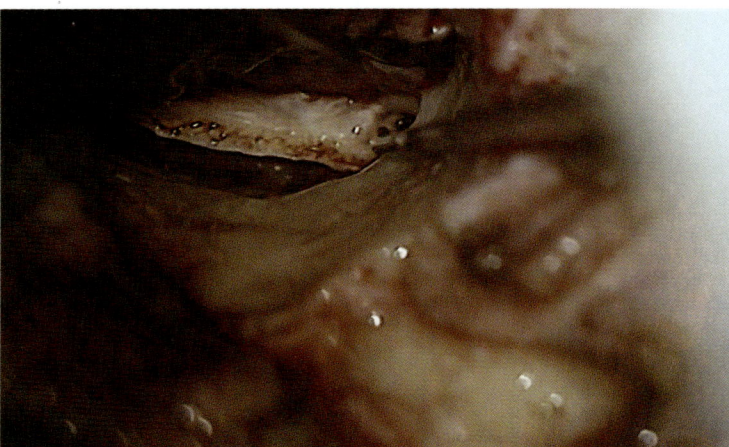

Fig. 26j18 Cartilage is placed horizontally in the middle ear with its lower end resting over the groove at the inferior sulcus and the upper end lying under the necrosed long process of the incus touching the stapes head.

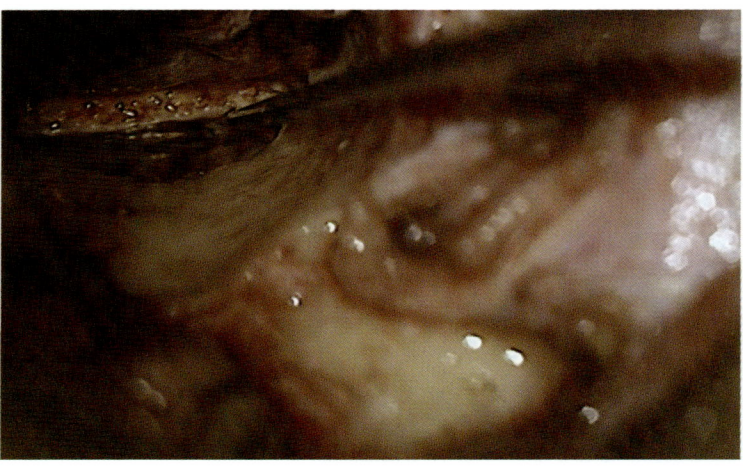

Fig. 26j19 Cartilage is lifted up to see the stapes head below. Cartilage is not touching the promontory. There is enough middle ear space medial to the cartilage.

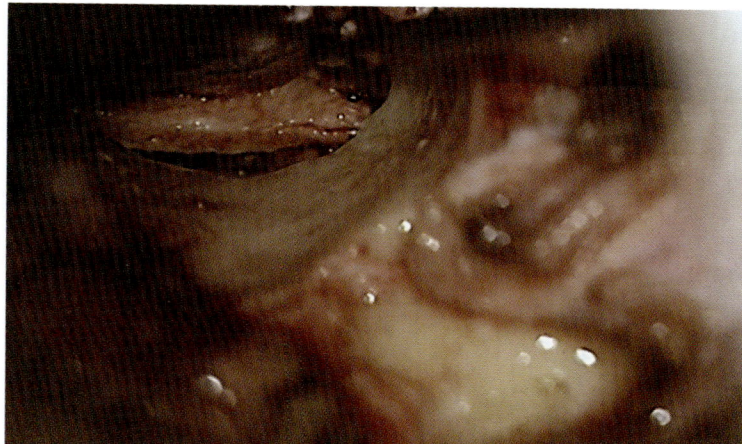

Fig. 26j20 Cartilage is in contact with the stapes head and pressure of the long process of the incus is keeping this cartilage in good contact with the stapes head. Cartilage is not touching the promontory. There is enough middle ear space medial to the cartilage.

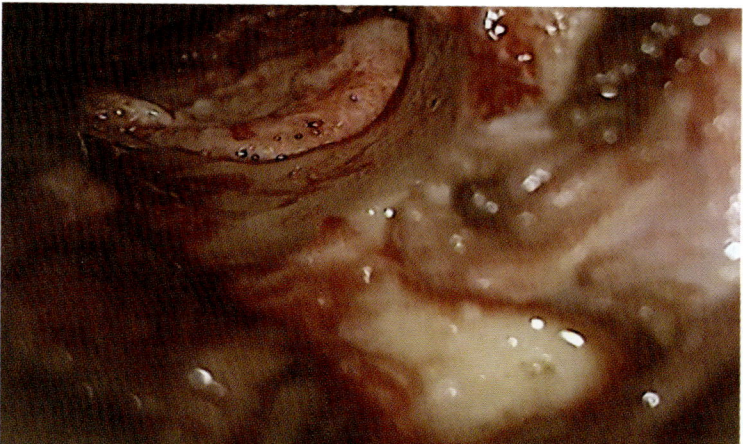

Fig. 26j21 The posterior part of the tympanic cavity is covered (reinforced) by the perichondrium to prevent future retraction pocket.

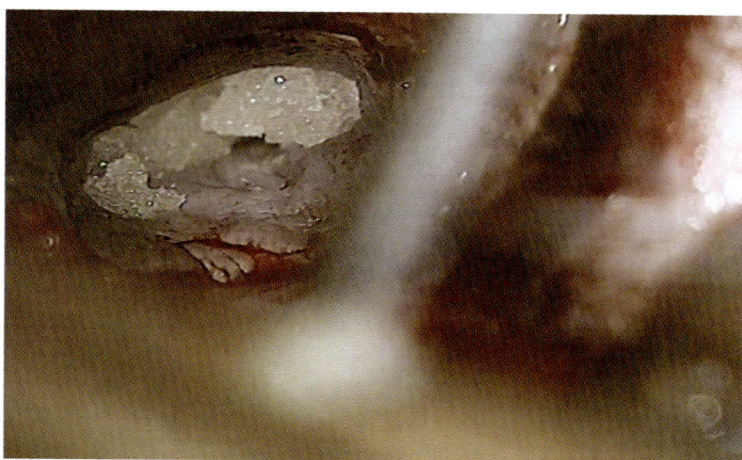

Fig. 26j22 The tympanomeatal flap is reposited back and Gelfoam is packed in the external auditory canal. One or two stitches are required to close this small endaural incision.

26k: Causes of Failure of Autograft Ossicles

Delayed or late failure in ossiculoplasty with autograft ossicle is very high. This failure with autograft ossicle is due to gradual healing, which takes place in the middle ear associated with fibrosis.

- *Displacement*: The problem of displacement of the ossicle is more when the incus is transposed between the stapes footplate and the malleus handle or the tympanic membrane. The incus moves away from the stapes footplate due to healing with fibrosis, causing retraction of the tympanic membrane or the handle of the malleus.

  This displacement problem is least when the incus is placed between the malleus handle and the stapes head. Here, the transposed ossicle is more stable and least vulnerable for displacement.

  The distance between the malleus handle and the stapes head is measured accurately and the transposed incus of proper length is placed, which fits accurately. The transposed incus is more stable when it is of proper length. Chances of displacement is more when the ossicle is smaller than what is required and assembly is loose.

- *Adhesions*: Healing with fibrosis causes fibrous adhesions in the middle ear, between the incus and the fallopian canal, promontory, and tympanic membrane. This fibrosis is associated with displacement of the autograft ossicle.

- *Atrophy*: The ossicle may undergo atrophy due to failure of neovascularization of the transposed ossicle. This atrophied ossicle shrinks in size and is not useful in transmitting sound.

- *Dislocation of the stapes footplate*: Very rarely the stapes footplate gets dislocated, causing sensorineural hearing loss. This dislocation of the stapes footplate is due to retraction of the tympanic membrane or malleus associated with eustachian tube block with negative pressure in the middle ear. This transposed ossicle exerts pressure over the stapes footplate. This is common with titanium prosthesis.

26l: Advantages of Cartilage Ossiculoplasty

As discussed earlier, there are many disadvantages of the transposed ossicle. These disadvantages are not there with cartilage. Cartilage is a very stable ossiculoplasty material and is very useful with a very high success rate.

- It supports the graft, preventing its retraction, hence maintaining the path of good aeration to the footplate area and the mastoid.

- *No fixation:* The cartilage will not get fixed to the middle ear bone, the point where it is resting or in touch. It remains free.

- There is no displacement, as the cartilage assembly is very stable.

- There is no pressure over the footplate of the stapes as cartilage is soft and elastic.

- No cost. It is freely available.

- It does not get absorbed if the perichondrium is intact.

- Success rate in situations 1 and 2 is more than 90%.

Hence, make more and more use of cartilage for ossiculoplasty. Your patients will be happy and satisfied.

26m: Titanium Prosthesis for Ossiculoplasty

Titanium is the most favorable metal for ossiculoplasty. Titanium prosthesis is available in the form of TORP or PORP. It is corrosion free and biocompatible, has good strength, and easily joins with the bone and other tissue (osteointegration). It is the ideal metal for perfect sound conduction from the outer ear to the inner ear; hence, it is a metal of choice for ossiculoplasty.

There is no foreign body reaction with titanium. These patients can undergo magnetic resonance imaging (MRI) investigation without any adverse effect.

Problems with titanium is that it is costly and, being a foreign body, chances of its extrusion are there. This can be minimized by placing a piece of cartilage between the titanium prosthesis and the tympanic membrane.

Another big problem with titanium is that being rigid it can subluxate the stapes footplate if pressure is exerted from outside the drum or drum is pulled in due to some negative pressure in the middle ear due to eustachian tube block causing medialization of prosthesis (**Fig. 26m1**).

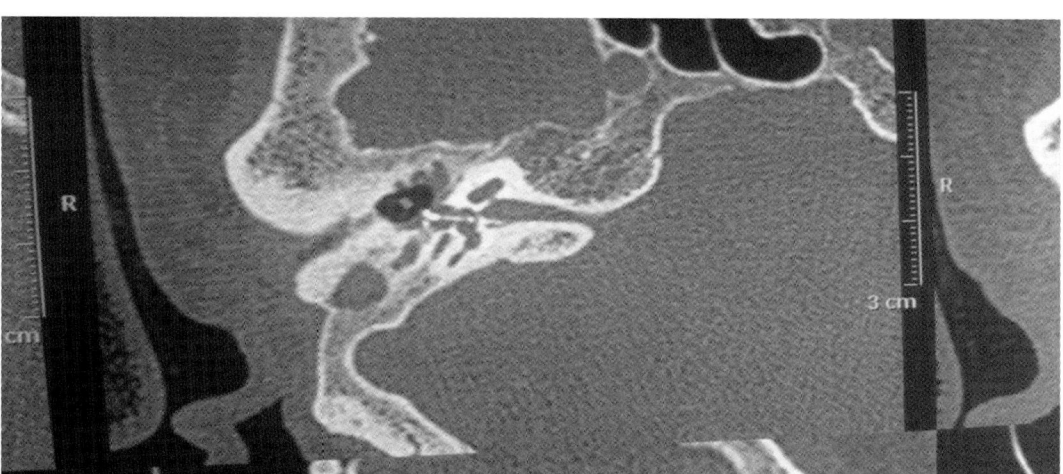

Fig. 26m1   Titanium prosthesis enters the inner ear.

26n: Hints for Ossiculoplasty

- Ossiculoplasty does not give the same results as stapedectomy. Usually, some air–bone gap remains after surgery.

- In very few cases, incus transposition gives good results with complete closure of the air–bone gap.

- Ossiculoplasty results are very good with cartilage.

- Ossiculoplasty assembly is more stable when the handle of the malleus is present and the stapes superstructure is also present and mobile. This handle of the malleus gives additional support to the transposed ossicle.

- The ossicle placed should be of perfect length. The length of the prosthesis should be slightly more than what is required. Short prosthesis will not fit perfectly, will not transmit the sound adequately, and some air–bone gap remains. Excessively short prosthesis may get displaced easily, leading to failed ossiculoplasty. Excessively long prosthesis will be tight enough to decrease sound transmission due to pressure over the stapes or its footplate and worsen the hearing results.

- The angle between the ossicle and the tympanic membrane or the malleus should not be more than 45 degrees. If it is more than 45 degrees, the results are not good. As already mentioned, incus transposition is difficult and the results are not satisfactory when the malleus is very much anterior to the stapes.

- The ossicle or prosthesis should be in contact with the center of the drum or with the handle of the malleus for its maximum benefit. Placement of the prosthesis close to the periphery of the tympanic membrane decreases sound transmission.

- Eustachian tube should function normally, and adequate middle ear space should be maintained for proper functioning of the ossicular chain.

- In the presence of active infection and when eustachian tube function is doubtful, do not use titanium.

- Ossiculoplasty results are better when performed as a second-stage operation, when the middle ear has completely healed up and has taken the final shape.

- Whatever ossicle is placed over the stapes superstructure, it should not touch the promontory and the fallopian canal. It should be exactly at right angle to the stapes. It should point anteriorly rather toward the hypotympanum.

26o: Second-Stage Ossiculoplasty

- Ossiculoplasty performed as a second-stage surgery gives better hearing results. Patients will definitely accept second-stage surgery if they know that this will offer them better hearing results.

- Wait for 6 to 8 months for the second-stage operation to obtain the following:

  o Complete stabilization of the drum.

  o Complete healing of the middle ear mucosa.

○ Complete assessment of the eustachian tube function.

Here eustachian tube function is very important. If the eustachian tube is blocked, retraction of the tympanomeatal flap leads to poor hearing results following ossiculoplasty. The patient can be informed of this before the second-stage surgery.

If everything is favorable, the ossiculoplasty results are very good.

26p: Revision Ossiculoplasty

The need of revision ossiculoplasty arises when the first ossiculoplasty fails and there is a persistent air–bone gap despite good tympanic membrane reconstruction. The purpose of revision ossiculoplasty is to find out the cause of failure and correct it.

These cases can be done under local anesthesia with limited incision, either endomeatal or endaural. The middle ear is exposed after elevating the tympanomeatal flap. If the exposure is not sufficient, the posterosuperior bony overhang is removed. Good exposure is highly essential for perfect working. All the ossicles are examined one by one. The autograft incus, which has been transposed between the stapes head and the malleus handle, is examined for any displacement or for any contact with the surrounding structure.

The incus may get displaced if it has become short, due to atrophy in due course of time.

At times, the incus may develop adhesions with the fallopian canal or with the promontory or posterior canal wall due to fibrosis.

Many a time, the incus is displaced due to retraction of the tympanic membrane caused by eustachian tube block.

The position of the incus or other prosthesis placed between the stapes head or stapes footplate and handle of the malleus or tympanic membrane may change in due course of time due to healing with fibrosis, especially when the handle of the malleus is absent.

Ossiculoplasty is more stable when the handle of the malleus is present and when the stapes superstructure is present. All these problems do not occur when ossiculoplasty is performed as a second-stage procedure where the middle ear is completely stabilized.

At times, the incus is extra-long and may exert undue pressure over the stapes with the displacement of the stapes footplate leading to sensorineural hearing loss (SNHL). This generally happens when the eustachian tube gets blocked due to persistent upper respiratory infection.

All these cases should be revised. Cartilage with perichondrium is found to be the most suitable ossiculoplasty material for revision ossiculoplasty, with no chance of its displacement, atrophy, and absorption. As it is soft and elastic, it does not exert any undue pressure over the stapes footplate. Finally, it is available free of cost. This cartilage with perichondrium gives very good long-term hearing results.

The chances of extrusion are high with alloplast material like titanium or hydroxylapatite. This extrusion can be prevented by keeping a cartilage with perichondrium between the prosthesis and the tympanic membrane.

The most important step in ossiculoplasty surgery, before repositing the tympanomeatal flap, is to check and recheck the placement of the ossicle, for its perfect positioning, not touching the surrounding tissues as already mentioned, and it should be stable, exactly at right angle to the stapes head or footplate.

26q: Results of Ossiculoplasty

- Immediate results are more than 90%.

- Results depends upon proper preoperative preparation of the patient, proper technique, and proper postoperative care of the patients.

- Results of ossiculoplasty are decided by closure of the air–bone gap.

- In situation 1, 80% of patients get closure of the air–bone gap up to around 20 dB with cartilage and incus transposition.

- In situations 2 and 3, around 60% patients get closure of the air–bone gap up to 20 dB with cartilage.

- Ossiculoplasty results are best when the stapes superstructure is present.

- Few patients develop delayed perforation of the tympanic membrane in spite of all possible care. The cause for this delayed failure is not known.

26r: Conclusion

Tympanoplasty has a high rate of success in closing the tympanic membrane perforation and improving the hearing results, but all the cases where grafting is successful are not necessarily associated with improvement in hearing.

Various factors responsible for nonimprovement in the hearing following tympanoplasty are as follows:

- Associated ossicular chain pathology, which was missed during the first surgery

- Final position of the tympanic membrane like blunting of the anterior sulcus and lateralization of the graft, which is common with overlay technique and is not common with the underlay graft:

  o Patients should be chosen carefully based on the indications discussed, and attempts should be made to dry the ear prior to the surgery.

  o Patients should be thoroughly counseled before surgery about their expectations and goals of the surgery.

  o For sure success in tympanoplasty, technique is very important. Just elevating the posterior tympanomeatal flap and placing the underlay graft under the margins of the perforations with very limited overlapping of the perforation margins and the graft is most likely to get displaced with the slightest of pull or push from the middle ear side.

  o For sure success in tympanoplasty, the graft should be well supported by the bony meatal wall on all sides and for that there should be complete 360-degree elevation of the tympanomeatal flap. Also, while replacing this 360-degree elevated tympanomeatal flap, the annulus should be placed into its original position so that normal anatomy of the tympanic membrane is achieved.

  o The anterior and inferior tympanomeatal angle should be less than 90 degrees, and it should be skin lined to prevent blunting. If all these precautions are taken, good hearing improvement with good closure of air–bone gap can be achieved.

○ Unlike stapedectomy, results of revision tympanoplasty are good. When required, it should be done with all possible precautions. Cartilage tympanoplasty plays a very important role in getting better results in revision cases with equally good closure of the air–bone gap.

Ossiculoplasty does not give the same results as stapedectomy. Usually, some air–bone gap remains after surgery.

- Incus transposition gives good results with complete closure of the air–bone gap in 90% of cases.

- Ossiculoplasty results are very good with cartilage.

- Ossiculoplasty is more stable when the handle of the malleus is present. This handle of the malleus gives additional support to the transposed ossicle.

- Ossiculoplasty results are very good when the stapes superstructure is present and the footplate is mobile.

- Ossiculoplasty performed as a second-stage surgery gives better hearing results. Patients will definitely accept second-stage surgery if they know that this will offer them a better hearing result.

- Titanium is the most favorable metal for ossiculoplasty. It is an ideal metal for perfect sound conduction from the outer ear to the inner ear. Hence, it is a metal of choice for ossiculoplasty. Chances of its extrusion are there, but this can be minimized by placing a piece of cartilage between the titanium prosthesis and the tympanic membrane.

- Remember long-term results are more important than the immediate results with tympanoplasty and ossiculoplasty. Hence, all efforts should be taken to make it successful in the long run.

Index